PROCEDURES IN WOMEN'S HEALTH

PROCEDURES IN WOMEN'S HEALTH

Roger P. Smith, M.D.

Professor
Chief, Section of General Gynecology and Obstetrics
Department of Obstetrics and Gynecology
Medical College of Georgia
Augusta, Georgia

Frank W. Ling, M.D.

Faculty Professor and Chairman
Department of Obstetrics and Gynecology
University of Tennessee, Memphis
Memphis, Tennessee

SANS TACHE

Williams & Wilkins
A WAVERLY COMPANY

BALTIMORE • PHILADELPHIA • LONDON • PARIS • BANGKOK
BUENOS AIRES • HONG KONG • MUNICH • SYDNEY • TOKYO • WROCLAW

Editor: Charles W. Mitchell
Managing Editor: Grace E. Miller
Marketing Manager: Lorraine A. Smith
Production Coordinator: Cindy Park
Book Project Editor: Karen M. Ruppert
Designer: Elizabeth Sanders
Illustration Planner: Cindy Park
Cover Designer: Elizabeth Sanders
Typesetter: Peirce Graphic Services, Inc.
Printer: Maple Press
Digitized Illustrations: Peirce Graphic Services, Inc.
Binder: Maple Press

351 West Camden Street
Baltimore, Maryland 21201-2436 USA

Rose Tree Corporate Center
1400 North Providence Road
Building II, Suite 5025
Media, Pennsylvania 19063-2043 USA

Accurate indications, adverse reactions and dosage schedules for drugs are provided in this book, but it is possible that they may change. The reader is urged to review the package information data of the manufacturers of the medications mentioned.

Printed in the United States of America

First Edition,

Library of Congress Cataloging-in-Publication Data
Smith, Roger P. (Roger Perry), 1949–
Procedures in Women's Health / Roger P. Smith, Frank W. Ling.
p. cm.
Includes bibliographical references and index.
ISBN 0-683-18219-6
1. Women—Medical care. 2. Primary care (Medicine) 3. Medical protocols. 4. Gynecology.
I. Ling, Frank W. II. Title. [DNLM: 1. Gynecology—methods. 2. Primary Health Care.
3. Women's Health. WP 100 S658p 1997]
RC48.6.S65 1997
618.1—dc21
DNLM/DLC
for Library of Congress 96-39955
CIP

The publishers have made every effort to trace the copyright holders for borrowed material. If they have inadvertently overlooked any, they will be pleased to make the necessary arrangements at the first opportunity.

97 98 99 00
1 2 3 4 5 6 7 8 9 10

This book is dedicated to those who serve on the "front line" of women's health care.

PREFACE

Many forces have come to influence the practice of medicine, and physicians have responded by making fundamental changes in their mode of practice. Gynecologists have always acted as entry points to medical care for women. In this mode we have often acted to triage patients to other specialists for care. Growing economic pressures from changing practice patterns, managed care contracts, and restrictive contracts have forced many gynecologists to re-evaluate the services they supply in the office setting. In many cases, this has meant that gynecologists are now offering diagnostic and therapeutic services that have always been within their capability but were traditionally referred to someone else. This book is directed toward that changing view of office gynecology.

In this book we have sought to provide the reader with a common sense guide to many primary care procedures that gynecologists might consider offering to their patients. Each chapter offers lists of equipment that will be required, a suggested technique to follow, and the appropriate billing codes that may be used for the procedure. Special considerations, hints, and pitfalls are also highlighted. While not all physicians will want to perform all of the procedures addressed here, we hope that we have provided sufficient depth and breadth that those considering adding these services will do so.

Roger P. Smith, M.D.

Frank W. Ling, M.D.

ACKNOWLEDGMENTS

The authors are once again indebted to Mr. Charles Mitchell and Mrs. Grace Miller of Williams & Wilkins for their invaluable advice, support, encouragement, and patience. They have guided us smoothly through the complex process that brings a work to publication. Thanks must also go to the many Williams & Wilkins authors who have generously allowed many excellent drawings and illustrations to be taken from their works.

Obstetrics and Gynecology, Second Edition—Charles R.B. Beckmann, Frank W. Ling, Barbara M. Barzansky, William G. Bates, William N.P. Herbert, Douglas W. Laube, Roger P. Smith

Photographic Manual of Regional Orthopaedics and Neurological Testing, Second Edition—Joseph J. Cipriano

Office Gynecology, Fourth Edition—Robert H. Glass

Novak's Textbook of Gynecology, Eleventh Edition—Howard W. Jones III

The Female Breast and Its Disorders—George W. Mitchell, Jr., Lawrence Bassett

The Art and Science of Bedside Diagnosis—Joseph D. Sapira, Jane M. Orient

Emergency Procedures and Techniques, Third Edition—Robert R. Simon, Barry E. Brenner

Physical Diagnosis—Janice L. Willms, Henry Schneiderman, Paula S. Algranati

Diagnostic Imaging in Infertility, Second Edition—Alan C. Winfield, Anne Colston Wentz

CONTENTS

VIII Orthopedic Procedures and Evaluations

IX Urologic Procedures

Section I

INTRODUCTION

Chapter 1

GENERAL CONSIDERATIONS

Gynecology has always consisted of a mixture of the cognitive and procedural, with a rich tradition of operative care that ranges from minor to major. Despite this technical experience and expertise, many gynecologists have elected not to carry out simple primary care procedures or procedures that were perceived to lie in the province of other specialties, choosing instead to refer patients to colleagues for this care. As the character of ambulatory practice has changed in response to forces such as managed care, more and more gynecologists are choosing, or are being pushed, to perform procedures that they would have referred to other physicians in the past. This may be caused by a physician's designation as a primary provider (which results in a contractual obligation to provide a wider range of services), by capitation that favors retaining control over costs by limiting referrals, or by a desire to maintain a market share in a changing economic environment.

As the practitioner considers adding new procedures to those offered in the office or ambulatory care setting, several considerations come to mind: the time required, credentialing and training, specialized personnel, specialized equipment, and reimbursement. Most of the procedures discussed in this book will create minimal disruption to the normal office routines, require skills that are already a part of gynecologic practice or are easily acquired, do not require skilled personnel, and may be performed with a minimum of specialized equipment.

TIME

Concerns about the time a task requires have taken on new significance as economic and other pressures have reshaped office practice. Most physicians are reluctant to consider the addition of a procedural service, whether it be flexible sigmoidoscopy, urodynamics testing, or ear piercing, without some consideration of the impact on their time. Almost all of the procedures covered in this book take less than 30 minutes to perform; most require significantly less. A few require more extensive set-up or procedure times and may be best suited to an ambulatory surgery center. Some of the procedures discussed can be completed in an appropriate time slot reserved at the end of the morning or afternoon, whereas others will have to be integrated into the normal flow of care.

CREDENTIALS

Most of these procedures are well within the expertise and training of any gynecologist and as such require no extra training or credentials. For procedures that are best suited for the ambulatory surgery center, hospital emergency department, or operating room, a more formal credentialing process is usually involved. Although this process varies greatly from one location to another and depends on the type of credentials being sought, most privileges require some evidence of training, experience, or both. This training or experience is often desirable for more advanced procedures that may be performed in the office setting, where no formal credentialing process is involved. Training in office procedures is frequently available as part of continuing education programs offered by academic centers or by the American College of Obstetricians and Gynecologists. Preceptorships with colleagues or other specialists can often be arranged on an individual basis and should be explored as the practitioner gains experience.

PERSONNEL

The inclusion of primary care procedures in a gynecologic practice seldom requires any change in the number or type of personnel available. For many procedures, the presence of an assistant is desirable; such procedures are noted throughout the text. For the most part, these assistants need not have any skills or expertise greater than those normally available in a gynecologic office setting. If a procedure is to be offered on a frequent or recurring basis, such as flexible sigmoidoscopy, the use of a specific person to act as technician or assistant can be advantageous. This person will be more familiar with the equipment and its function and maintenance, thereby allowing for smoother performance of the procedure. In some cases, the assistant may be able to perform portions of the procedure independently or with supervision, freeing the physician for other duties.

SPECIALIZED EQUIPMENT

As with personnel, the inclusion of many primary care procedures in a gynecologic practice seldom requires a great expenditure for additional equipment. Most of the procedures discussed in this book can be performed with equipment drawn together from normal office supplies. In some cases, advance preparation of a collection of instruments or supplies for a frequently performed procedure can expedite its performance. In even fewer instances, such specialized equipment as lighting supplies, endoscopes, electrosurgical generators, or ultrasound equipment will be needed. The cases in which this type of investment in equipment is needed are obvious and are generally associated with a decision to offer a given procedure on a regular basis.

A few simple supplies will suffice for most office primary care procedures: skin disinfecting solutions; a selection of local anesthetics; a selection of hemostatic agents; a simple utility tray or pack of instruments; sterile gloves; a few sterile drapes of paper or cloth; and simple sterile bandaging such as self-adhesive bandages, gauze pads, and adhesive tape. In many cases, improvisation can be brought to bear. For example, if care is exercised in donning sterile gloves, the inner glove wrapper may be used as a make-shift sterile field; a general utility instrument kit may be used to suture wounds, remove contraceptive rods, or perform skin biopsy. A list of instruments that may be packaged to form a utility kit for most minor procedures is shown in Table 1.1. Local anesthetic and hemostatic agents are discussed in subsequent chapters.

REIMBURSEMENT

Reimbursement for procedures discussed in this book will generally be independent of the setting in which they are performed. Although every effort has been made to sup-

TABLE 1.1. Instruments Commonly Included in a Utility Kit for Primary Care Procedures

Knife handle with #15 or #11 blade (or disposable scalpel)
Short needle holder
A straight and a curved hemostat (more than one of each may be included but both should be represented); those with fine points are the most useful
Pair of fine scissors
Pair of suture scissors
Pair of thumb forceps (smooth-tipped are most universal but those with teeth may also be included)
2–3 2-inch × 2-inch or 4-inch × 4-inch gauze pads
1–2 small skin retractors (optional)
Suture may be included but is generally made available separately to accommodate the needs of the procedure

ply relevant charge codes based on the Physician's Current Procedure Terminology: CPT 97, published by the American Medical Association, codes change and may be modified by many factors. Care in coding and documentation is required to ensure appropriate reimbursement for any procedure performed. In addition, care must be taken that appropriate notations in the patient's medical record are made to support the indications, to document the counseling and consent process and the procedure performed, and to record an assessment of the immediate outcome of the procedure. The issue of informed consent is discussed more fully in Chapter 2, Informed Consent.

It is important to recognize that under many forms of managed care, no reimbursement will be made if precertification is not obtained. In many instances, precertification may be obtained from the patient's designated primary care provider. In a few cases, the patient's primary care provider may be her gynecologist and may therefore be able to authorize the procedure directly. Even in such a case, procedural care often still requires direct contact with the patient's insurer.

Suggested Readings

Kirschner CG, Davis SJ, Jackson JA, et al. *Physician's Current Procedure Terminology: CPT 96.* Chicago: American Medical Association; 1996.

Chapter 2

INFORMED CONSENT

Before any procedure is performed, the patient and the physician must have discussed the nature of the procedure, the reasons for the procedure, alternatives (including the possibility of not performing the procedure), and the adverse outcomes that may result from the decision to perform or not perform the proposed procedure.

Equipment

- No specific equipment needed
- Many offices augment the traditional methods of informed consent with videotapes or computer-based teaching or consent aids (optional)

Training/Credentialing

No special credentialing needed.

Coding

No special code for obtaining informed consent is used. The inclusion of special counseling and discussion may justify or support a higher acuity for the other services rendered.

General Considerations

The right to control one's fate (the ethical principle of autonomy) underlies the need to establish consent for all procedures performed on a patient, whether in the office, ambulatory surgery area, emergency department, or operating room. For much of the care delivered in the office, consent is an informal, verbal process. This is exemplified by the performance of the physical examination, many portions of which involve discomfort, minimal risk, or special access. (For example, the pelvic examination performed under other circumstances would be grounds for arrest.) When more involved or invasive procedures are contemplated, such as those described in this book, a somewhat more formal process of informed consent should be used.

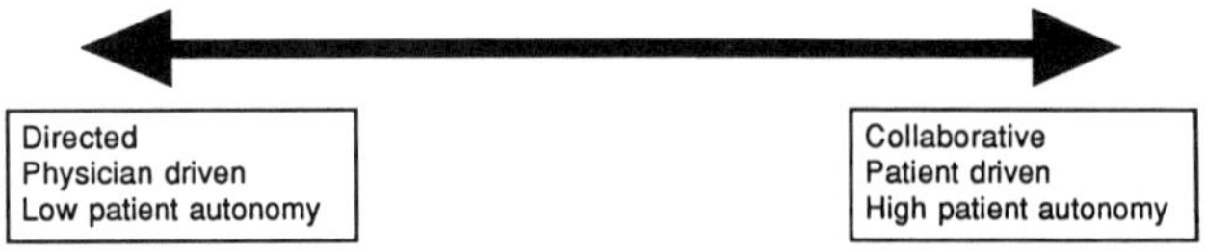

FIGURE 2.1.

There has traditionally been a continuum of patient and physician involvement in the process of medical decision making (Fig. 2.1). The general principles governing informed consent remain the same no matter where on this continuum a particular consent or encounter falls. The general principles of any informed consent are summarized in Table 2.1. For the more invasive procedures and tests outlined in this book, care should be taken that these elements are included in the verbal or written consent obtained.

All consent should be based on the principles of providing the patient with all the information required by a "reasonable person" under similar circumstances to make an informed decision. The amount, character, and detail of this information varies with the proposed procedure, its risks, and the ability of the patient to assimilate the information. Legal guidelines beyond these broad statements are lacking. No legal precedent requires that all possible alternatives or risks be disclosed, but it is expected that any that are probable to or might influence the patient's decision to grant permission will be discussed. This discussion, as well as its outcome, should be documented in the patient's medical record, independent of any written consent document that may have been created.

Written consent forms do not relieve the provider of the obligation to provide counseling and education. Although the written consent may act as a witness to part of the process should a legal challenge occur, it does not provide incontrovertible evidence. For this reason, many practitioners do not use a written consent form for most office-based procedures or testing, believing that it is an unnecessary step that provides little legal protection. What may be a more reasonable "middle ground" is to use a written consent form for any procedure that requires the use of sedation or local anesthetic and to rely on medical record notations to document the consent process for all other procedures. Even when written permission is obtained, the medical record should reflect the character, duration, and depth of the discussion on which the consent was based.

Whether the consent obtained is written or verbal, it should be based on some degree of education provided to the patient. For the simplest procedures or tests, this may be a brief verbal review of the procedure, what is involved, and what is expected. For more involved tests or procedures, many providers have turned to videotaped education or computer-based consent systems to ensure consistency. These resources provide reproducible, in-depth discussions that provide a starting point for counseling while freeing medical personnel for other tasks. The decision to use such an adjunct is usually based on the frequency with which a procedure is performed and the complexity of the teaching required. The use of such adjuncts does not relieve the requirement that the patient be allowed to freely ask questions.

TABLE 2.1. Elements of Informed Consent

Disclosure of information
Patient competence
Patient understanding
Freedom of choice

Special Notes

Some legal jurisdictions have more specific rules about informed consent or guidelines for consent for specific procedures. If present, these rules should be rigorously followed. State or local medical societies can provide information or copies of required forms when appropriate.

Most states require that a written consent form be witnessed by a third party. This is usually a member of the physician's office staff. The addition of a member of the patient's family as an additional witness will avoid the possibility of allegations of conflict of interest should the consent be contested. A copy of the written consent, with the patient's signature, should be given to the patient for further reference.

Consent that requires the evaluation of complex issues, significant risk, or threatening information should be obtained in stages whenever possible. This allows the patient time to consider her decision and permits questions to be answered. Only under emergency conditions (unlikely for the procedures discussed in this book) should this need for thoughtful consideration be circumvented.

Suggested Readings

Caterine JM, Miller B. Informed consent: procedure specific. *Iowa Med* 1989;79:231.

Green JA. Minimizing malpractice risk by role clarification: the confusing transition from tort to contract. *Ann Intern Med* 1988;109:234.

Lidz CW, Appelbaum PS, Meisel A. Two models of implementing informed consent. *Ann Intern Med* 1988;148:1385.

Mazur DJ. What should patients be told prior to a medical procedure? Ethical and legal perspectives on medical informed consent. *Am J Med* 1986;81:1051.

Sprung CL, Winick BJ. Informed consent in theory and practice: legal and medical perspectives on the informed consent doctrine and a proposed reconceptualization. *Crit Care Med* 1989;17:1346.

Chapter 3

TOPICAL AND LOCAL ANESTHETICS

Many office and ambulatory procedures benefit from some form of topical or local anesthesia. Understanding the options available and the advantages and disadvantages of each allows the clinician to choose the best anesthesia for a given situation.

Equipment

The most common topical and local anesthetic agents are summarized in Tables 3.1 and 3.2, respectively. The following are agents appropriate to have on hand in a gynecologic office practice:

- Ice or ethyl chloride spray
- Single-agent local anesthetics such as lidocaine (0.5–2% solution, with and without epinephrine), procaine (2%), and chlorprocaine (2%)
- 25-, 27-, or 30-gauge needle, 2.5- to 10-mL syringe for anesthetic infiltration, and an 18-gauge needle if a multidose vial is used
- Skin cleansing solutions if injection is used
- Sodium bicarbonate 7.5% solution (optional)

Training/Credentialing

No special credentialing is needed. A familiarity with the possible side effects of the agents used, along with therapies for those side effects, is advisable.

Coding

For most office and ambulatory care procedures, the use of a topical anesthetic is included in the coding and charge structure of the procedure itself. If the anesthetic is administered by a physician other than the surgeon, separate billing is permissible. In special cases the following code may be used:

64450 Introduction or injection of anesthetic agent (nerve block), diagnostic or therapeutic

TABLE 3.1. Topical Anesthetic Agents

AGENT AND METHOD	FORM	APPLICATION	COMMENTS
Physical agents			
Pressure		Before injection, for removal of small lesions	
Cold			
Ice	Water ice	Before injection, for removal of small lesions, incision, and drainage of abscess	Anesthesia lasts only a few seconds
Ethyl chloride	Spray		Care must be used to avoid frostbite and blistering
Skin-freezing spray	Compressed gas		
Single pharmacologic agents			
Benzocaine	1–5% cream, 20% ointment, spray	Skin and mucous membrane	
Cocaine	4% solution	Ear, nose, throat	Provides vasoconstriction, restrictions on use and storage limit clinical utility
Dibucaine	0.25–1% cream, ointment, solution, spray	Skin or ear	Slow onset of action (15 min) but long duration (3–6 h), high toxicity
	2.5% suppository	Rectum	
Cyclonine	0.5–1% solution	Skin, mucous membranes (including urethra and rectum)	Not as effective as others listed
Lidocaine	2–4% solution, jelly, viscous solution	Skin, mucous membranes (including urethra and rectum), respiratory tract	Produces rapid, intense anesthesia
	5–10% ointment, suppository	Mucous membranes, rectum	
Tetracaine	0.25–1% solution, cream, ointment	Skin, mucous membranes (including rectum), nose, respiratory tract	Toxic when injected
Combination pharmacologic agents			
EMLA (eutectic mixture of local anesthetic)	Cream	Skin	Intact skin only, requires 60–90 minutes to be effective
TAC (tetracaine, 2.5 mg; adrenaline, 1:1000; 2.5 mL; cocaine, 0.59 g; in sterile water to make 5 mL)	Solution	Best for face, scalp, proximal extremity	May not be used on mucous membranes or open or damaged skin

Agents and Their Use

In both the physical and pharmacologic approaches, all topical or local anesthesia is directed toward reducing or blocking nerve conduction to reduce or eliminate sensation. Topical techniques do not require perforation of the skin and do not distort cutaneous landmarks, but they provide more transient effects and often require longer exposure times to be effective. Local anesthesia techniques can provide anesthesia over an area as limited as a field block or as large as the distribution of a major nerve bundle. The

TABLE 3.2. Local Anesthetic Agents

AGENT	EQUIVALENT CONCENTRATION	SPEED OF ONSET, MIN	DURATION OF ACTION, MIN[a]	MAXIMAL DOSE, MG[b]
Amides				
Bupivacaine	0.25%	5	120–240	175 (2.5 mg/kg per hour)
Etidocaine	0.5%	3–5	120–240	300
Lidocaine	0.5–2%	1	30–120	350 (4.5 mg/kg per hour)
Mepivacaine	1%	3–5	30–120	500 (7 mg/kg per hour)
Esters				
Chloroprocaine	2%	1–3	15–30	1000 (20 mg/kg per hour)
Procaine	2%	3–5	15–30	500 (7 mg/kg per hour)
Tetracaine	0.25%	3–5	120–240	50

[a]If epinephrine is included in the preparation, these times are increased by twofold to threefold.
[b]Based on a patient weighing 70 kg. If epinephrine is included in the preparation, these doses may be increased by 25 to 50%.

choice of agent and techniques will be based on the type, location, and duration of the planned procedure, preferences of the patient, and the experience of the operator.

PHYSICAL METHODS

Some of the simplest ways to create transient anesthesia are through physical methods such as pressure or cold. Gentle but firm pressure, as with a finger, applied for several seconds provides some measure of analgesia. Although this analgesia lasts only a few seconds, it may be sufficient for removing a skin tag, unroofing a cyst, or reducing the discomfort of needle punctures or skin weals. In a similar manner, applying ice to the skin for 10 to 15 seconds, or exposing the skin to a skin-cooling spray such as ethyl chloride or a compressed gas skin-freezing agent for 2 to 3 seconds, may be used to produce slightly more profound analgesia or anesthesia. The duration of analgesic effects is short but proportional to the degree of skin cooling obtained. When skin-freezing sprays are used, care must be taken to ensure that tissue damage does not result.

TOPICAL AGENTS

Many local anesthetics may be applied directly over the site of a planned procedure to provide an alternative to parenteral techniques. Most agents are commercially available in forms and concentrations appropriate to this use (Table 3.1). When agents are used in this way, effectiveness is greatest on mucous membranes or in areas where the skin is thin. The single agents most commonly used for this purpose are lidocaine (2–4%), cocaine (4–10%), and tetracaine (1–2%). Procaine and mepivacaine do not penetrate tissues in concentrations sufficient to create anesthesia and thus are not used for this purpose. Similarly, most vasoconstrictors do not penetrate tissue well. If vasoconstriction is desirable, cocaine should be used because of its simultaneous vasoconstriction action.

Combination agents such as TAC (tetracaine, 2.5 mg; adrenaline 1:1000, 2.5 mL; cocaine, 0.59 g; in sterile water to make 5 mL) or EMLA (eutectic mixture of local anesthetic) are somewhat more effective but carry restrictions on dosage and location. Before EMLA cream is applied, the skin must be prepared by cleansing and degreasing; after the cream is applied, an occlusive dressing is placed for up to 90 minutes before the procedure. The anesthesia obtained through the use of EMLA may last for as long as 2 hours after the cream is removed.

Depending on the agent and the amount of time it is left in contact with the skin, topical agents provide anesthesia to a depth of 3 to 5 mm. Procedures that involve

TABLE 3.3. Contraindications to the Use of Parenteral Local Anesthesia

Anticoagulant therapy (relative)
Blood dyscrasia
Cholinesterase deficiency (especially for ester type agents)
Hepatic failure or significant damage (relative)
Hypersensitivity to local anesthetic agents or paraben preservatives
Infected operative or injection site
Pre-existing neurovascular disease (relative)
Septicemia

deeper tissues or large surfaces generally require the use of a parenteral technique. Topical agents are best suited for such procedures as removal of foreign bodies, excision of skin lesions or tags, and repair of traumatic wounds or as a preparation of parenteral anesthetics.

INJECTABLE AGENTS

Many clinically useful local anesthetic agents are available (Table 3.2). The choice of agent should be based on the body site and procedure, the speed of onset, and the duration of effect the agent provides. Some agents provide better tissue permeation (e.g., lidocaine), which allows for more effective field blocks or for effective nerve blocks when the exact location of the nerve is not infiltrated. Other agents provide much longer duration of action (e.g., bupivacaine); this property makes them better suited to such applications as trigger point injection, for which a long duration of anesthesia is desirable. Parenteral local anesthesia of any sort is contraindicated in several situations, as shown in Table 3.3.

VASOCONSTRICTORS

The addition of epinephrine or other vasoconstrictor to a local anesthetic is useful for some procedures. The inclusion of a vasoconstrictor results in reduced bleeding, reduced systemic absorption, and prolonged anesthetic effect. Vasoconstrictor agents are contraindicated in settings in which the vascular supply is compromised or limited (such as microvascular disease or in the distal extremities, skin flaps, nose, or ear). Additional contraindications to the use of vasoconstrictors are shown in Table 3.4.

TABLE 3.4. General Contraindications to the Use of Vasoconstrictors in Local Anesthesia

Arteriosclerosis
Cerebral vascular disease
Diabetes
Heart block
Hypertension
Hypotension
Peripheral vascular disease
Thyrotoxicosis

TABLE 3.5. General Principles of Parenteral Anesthesia

If a multidose vial is used, the top must be cleansed before each use and withdraw should be performed with a needle that has a larger gauge (e.g., 18-gauge) than that used to inject the agent. This needle must then be disposed of safely (generally without being recapped)

Intradermal injection produces anesthesia more quickly than subcutaneous infiltration

No local anesthetic should be injected until the plunger of the syringe has been withdrawn slightly to test for blood return. If blood is present, the needle must be withdrawn and repositioned to avoid intravascular injection

If a field-block is to be used, the anesthetic agent should only be injected as the needle is withdrawn

The absence of an anesthetic effect is most often related to an inadequate time interval from infiltration

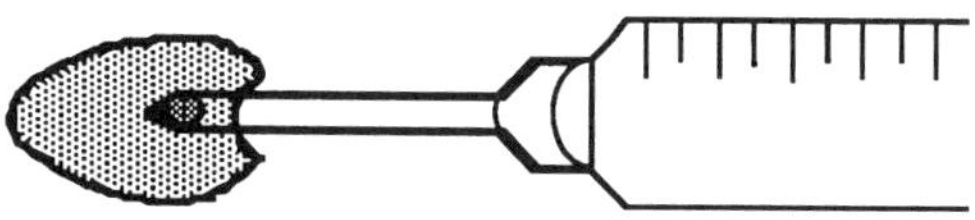

FIGURE 3.1.
Local infiltration of anesthetic agent should be performed with the smallest needle practical, inserted just below the skin surface with the bevel facing upward. The plunger of the syringe should always be slightly withdrawn to check for vessel perforation before the anesthetic is injected.

PARENTERAL ANESTHETIC TECHNIQUES

Parenteral anesthesia may be achieved by local infiltration, field block, or nerve block techniques. The choice of method is based on the location and type of procedure planned. All techniques must follow the general principles outlined in Table 3.5.

Infiltration and Field-Block

The simplest form of parenteral anesthetic is local infiltration. In this technique, a skin weal slightly larger than the planned operative site is raised by direct injection of the anesthetic agent (Fig. 3.1). The amount of agent used should be restricted to the smallest amount possible, consistent with effective analgesia. This minimizes the discomfort of injection and causes the least amount of tissue distortion.

A field block is used when a larger area must be anesthetized but the area is not served by a single nerve bundle. The boundaries of the site to be numbed are infiltrated in a series of local injections (Fig. 3.2) that block sensations from the area. Field blocks provide good anesthesia without distorting the operative site. Just as in other forms of local infiltration, care must be used to avoid intravascular injection by periodically aspirating to check for blood return and only injecting anesthetic agent as the needle is withdrawn. Because of the relatively larger amounts of agent used, care must also be exercised to avoid inadvertent administration of a toxic dose of medication.

Nerve-Block

When the area to be anesthetized is served by one or more clearly defined nerve bundles, a nerve block may be the most appropriate technique. An example of this is the digital block used for procedures involving the fingers or toes (see Chapter 37, Digital Block

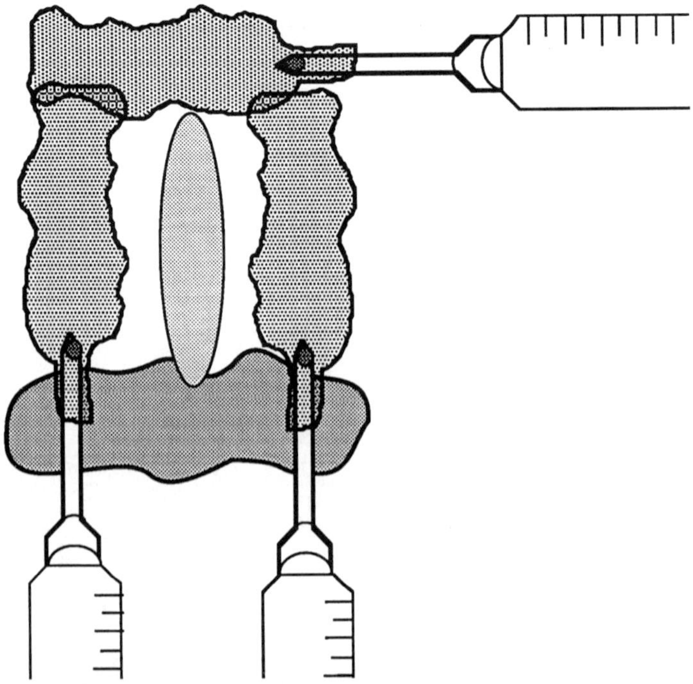

FIGURE 3.2.
A field block is created when the area to be numbed is surrounded by local anesthetic infiltration. Each side of the field is defined by inserting the needle to its greatest extent; the anesthetic is infused as the needle is withdrawn.

Anesthesia). Before a nerve block is performed, a careful neurologic evaluation of the area to be numbed should be done. Any deficiencies present before the injection of local anesthetic should be carefully documented in the medical record. The location of the nerve bundle to be blocked should be identified, the skin cleansed, and the chosen local anesthetic agent injected using a 25- to 30-gauge needle. The amount of agent required varies according to the site but is often as little as 1 or 2 mL. Because vessels often accompany neural bundles, extra care should be taken to avoid an intravascular injection. If the patient experiences paresthesia when the needle is initially inserted, it should be withdrawn 2 mm before anesthetic is injected. The goal is perineural deposition of the agent, not direct injection into the nerve itself. Because of the risk for ischemia, vasoconstrictors should not be used when a nerve block involves the fingers, toes, ear, or penis.

Special Notes

Although true allergies to local anesthetic agents are rare, they are most common with the amino esters, such as procaine. A history of true allergy to local anesthetic agents is a relative contraindication to further use. If these agents must be used, an anesthesiologist or allergist should be consulted. Because cross-reaction between esters and amides is unlikely, an appropriate agent that safely achieves anesthesia can often be found. As with any patients in whom an allergic reaction is possible, preparations for such an allergic event should be made before any agent is given.

Multidose vials of local anesthetic generally contain a paraben preservative. This substance is chemically similar to the ester anesthetics and may cause a cross-reaction in ester-sensitive patients. For these persons, a single-dose vial that does not contain the preservative should be used.

The discomfort of injection caused by parenteral local anesthetics can be reduced by using a mixture of 10 mL of agent with 1 mL of a 7.5% sodium bicarbonate solution. This mixture buffers the usually acidic agent, significantly reducing the pH-induced pain of injection without altering the effectiveness of the anesthetic.

Central nervous system toxicity caused by local anesthetic agents may be difficult to differentiate from vasovagal effects. Symptoms may include anxiety, lightheadedness, blurred vision, drowsiness, altered or slurred speech, or a metallic taste in the mouth. Restlessness, tremors, convulsions, coma, respiratory arrest, and death are rare but possible. Arrhythmias and cardiovascular or cerebrovascular changes may occur if a vasoconstrictor such as epinephrine is used to excess, if intravascular injection occurs, or if systemic absorption is accelerated.

Before any nerve block is attempted, the pertinent anatomy should be carefully reviewed.

Suggested Readings

Abott K, Fowler-Kerry S. The use of a topical refrigerant anesthetic to reduce injection pain in children. *J Pain Sympt Mangmt* 1995;10:584.

Adriani J. Local and regional anesthesia for minor surgery. *Surg Clin North Am* 1951; 31:1507.

Atkinson RS. Regional anesthesia in obstetrics. *Surg Gynecol Obstet* 1962;31:423.

Bonadio WA, Wagner V. Efficacy of TAC topical anesthetic for repair of pediatric lacerations. *Am J Dis Child* 1988;142:203.

Brooks-Gunn J, McCarton C, Hawley T. Effects of in utero drug exposure on children's development. Review and recommendations. *Arch Pediatr Adolesc Med* 1994;148:33.

Brown DL, Ransom DM, Hall JA, et al. Regional anesthesia and local anesthetic-induced systemic toxicity: seizure frequency and accompanying cardiovascular changes. *Anesth Analg* 1995;81:321.

Covino BG. Local anesthesia. *N Engl J Med* 1972;286:975.

de Waard-van der Spek FB, van den Berg GM, Oranje AP. EMLA cream: an improved local anesthetic. Review of current literature. *Pediatr Dermatol* 1992;9:126.

Doyle DJ. A closer look at local anesthesia. *Emerg Med* 1991;23:147.

Fox CH. Cocaine use in pregnancy. *J Am Board Fam Pract* 1994;7:225.

Grekin RC, Auletta MJ. Local anesthesia in dermatologic surgery. *J Am Acad Dermatol* 1988;19:599.

Hogan Q, Dotson R, Erickson S, et al. Local anesthetic myotoxicity: a case and review. *Anesthesiology* 1994;80:942.

Homes HS. Options for painless local anesthesia. *Postgrad Med J* 1991;89:71.

Juhlin L, Evers H. EMLA: a new topical anesthetic. *Adv Dermatol* 1990;5:75.

Kalichman MW. Physiologic mechanisms by which local anesthetics may cause injury to nerve and spinal cord. *Region Anesth* 1993;18:448.

McKay W, Morris R, Mushlin P. Sodium bicarbonate alleviates pain on skin infiltration with lidocaine, with or without epinepherine. *Anesth Analg* 1987;66:572.

Middleton RM, Kirkpatrick MB. Clinical use of cocaine. A review of the risks and benefits. *Drug Safety* 1993;9:212.

Moore DC, Fridenbaugh LD, Bridenbaugh PO, et al. Bupivacaine. A review of 2,077 cases. *JAMA* 1970;214:713.

Murphy MF. Local anesthetic agents. *Emerg Med Clin North Am* 1988;6:769.

Om A. Cardiovascular complications of cocaine. *Am J Med Sci* 1992;303:333.

Rodriguez LF, Smolik LM, Zbehlik AJ. Benzocaine-induced methemoglobinemia: report of a severe reaction and review of the literature. *Ann Pharmacother* 1994;28:643.

Rowlingson JC. Toxicity of local anesthetic additives. *Region Anesth* 1993;18:453.

Sadove MS, Kobak AJ, Morch ET. Regional analgesia in obstetrics. *Med Clin North Am* 1961;45:1743.

Wilds PL. Transvaginal pudendal nerve block. *Obstet Gynecol* 1956;8:385.

Wootton J, Miller SI. Cocaine: a review. *Pediatr Rev* 1994;15:89.

Chapter 4

HEMOSTASIS

Many of the procedures described in this book involve the loss of small amounts of blood. Minimizing blood loss decreases wound complications and improves patient comfort and acceptance. Although topical hemostatic agents are not a substitute for good surgical technique, a familiarity with their use is essential.

Equipment

The most common topical hemostatic agents are summarized in Table 4.1. The following is a practical list of agents appropriate to have on hand in a gynecologic office practice:

- Sliver nitrate sticks
- Ferric subsulfate solution (20%) (Monsel's solution)
- Trichloracetic acid (50–85%)
- Absorbable gelatin sponge (Gelfoam)

Training/Credentialing

No special credentialing needed.

Coding

Not applicable.

Agents and Their Use

The first line of hemostasis should be physical measures such as pressure, cold, or suture ligation. Procedures performed in the office setting may produce bleeding sufficient to require adjuncts to pressure or cold but insufficient to justify the cost or bulk of suture ligature. The ease and speed of action of topical hemostatic agents make them attractive for this setting. An agent should be chosen on the basis of its mode of action, the location and type of wound involved, and the agent's efficacy. The relative cost and efficacy of common topical hemostatic agents are shown in Table 4.1.

TABLE 4.1. Topical Hemostatic Agents[a]

FAMILY OR AGENT	EFFICACY	COST
Vasoconstriction, occlusion, and denaturation		
Aluminum chloride (30%)	+++	$$
Cocaine hydrochloride	+++	$$$
Ferric subsulfate (Monsel's solution, 20%)	+++	$$
Hydrogen peroxide (3%)	+	$
Phenol (50%)	++	$$
Silver nitrate sticks	+++	$$
Trichloroacetic acid (50%–85%)	++	$$
Zinc chloride paste	++	$$
Physical meshwork for coagulation		
Absorbable gelatin sponge (Gelfoam)	+++	$$$
Microfibrillar collagen (Avitene)	+++++	$$$$$
Oxidized cellulose (Surgicel)	++++	$$$
Physiologic agents		
Epinephrine	+++	$
Fibrin sealant (tissue glue)	+++++	$$$$$
Thrombin spray (Thrombostat)	+++++	$$$$$

[a]Efffectiveness and cost are rated on a scale from 1 to 5.

In general, agents that act by denaturing protein, causing vasoconstriction, or occluding the bleeding vessels are the least expensive and most commonly used. Physical meshwork agents provide a skeleton on which the normal clotting process may proceed, but the presence of these agents in a wound may slow healing or be a nidus for infection. Agents that augment or replace physiologic mechanisms are the most effective but are also the most expensive and cumbersome to use. A passing familiarity of the specific characteristics of one or more agents from each group will facilitate the selection of the best agent for a given situation.

VASOCONSTRICTORS AND OCCLUDING AND DENATURING AGENTS

Agents that denature protein, cause vasoconstriction, or occlude bleeding vessels are applied topically. These agents are not used in wounds that are to be closed surgically or those that involve a clinically significant cavity.

Aluminum Chloride

Aluminum chloride (alum) may be applied as a 30% solution or in the form of a solid stick (styptic pencil). Once common for shaving cuts, the latter is less frequently used today because of concerns about cross contamination. When applied to a relatively dry wound, the aluminum chloride hydrolyzes to form hydrochloric acid, which denatures protein and prompts vasospasm. This agent produces mild burning and tissue damage if applied to normal skin. Because this agent is colorless, it is appealing for areas where a wound may be visible and avoids the slight risk for tattooing associated with pigmented agents such as silver nitrate or ferric subsulfate.

Ferric Subsulfate (Monsel's Solution)

First described in 1856, Monsel's solution is widely used for its hemostatic properties. Monsel's solution is a 20% solution of ferric subsulfate. It is readily available from several suppliers, including many local or hospital pharmacies. Applied using an applicator swab or the tip of a gauze sponge, Monsel's solution denatures protein and occludes blood vessels by virtue of its pH and the action of the subsulfate moiety.

Monsel's solution is most effective for capillary bleeding. It should be applied to a relatively dry surgical field. Effectiveness can be enhanced by allowing the solution to settle or evaporate to form a thick or paste-like consistency. Because of a slight risk for tattooing, Monsel's solution should not be used in areas where cosmetic considerations are important. Because iron may be incorporated into local macrophages after the application of Monsel's solution, the solution should not be used in areas where later excision and histologic examination of the tissue are anticipated.

Silver Nitrate

Silver nitrate is most often encountered in the form of applicator sticks coated with the agent on one end. These silver nitrate sticks are inexpensive, easy to use, and have a long shelf-life. Silver nitrate may also be applied as a 20 to 50% solution, but these solutions are harder to apply with precision. When silver nitrate is applied in the presence of moisture, liberated silver ions cause proteins to precipitate, thereby destroying tissue and occluding small blood vessels. The eschar of precipitated protein inhibits the further diffusion of silver into the tissue, which provides a self-acting limit to the depth of tissue effect achieved. Because of the deposition of silver salts, tissues treated with silver nitrate will be stained black. Although this color generally fades with time, tattooing is possible and should be kept in mind when this agent is considered.

Trichloroacetic Acid

Most often associated with the destruction of lesions such as condyloma, trichloroacetic acid is an efficient topical hemostatic agent. When applied to tissue, trichloroacetic acid rapidly coagulates protein, resulting in an eschar that occludes vessels. When the agent is used for this purpose, solutions of 50 to 85% are used. Problems with controlling the depth of tissue damage, spillage onto adjacent tissues, and the pain associated with the use of this agent have generally limited it to tissue destruction rather than hemostasis.

Other Agents

When applied topically, cocaine has both anesthetic and vasoconstrictive actions that make it useful for procedures involving mucosal surfaces. Although most often used in this manner for procedures that involve the nasal passages, cocaine can be used on vulvar or vaginal tissues to produce hemostasis and analgesia. Cost, the potential for abuse, and the need for careful (locked) storage and extensive record keeping generally limit the use of cocaine for these purposes.

Phenol, in a 50% solution, may be used to cauterize a wound and produce hemostasis. Inexpensive and readily stored for use, phenol produces moderate tissue damage in addition to hemostasis. For this reason, it should be used sparingly.

Such household agents as zinc chloride paste or hydrogen peroxide have moderate hemostatic properties. Zinc chloride paste leaves a residue that may interfere with healing, and hydrogen peroxide produces mild tissue damage in addition to its germicidal action.

PHYSICAL MATRIX AGENTS

Agents in this group provide a structural matrix on which the body's normal clotting mechanism can act to stop further bleeding. All must be placed and retained in proximity to the source of bleeding. The patient's clotting mechanisms, including platelet function, must be intact for these agents to prompt hemostasis. As do the other agents discussed in this chapter, these agents work best on bleeding that is capillary; however, small-vessel bleeding may respond if the agents are combined with pressure or suture ligation.

Absorbable Gelatin

Available in both powder and foam sponge forms, absorbable gelatin is made from purified gelatin. Both forms hold blood and clotting proteins while a clot forms. These agents stimulate an inflammatory response that may lead to granulation tissue. For this reason, they should be used with caution around delicate tissues or nerve and tendon sheaths. The solid forms may be "glued" in place with the addition of thrombin solutions.

Microfibrillar Collagen

Microfibrillar collagen is made from bovine collagen and supplied as granules or fibers. More effective and closer to the normal physiology of wound healing than are other agents in this class, microfibrillar collagen stimulates the aggregation of platelets and the induction of the clotting cascade. This material readily adheres to damp surfaces, including surgical instruments and gloves, and must therefore be carefully applied with dry instruments. Although microfibrillar collagen leaves less of a residue as a nidus for infection, the material still interferes with wound healing and revascularization if it is interposed between tissues or wound edges. Cost and ease of use tend to restrict the use of these agents to general surgery settings, but they may still be used for procedures in the primary care setting.

Oxidized Cellulose

Readily available, oxidized regenerated cellulose meshwork may be cut to size and applied to irregular surfaces to help provide hemostasis. As do gelatin- and collagen-based agents, oxidized cellulose provides a scaffold on which coagulation can take place. In addition to this function, oxidized cellulose produces a mild vasoconstriction that slightly increases its effectiveness. Because foreign-body reactions at the site of application are not uncommon, the areas where oxidized cellulose may be used are limited.

PHYSIOLOGIC AGENTS

Agents in this group derive their hemostatic action from their ability to either imitate or augment processes normally involved in clotting and the response to tissue trauma.

Epinephrine

A potent initiator of vasoconstriction, epinephrine is often combined with local anesthetics to prolong anesthetic action and reduce blood loss. When used in small amounts, excessive vasospasm or rebound vasodilatation (which could delay wound healing) are uncommon. Epinephrine may cause cardiac arrhythmias if excessive amounts are used, direct intravascular injection occurs, or significant absorption occurs. Other topical vasoconstrictive agents, such as those listed above, may damage tissue in the base of the wound. This is not the case with epinephrine. Epinephrine is not generally used for procedures involving the digits or any area supplied by a single vascular supply.

Fibrin Paste

Probably the most effective of any topical hemostatic agent, fibrin paste (also known as tissue glue) is made by mixing clotting factors just before application. The resultant paste is quickly applied directly to the wound as a fibrin clot forms. Although rapid acting, this product is expensive, must be mixed at the time of use, and carries some of the risks (particularly hepatitis) associated with the human blood products from which it is derived.

Thrombin

Thrombin, in the form of activated prothrombin, may be applied as a powder or spray. When applied to a relatively dry wound, thrombin supplements the body's normal clotting mechanism, leaving little residue or tissue damage. Unlike fibrin paste, which must be used immediately, thrombin may be mixed and used as long as 6 hours later. High cost generally restricts the use of thrombin products to major surgical procedures.

Special Notes

Most techniques for controlling bleeding are most effective when the surgical field is relatively dry. This may be accomplished by blotting the wound with a suitable gauze or towel immediately before the agent is applied. Placing the tissues involved under mild stretch or applying pressure adjacent to the wound may also transiently reduce bleeding while long-term hemostasis obtained.

Most topical agents that result in vasoconstriction or occlusion as a mechanism of action will slightly delay the rate of wound healing. As a result, these agents should be used only when needed and should not be applied in a prophylactic manner.

Suggested Readings

Armstrong RB, Nichols J, Pachance J. Punch biopsy wounds treated with Monsel's solution or a collagen matrix: a comparison of healing. *Arch Dermatol* 1986;122:546.

Baden HP. Rapid hemostasis with Monsel's solution. *Arch Dermatol* 1984;120:708.

Briggs TP, Parker C, Anson K, Miller RA. Haemostasis in urology: mechanism and pharmacology. *Br J Urol* 1992;70:225.

Camisa C, Roberts W. Monsel's solution tatooing. *J Am Acad Dermatol* 1982;7:753.

Chang H, Wu GJ, Perng WL, et al. Effects of fibrin glue on hemostasis. *J Formosan Med Assoc* 1992;91:601.

Hill RC, Kalantarian B, Jones DR. Use of microfibrillar collagen hemostat (Avitene) and thrombin to achieve hemostasis after median sternotomy. *J Thoracic Cardiovasc Surg* 1994;108:1151.

Jetmore AB, Heryer JW, Conner WE. Monsel's solution: a kinder, gentler hemostatic. *Dis Colon Rectum* 1993;36:866.

Kohno H, Nagasue N, Chang YC, et al. Comparison of topical hemostatic agents in elective hepatic resection: a clinical prospective randomized trial. *World J Surg* 1992;16:966.

Landry JR, Kanat IO. Considerations in topical hemostasis. *J Am Podiatr Med Assoc* 1985;75:581.

Larson PO. Topical hemostatic agents for dermatologic surgery. *J Dermatol Surg Oncol* 1988;14:623.

Sheppard BB, De Virgilio C, Bleiweis M, et al. Inhibition of intra-abdominal adhesions: fibrin glue in a long term model. *Am Surg* 1993;59:786.

Smith KJ, Skelton HG, Turiansky G, et al. Bovine collagen hemostatic agent used in removal of a basal cell carcinoma of the nose with a good cosmetic result. *Dermatol Surg* 1995;21:907.

Spence RK. Bleeding and the vascular surgery patient. *Semin Vasc Surg* 1994;7:104.

Takeuchi H, Konaga E, Kashitani M, et al. The usefulness of Avitene for the control of oozing in laparoscopic cholecystectomy. *Surg Gynecol Obstet* 1993;176:495.

Tawes RL Jr, Sydorak GR, DuVall TB. Autologous fibrin glue: the last step in operative hemostasis. *Am J Surg* 1994;168:120.

Chapter 5

ELECTROSURGERY AND CAUTERY

Although many associate electrosurgery and cautery with major surgery, these methods are extremely useful in the performance of the type of office and minor surgical procedures covered in this book.

Equipment

- Electrosurgical generator (with return electrode or "ground pad," active electrode with control switches or a foot switch)
- "Hot cautery" device
- Chemical cautery agents (e.g., trichloroacetic acid and silver nitrate)
- Cryocautery device
- Office laser (CO_2)

Training/Credentialing

No special credentialing is needed when performed in the office. If photocautery (laser) is used in an ambulatory surgery area of a hospital operating room, special credentialing is generally required. This is most often obtained by supplying proof of didactic course work on the safety and action of lasers and by submitting evidence of clinical experience. In the absence of such experience, many institutions require a period of proctored probation before full privileges are granted.

Coding

Some procedure codes differ depending on the method used. No codes relate solely to cautery or electrosurgery independent of the procedure in which either is used.

TABLE 5.1. Types of Cautery[a]

Actual (hot cautery)
Button
Chemical
Cold or cryocautery
Electric
Galvanic
Paquelin's
Photocautery or photocoagulation (laser)
Potential
Solar
Souttar's (steam)
Virtual

[a]Items in bold face are commonly used in current clinical practice.

Technique

PRINCIPLES OF CAUTERY

Technically, "cautery" involves the application of a caustic substance, hot instrument, electric current, or other agent to destroy tissue (Table 5.1). As a result, electrosurgical generators (often incorrectly referred to as "the cautery") are only one way of applying the principles of cautery. Other forms of cautery are also useful in the office setting. As a result, the final decision as to what type or types of cautery to have available in the primary care setting and when to use them will be based on such factors as anticipated procedure volume, provider preference, and cost. Most gynecologic care settings have on hand one or more chemical cautery agents, and a high percentage have access to cryocautery devices. Fewer have access to office electrosurgical generators or lasers, although reductions in equipment costs and the more widespread acceptance of office cervical excision procedures (loop electrosurgical excision procedure and large loop excision of the transformation zone) is changing this to some extent.

The effects of heat transfer (actual or hot cautery) or heat induction (electrosurgery, laser) on tissue depend on the temperature created and the duration of transfer or induction (Table 5.2). Knowledge of these effects may be applied to tailor the techniques used to the need at hand. For example, the application of less energy results in a more gradual increase in tissue temperature. More time is required to destroy tissue, but the area affected will be larger because of the diffusion of heat. High levels of energy result in rapid but more superficial effects.

For most clinicians, cautery is associated with the control of bleeding. For this purpose, the most common methods are electrosurgery, actual (hot) cautery, and selected

TABLE 5.2. Effects of Heat on Tissue with Time

TEMPERATURE, °C	MECHANISM	TIME REQUIRED TO DAMAGE TISSUE
40–45	Accelerated metabolism	>2 hours
50	Protein denaturation	10 minutes
70	Desiccation and coagulation	<1 second
100	Vaporization	Milliseconds

TABLE 5.3. Characteristics of Cautery

- Direct heat transfer (hot or cold)
  - Denatures protein (heat)
  - Disrupts cellular ultrastructure (cold)
  - Causes cell death
  - Creates eschar and necrosis
  - Hard to control depth of effect
- Induction of heat (electrosurgery, laser)
  - Denatures protein
  - Causes cell death
  - Creates eschar and necrosis
  - Somewhat more easily controlled
  - High levels of heat transfer may be used to cut or part tissues
- Chemical cautery (e.g., trichloroacetic acid, silver nitrate, phenol)
  - Denatures protein
  - Causes cell death
  - Hard to control depth of effect but generally superficial

hemostatic chemical cautery agents. The application of cold or the use of intense light energy (generally from a laser) may also be used for this purpose, but both have practical drawbacks that limit their use for this intent. In many cases, the choice of which cautery to use may be driven by the characteristics of the method itself (Table 5.3).

ELECTROSURGERY

Electrosurgical generators are very useful for major surgical procedures but are also useful for minor procedures (Fig. 5.1). Electrosurgical generators create high (radio)-frequency, high-voltage (6000–8000 volts) currents that induce heat in proportion to the current flowing through tissue. The shape of the electrical wave is generally sinusoidal, but the duty cycle (proportion of time that the current flows) varies for cutting and coagulation applications. When the unit is set to "cutting," the current flows continuously when the switch is pressed and the active electrode is in contact with tissue, thereby completing the electrical circuit. In contrast, when the unit is set to "coagulating," the current flows in short bursts of a few cycles of current followed by a short period with no current flow. This "on-off-on-off" pattern is repeated very rapidly

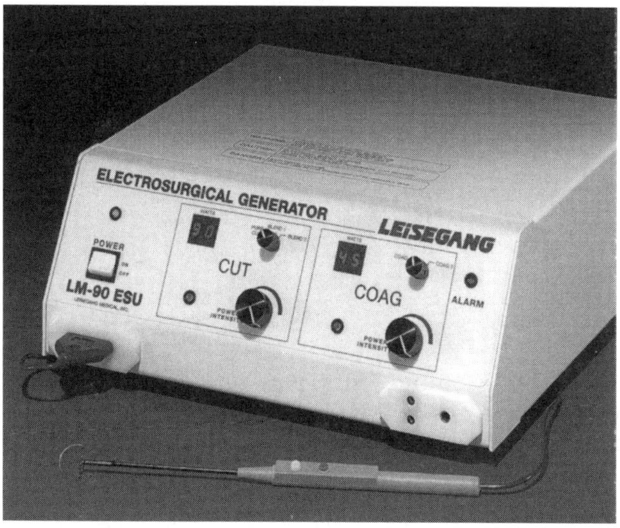

FIGURE 5.1. *Small electrosurgical units such as this one are well suited to the primary care setting. Courtesy of Leisegang Medical, 6401 Conress Avenue, Boca Raton, FL 33487.*

TABLE 5.4. Do's and Don't's of Return Electrodes

Do not
Place electrode over bony projections
Place electrode over scar tissue
Place electrode on pressure point or area with poor vascular supply
Place electrode where it may come into contact with any part of the operating table or other electronic equipment
Do
Place long edge toward incision or surgical site
Maintain good skin contact
Avoid solutions, blood, and fluids that may come into contact with the electrode (pad)

and is not apparent to the user. This pattern causes a relatively slower build-up of heat and results in coagulation of proteins and hemostasis. When the current flow is continuous, heat is built up rapidly, steam is liberated, and tissue is disrupted, yielding "cutting" effects. A "blended" setting combines these two effects by modifying the relative balance between current flow and "off" time in the coagulation setting.

When an electrosurgical generator is used, whether in the main operating room, ambulatory surgery center, or primary office, several safety issues must be addressed. Care must be taken that the return electrode ("ground plate") be placed properly to ensure that the electrical circuit completed is controlled and safely directed. This involves not only ensuring that good skin contact is maintained but also that no extraneous fluids come in contact with this return electrode during the process of skin preparation or the performance of the procedure itself. Additional considerations in the placement of the return electrode are shown in Table 5.4.

The choice of active electrode to be used is based on the procedure proposed: Fine tips are excellent for cutting or very superficial cautery; loops are best suited to excising tissue; and balls or broad tips are good for coagulating the destruction of large areas of tissue. The power setting used varies with the tip used and the electrosurgical generator. The manufacturer's operating manual should be consulted for setting guidelines.

ACTUAL (HOT) CAUTERY

Although a much older method, actual or "hot" cautery is still a very useful tool in clinical practice. Born of the red-hot iron bar, the most common form of actual cautery in use today is the heated wire cautery. Somewhat analogous to an electrical soldering iron, these devices generate an electrical current (often a low voltage) that flows through the resistance of the cautery tip, heating it to incandescence. This hot tip is then applied to the tissue to be treated, transferring heat to the tissue to destroy the tissue or provide hemostasis. Both plug-in and portable units are available (Fig. 5.2). Procedures for which this method is most commonly used are cervical cautery and the opening of a loop colostomy. Because radiant heat transfer occurs even without direct physical contact, the use of actual cautery near heat-sensitive tissues (e.g., the vulva) limit patient acceptance.

CRYOCAUTERY

Although the techniques of cryocautery are more fully discussed in Chapter 15, Cryosurgery, it should be recognized that the application of intense cold is a form of cautery. Intense cold freezes cells, resulting in cellular organelle disruption and cell death—part of the definition of cautery. The application of cold (or the removal of heat) may also be used to slow bleeding by causing vasospasm and inducing the clotting cas-

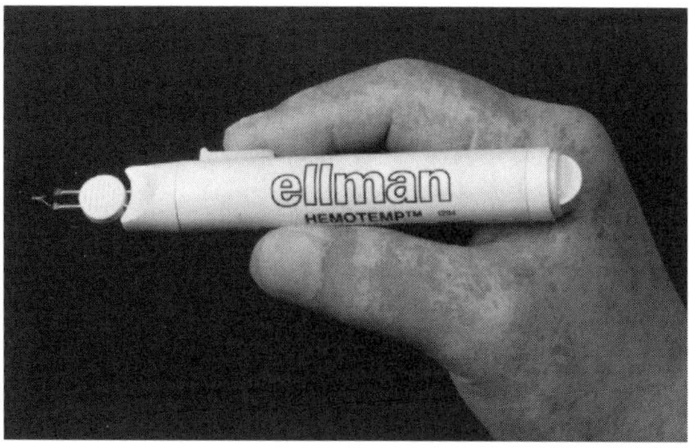

FIGURE 5.2.
Portable battery-operated cautery units are useful for small lesions or situations in which single use may be desirable. Courtesy of Ellman International, 1135 Railroad Avenue, Hewlett, NY 11557.

cade. Because cold slows most biochemical reactions, extreme cold inhibits inflammation and the vasoactive responses involved in trauma, infection, or allergy.

CHEMICAL CAUTERY

Several caustic substances are used in clinical medicine as chemical cautery agents. The most commonly used agents are trichloroacetic acid, silver nitrate, and phenol. Each of these substances acts to denature and coagulate cellular proteins, resulting in tissue destruction. These agents may be used as topical hemostatic agents (see Chapter 4, Hemostasis) or to destroy tissue, as when they are used to treat condyloma.

PHOTOCAUTERY AND PHOTOCOAGULATION (LASER)

The techniques of using laser-created light energy as a cauterizing agent are more fully discussed in Chapter 19, Laser Ablation. In a manner similar to that of electrosurgery, when less intense light energy is delivered to tissues or is delivered during a prolonged period, the subsequent build-up of heat destroys tissue. When more energy is delivered during a shorter period, the liberation of steam and pyrolytic products results in the physical disruption of cells and tissue, thereby causing tissue vaporization and "cutting."

Special Notes

The formation of eschar (char) on the tip of an electrosurgical active electrode indicates the presence of a power setting that is too low, a surgical field that is excessively dry, or movement of the active electrode that is too rapid.

To provide the best hemostasis, the electrosurgical instrument should be applied to the bleeding site and then activated. When the device is activated before it is in contact with the tissue, initial arcing of current will occur when the tip approaches the surface. This results in a superficial scar but does not cause deep coagulation of the vessels, which would lead to continuing or late bleeding. When the tip is placed against the bleeding site and then activated, the current tends to propagate up the vessel, providing superior hemostasis.

Suggested Readings

Anonymous. Burns and fires from electrosurgical active electrodes. *Health Devices* 1993;22:421.

Anonymous. Electrosurgical units with accessory outputs. *Health Devices* 1993;22:601.

Anonymous. Risk of electrosurgical burns at needle electrode sites. *Health Devices* 1994;23:373.

Anonymous. Use of an incompatible footswitch with Aspen Excalibur, Birtcher 5000, and Valleylab Force electrosurgical units. *Health Devices* 22;593.

Baggish MS, Tucker RD. Tissue actions of bipolar scissors compared with monopolar devices. *Fertil Steril* 1995;63:422.

Chen RJ, Lee EF, Shih JC. Does the loop electrosurgical excision procedure adversely affect the histopathological interpretation of cervical conization specimens? *Acta Obstet Gynecol Scand* 1994;73:726.

Ferenczy A. Electroconization of the cervix with a fine-needle electrode. *Obstet Gynecol* 1994;84:152.

Ferris DG, Saxena S, Hainer BL, et al. Gynecologic and dermatologic electrosurgical units: a comparative review. *J Fam Pract* 1994;39:160.

Haag R, Cuschieri A. Recent advances in high-frequency electrosurgery: development of automated systems. *J Roy Coll Surg Edinburgh* 1993;38:354.

McLucas B, McGill J. Pure cutting current for loop excision of squamous intraepithelial lesions. *J Reprod Med* 1994;39:373.

Reidenbach HD. Fundamentals of bipolar high-frequency surgery. *Endoscop Surg All Technol* 1993;1:85.

Sebben JE. Modifications of electrosurgery electrodes. *J Dermatol Surg Oncol* 1992; 18:908.

Tucker RD, Hollenhorst MJ. Bipolar electrosurgical devices. *Endoscop Surg All Technol* 1993;1:110.

Tucker RD, Sievert CE, Kramolowsky EV, et al. The interaction between electrosurgical generators, endoscopic electrodes, and tissue. *Gastrointest Endos* 1992; 38:118.

Tucker RD, Voyles CR, Silvis SE. Capacitive coupled stray currents during laparoscopic and endoscopic electrosurgical procedures. *Biomed Inst Technol* 1992; 26:303.

Wicker P. Making sense of electrosurgery. *Nursing Times* 1992;88:31.

Wright VC. Contemporary electrosurgery: physics for physicians. *J Fam Pract* 1994; 39:119.

Section II

ADVANCED GYNECOLOGIC PROCEDURES

Chapter 6

AMNIOCENTESIS

The ability to obtain fluid samples from around the growing fetus has allowed substantial advances in prenatal biochemical and genetic diagnosis. What grew out of the management of Rh-factor hemolytic disease has become a common procedure. What was an uncommon hospital-based test has become a widespread office procedure. Despite its prevalence, amniocentesis remains an invasive test with the peril of complications if not performed with care.

Equipment

- Sterile gloves
- Skin preparation materials (e.g., povidone-iodine and 70% isopropyl alcohol)
- Sterile gauze pads (2 inches × 2 inches or 4 inches × 4 inches)
- Self-adhesive bandage
- 1% lidocaine without epinephrine, 5-mL syringe, 22-gauge needle (if not included in amniocentesis kit)
- Ultrasonography unit
- Fetal monitor or Doppler fetoscope
- Commercial amniocentesis tray

or

- 20- and 22-gauge spinal needles, 20-mL syringe, three sterile 10-mL specimen tubes with caps (plain, without additive), sterile drape (one with a small fenestration or multiple drapes)

Training/Credentialing

No special credentialing needed; office procedure only.

Coding

59000	Amniocentesis, any method
76946	Ultrasonic guidance for amniocentesis, physician supervision, and interpretation

Technique

Before amniocentesis is done, the indications, contraindications, risks, benefits, and complications should be reviewed and discussed with the patient and informed consent should obtained. In preparation, the patient should be placed in the supine position with the head elevated 20 to 30°. If the pregnancy is advanced, the patient may empty her bladder and be placed in a slight left decubitus position. Ultrasonography is used to assess fetal well-being, fetal lie, and placental position.

By using ultrasonography, a suitable pocket of amniotic fluid should be identified. Ideally, this pocket should be located away from the fetal face and placenta but should be accessible with a standard spinal needle. Areas around the fetal extremities are often best. The location of this pocket relative to the skin surface should be noted as a guide to needle insertion.

The skin of the abdominal wall over the chosen pocket of amniotic fluid should be disinfected with a suitable skin preparation solution and technique of the examiner's choice. If a local anesthetic is to be used, it is established at this point using sterile technique: A small skin weal of local anesthetic is placed and the proposed needle track is infiltrated with no more than 4–5 mL of anesthetic agent.

With the stilet in place, a 20- or 22-gauge spinal needle is passed perpendicularly

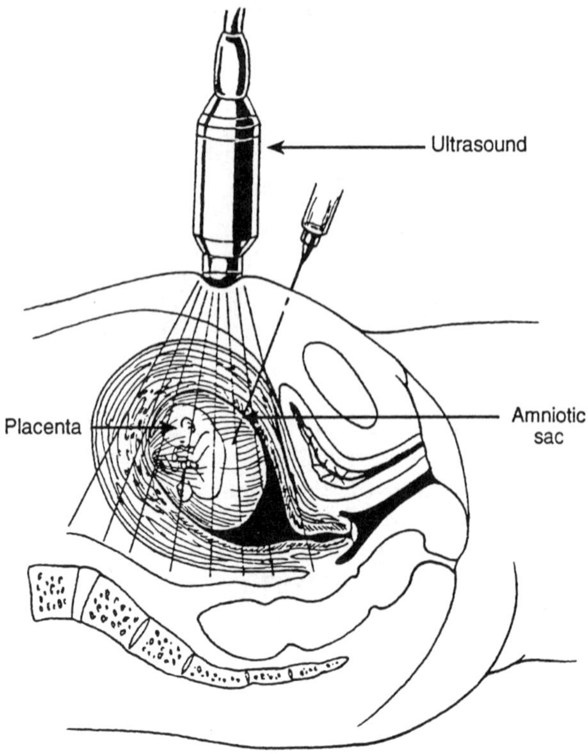

FIGURE 6.1. *Amniocentesis with ultrasound guidance; cross-section of uterus and fetus with the needle in a pocket of amniotic fluid is shown. (Reproduced with permission from Beckmann RB, Ling FW, Barzansky BM, et al.* Obstetrics and Gynecology. *2nd ed. Baltimore: Williams & Wilkins, 1995:20.)*

through the skin and abdominal and uterine walls into the amniotic sac. A slight pop or loss of resistance may be felt as the needle traverses the fascia. Once the pocket of fluid has been entered, the stilet is removed from the needle. Free flow of fluid should be demonstrated. If free flow is not found, the needle should be rotated or tipped and rechecked before being advanced further (with the stilet in place). Placement of the needle into the amniotic fluid pocket may be facilitated by using ultrasonography to guide the needle's advancement (Fig. 6.1). This can be especially helpful when amniocentesis is performed early in pregnancy.

Once free flow of fluid has been shown, a small syringe should be attached to the needle and 2–3 mL of fluid withdrawn. This fluid is discarded. Appropriate samples are now taken and placed in sterile specimen tubes. The amount of material needed and any special handling required for these specimens is dictated by the studies to be performed. If there is any doubt, consultation with the laboratory before the procedure can identify any special handling that must be used.

After samples have been obtained, the needle is withdrawn and a self-adhesive bandage is applied to the site of needle puncture. The fetus should be monitored for a short period after the procedure. If bloody fluid was obtained, this monitoring period should be extended to 1–2 hours or more, depending on other considerations. An appropriate procedure note should be entered into the patient's record.

Special Notes

None.

Suggested Readings

Bahado-Singh R, Schmitt R, Hobbins JC. New technique for genetic amniocentesis in twins. *Obstet Gynecol* 1992;79:304.

Bombard AT, Powers JF, Carter S, et al. Procedure-related fetal losses in transplacental versus nontransplacental genetic amniocentesis. *Am J Obstet Gynecol* 1995;172:868.

Bravo RR, Shulman LP, Phillips OP, et al. Transplacental needle passage in early amniocentesis and pregnancy loss. *Obstet Gynecol* 1995;86:437.

D'Alton ME. Prenatal diagnostic procedures. *Semin Perinatol* 1994;8:140.

Djalali M, Barbi G, Kennerknecht I, et al. Introduction of early amniocentesis to routine prenatal diagnosis. *Pren Diag* 1992;12:661.

Dombrowski MP, Isada NB, Johnson MP, et al. Modified stylet technique for tenting of amniotic membranes. *Obstet Gynecol* 1996;87:455.

Elliott JP, Sawyer AT, Radin TG, et al. Large-volume therapeutic amniocentesis in the treatment of hydramnios. *Obstet Gynecol* 1994;84:1025.

Giorlandino C, Gambuzza G, D'Alessio P, et al. Blood contamination of amniotic fluid after amniocentesis in relation to placental location. *Prenat Diag* 1996;16:180.

Giorlandino C, Mobili L, Bilancioni E, et al. Transplacental amniocentesis: is it really a higher-risk procedure? *Prenat Diag* 1994;14:803.

Henry GP, Miller WA. Early amniocentesis. *J Reprod Med* 1992;37:396.

Holzgreve W, Ganshirt-Ahlert D, Miny P. Indications and methods for antenatal chromosome analysis: more choices require more appropriate selection. *Curr Opin Obstet Gynecol* 1994;6:3.

Holzgreve W, Nippert I, Ganshirt-Ahlert D, et al. Immediate and long-term applications of technology. *Clin Obstet Gynecol* 1993;36:476.

Jorgensen FS, Bang J, Lind AM, et al. Genetic amniocentesis at 7–14 weeks of gestation. *Prenat Diag* 1992;12:277.

Kerber S, Held KR. Early genetic amniocentesis: 4 years' experience. *Prenat Diag* 1993;13:21.

Nicolaides K, Brizot M de L, Patel F, Snijders R. Comparison of chorionic villus sampling and amniocentesis for fetal karyotyping at 10–13 weeks' gestation. *Lancet* 1994;344:435.

Palo P, Piiroinen O, Honkonen E, et al. Transabdominal chorionic villus sampling and amniocentesis for prenatal diagnosis: 5 years' experience at a university centre. *Prenat Diag* 1994;14:157.

Petrikovsky BM, Kaplan GP. Fetal responses to inadvertent contact with the needle during amniocentesis. *Fetal Diagnos Ther* 1995;10:83.

Rousseau O, Boulot P, Lefort G, et al. Amniocentesis before 15 weeks' gestation: technical aspects and obstetric risks. *Eur J Obstet Gynecol Reprod Biol* 1995;58:127.

Schemmer G, Johnson A. Genetic amniocentesis and chorionic villus sampling. *Obstet Gynecol Clin North Am* 1993;20:497.

Stone JL, Lockwood CJ. Amniocentesis and chorionic villus sampling. *Curr Opin Obstet Gynecol* 1993;5:211.

Sundberg K, Bang J, Brocks V, et al. Early sonographically guided amniocenteses with filtration technique: follow-up on 249 procedures. *J Ultrasound Med* 1995; 14:585.

Sundberg K, Jorgensen FS, Tabor A, et al. Experience with early amniocentesis. *J Perinat Med* 1995;23:149.

Vaitkiene D, Bergstrom S. Management of amniocentesis in women with oligohydramnios due to membrane rupture: evaluation of a cervical adapter. *Gynecol Obstet Invest* 1995;40:28.

van Vugt JM, Nieuwint A, van Geijn HP. Single-needle insertion: an alternative technique for early second-trimester genetic twin amniocentesis. *Fetal Diagnos Ther* 1995;10:178.

Chapter 7

ASPIRATION OF A BREAST CYST

Simple cystic masses in the breast may be both diagnosed and treated by aspiration.

Equipment

- Skin preparation materials (alcohol, iodine- or hexachlorophene-based antibacterial solution [e.g., Betadine, Hibiclens])
- 10-mL disposable syringe
- 22–25-gauge needle
- Self-adherent bandage (optional)

Training/Credentialing

No special credentialing needed; office procedure only.

Coding

19000	Puncture aspiration of cyst of breast
19001	aspiration of each additional cyst

Technique

After adequate skin preparation, the cystic mass is stabilized by the nondominant hand (Fig. 7.1). This is accomplished by gently pinching the breast tissue below the mass between the thumb and fingers of the hand. A 22–25-gauge needle (attached to a 10-mL syringe) is inserted into the cyst cavity (Fig. 7.2). A small "pop" or loss of resistance is often felt as the cyst wall is breached. The cyst contents are aspirated by gentle suction from the syringe. No dressing or special breast care is required, although a self-adherent bandage may be used.

Fluid aspirated from patients with fibrocystic changes is usually straw colored. Dark brown or green fluid is found in cysts that have been present for a long time, but such

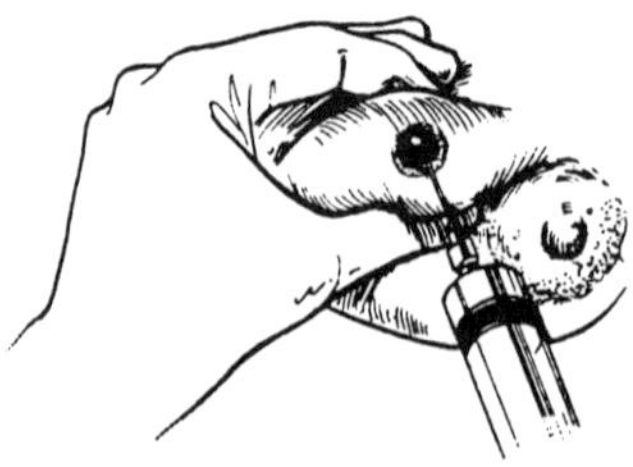

FIGURE 7.1.
The cystic lesion is stabilized by the nondominant hand while the needle is advanced. (Reproduced with permission from Mitchel GW, Bassett LW. The Female Breast and Its Disorders. *Baltimore: Williams & Wilkins, 1990:185.)*

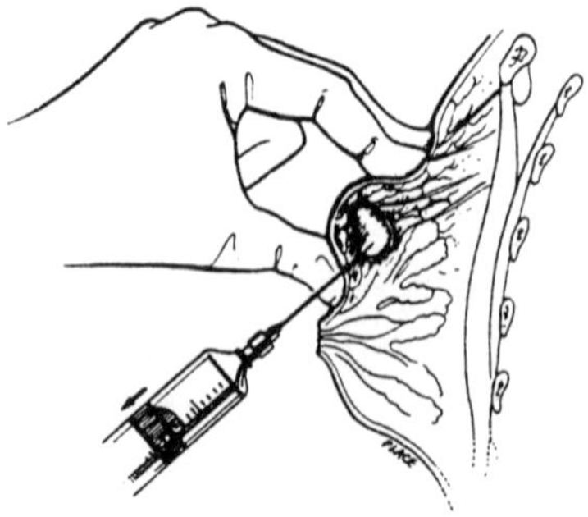

FIGURE 7.2.
Gentle pressure is maintained on the cyst while suction is applied to the syringe to aspirate the cyst contents. (Reproduced with permission from Mitchel GW, Bassett LW. The Female Breast and Its Disorders. *Baltimore: Williams & Wilkins, 1990:185.)*

fluid is equally innocuous. Because of high false–positive (up to 6%) and even higher false–negative rates (2–22%), cytologic evaluation of the fluid obtained is of little value.

Normal Findings

If the cyst disappears completely and has not reformed by the 1 month follow-up examination, no further therapy is required.

Selected Abnormal Findings

Bloody fluid requires further evaluation.

Special Notes

In women older than 35 years of age, mammography before aspiration should be considered because of the increased incidence of malignant neoplasms. Once aspiration has been attempted, mammography should be delayed several weeks because artifactual changes induced by the manipulation make mammograms difficult to interpret.

An evacuated test-tube of the type used for blood samples (Vacutainer), and its associated venipuncture needle, may be used instead of a syringe for aspiration of a breast cyst.

Suggested Readings

Marchant DJ. Diagnosis of breast disease and the role of the gynecologist. *Curr Opin Obstet Gynecol* 1993;5:67.

Palmer ML,Tsangaris TN. Breast biopsy in women 30 years old or less. *Am J Surg* 1993;165:708.

Parker SH, Stavros AT, Dennis MA. Needle biopsy techniques. *Radiol Clin North Am* 1995;33:1171.

Sneige N. Fine-needle aspiration of the breast: a review of 1,995 cases with emphasis on diagnostic pitfalls. *Diagnost Cytopathol* 1993;9:106.

Chapter 8

BREAST ULTRASONOGRAPHY

Thorough mammographic and sonographic work-up of lesions detected at screening reduces the number of biopsies performed and increases the true-positive biopsy rate. To this end, office ultrasonographic evaluation of the breast can provide direct management or facilitate needle aspiration or biopsy. Previous studies have indicated that breast ultrasonography used to differentiate between cystic and solid lesions has an accuracy rate of 95 to 100%. Palpable lesions may be most expediently managed by needle aspiration rather than ultrasonographic characterization. Ultrasonography is well suited to the evaluation of nonpalpable masses found on mammography.

Equipment

- Office ultrasonography equipment, with high-frequency, high-resolution ultrasound probe (dedicated breast units or special transducers designed for breast imaging are desirable)
- Water-soluble acoustic coupling agent
- Water-path acoustic offset, unless a transducer designed for breast imaging with a built-in offset is used (water-filled plastic bag or commercial water offset pad)

Training/Credentialing

No special credentialing needed; office procedure only. Experience with pelvic ultrasonography or transvaginal imaging is not sufficient for reliably performing ultrasonography of the breast without additional training or proctored experience.

Coding

76645	Echography, Breast(s) (unilateral or bilateral) B-scan and/or real time with image documentation

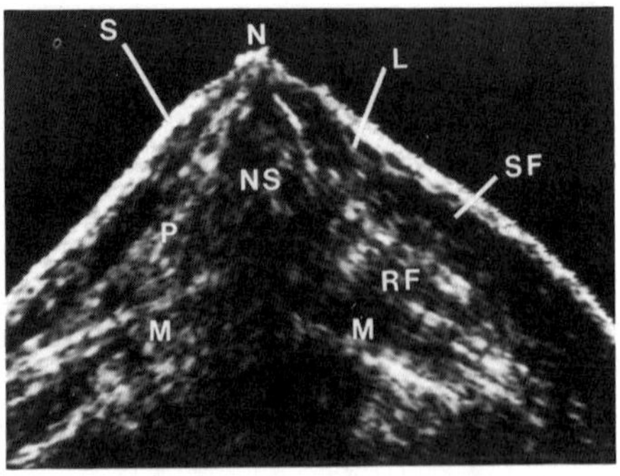

FIGURE 8.1.
Normal breast anatomy, automated whole-breast image. L, suspensory ligament; M, pectoral muscle; N, nipple; NS, shadowing from nipple; P, parenchymal tissue; RF, retromammary fat; S, skin; SF, subcutaneous fat. (Reproduced with permission from Mitchel GW, Bassett LW. The Female Breast and Its Disorders. *Baltimore: Williams & Wilkins, 1990;155.)*

Technique

Breast ultrasonography has evolved greatly since its introduction in 1952. Despite these improvements, technical factors, machine settings, and the technique used greatly influence the reliability of the results obtained. Care in the setting of power, time gain compensation, and gray scale adjustments is required.

The scanning technique must be chosen on the basis of the equipment available and the location and type of lesion being evaluated. Dedicated, water-path whole-breast scanners provide the best detail with the fewest artifacts. These devices produce a series of thin-section images of the entire breast (Fig. 8.1) and require a greater investment, space, time, and training than are generally available in the general gynecology setting. In the absence of such equipment, a hand-held unit may be used. Such transducers should have a sound frequency greater than 5 MHz and a depth of focus no greater than 2 cm. For this reason, even the transducers used for transvaginal ultrasonography are ill suited for breast examinations. Because the use of an incorrect transducer may result in artifacts or missed lesions, any attempt to use such a transducer should be regarded as "preliminary" or "screening," and no final clinical decisions should be based on the outcome of such an examination.

Hand-held transducers should be coupled to the skin with an acoustic coupling agent (e.g., Aquasonic) and an appropriate water path offset (if required). Care must be taken to avoid compressing or distorting the breast tissue by excessive pressure from the transducer. The breast must be examined from several angles to "look around" attenuation caused by the thicker skin of the nipple and areola, the suspensory ligaments of the breast, or excessive breast fat. Although these factors may lead to substantial attenuation of the sound beam, sonolucent masses (cysts) should be readily apparent.

As with most imaging techniques, care should be taken to examine all areas of the breast, the tissues around and behind the breast, and the contralateral breast. Appropriate documentation, including images, must be maintained.

Normal Findings

The normal ultrasonographic appearance of the breast is shown in Figure 8.1. It is common to be able to see the sonolucent ducts in the subareolar tissues (Fig. 8.2).

Selected Abnormal Findings

Single or multiple cysts are the most common and most easily recognized abnormality seen on breast ultrasonography (Figs. 8.3 and 8.4).

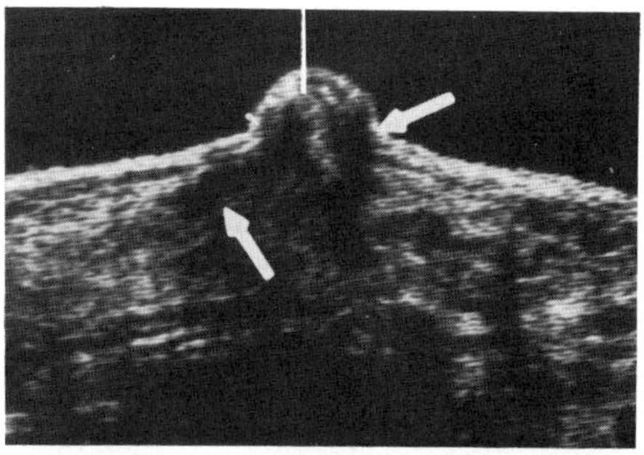

FIGURE 8.2.
Normal sonolucent ducts (arrows) in subareolar region. (Reproduced with permission from Mitchel GW, Bassett LW. The Female Breast and Its Disorders. *Baltimore: Williams & Wilkins, 1990;155.)*

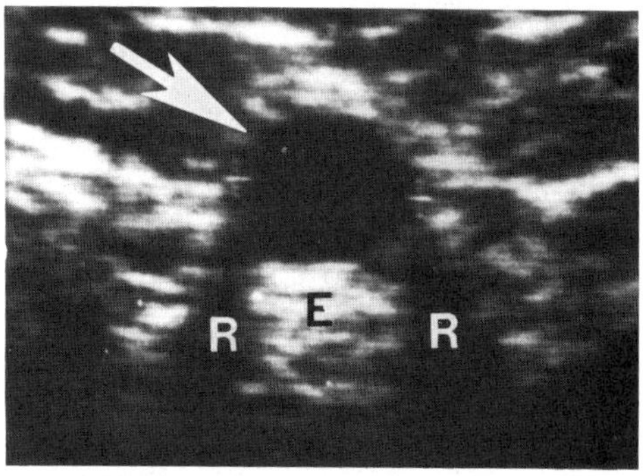

FIGURE 8.3.
Cyst (arrow). Hand-held examination shows typical cyst features: sharp anterior and posterior margins, round shape, anechoic interior, enhanced posterior echoes (E), and lateral edge refraction (R). (Reproduced with permission from Mitchel GW, Bassett LW. The Female Breast and Its Disorders. *Baltimore: Williams & Wilkins, 1990;155).*

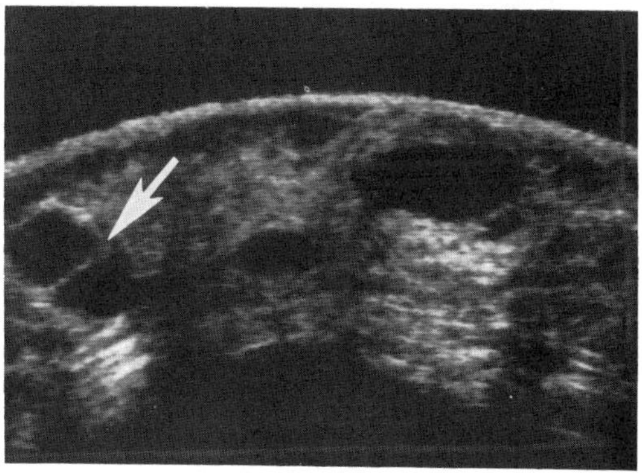

FIGURE 8.4.
Multiple cysts, one containing a septum (arrow). (Reproduced with permission from Mitchel GW, Bassett LW. The Female Breast and Its Disorders. *Baltimore: Williams & Wilkins, 1990;156.)*

Special Notes

Several technical problems make breast ultrasonography difficult. For example, the heterogeneous character of breast tissue results in many tissue interfaces that refract and reflect the ultrasound beam, resulting in artifacts, defocusing, and loss of signal. To overcome these problems, special high-frequency, tightly focused, large-aperture transducers are now available for breast evaluations. Even with these transducers, superficial breast masses may be missed unless fluid offset is used. This technique may take the form of a water bath into which the breast is suspended, a water-filled plastic bag, or a commercial offset pad. Transducers specifically designed for hand-held scanning of the breast often incorporate this offset into the design of the transducer itself.

Breast ultrasonography is less sensitive and specific for diagnosing breast cancer than is mammography. As a result, mammography remains the standard noninvasive diagnostic and screening method.

As is the case with mammography, imaging studies should be done before any attempt at needle aspiration or drainage because these procedures may produce artifacts (Fig. 8.5).

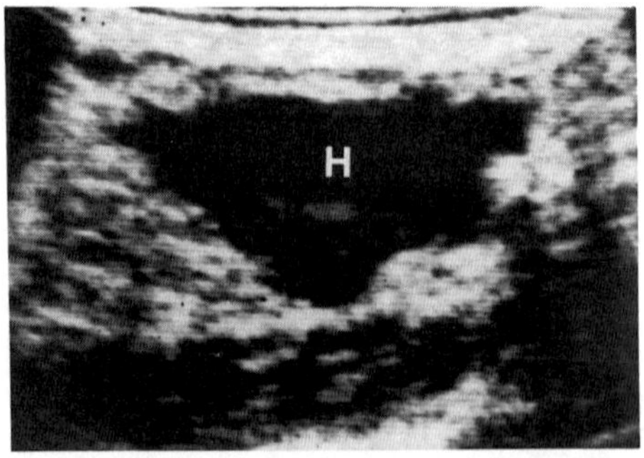

FIGURE 8.5.
Two weeks after biopsy, postsurgical hematoma (H) contains anechoic fluid above the echoic sediment. (Reproduced with permission from Mitchel GW, Bassett LW. The Female Breast and Its Disorders. *Baltimore: Williams & Wilkins, 1990;157.)*

Suggested Readings

Bassett LW. Breast sonography. In: Mitchell GW Jr, Bassett LW, eds. *The Female Breast and Its Disorders.* Baltimore: Williams & Wilkins, 1990:154.

Gordon PB, Goldenberg SL, Chan NH. Solid breast lesions: diagnosis with US-guided fine-needle aspiration biopsy. *Radiology* 1993;189:573.

Jokich PM, Monticciolo DL, Adler YT. Breast ultrasonography. *Radiol Clin North Am* 1992;30:993.

Nyirjesy I, Billingsley FS. Management of breast problems in gynecologic office practice using sonography and fine-needle aspiration. *Obstet Gynecol* 1992;79:699.

Phillips G, McGuire L, Clowes D. The value of ultrasound-guided fine needle aspiration in the assessment of solid breast lumps. *Aust Radiol* 1994;38:187.

Schepps B, Scola FH, Frates RE. Benign circumscribed breast masses. Mammographic and sonographic appearance. *Obstet Gynecol Clin North Am* 1994;21:519.

Shaw de Paredes E. Evaluation of abnormal screening mammograms. *Cancer* 1994;74:342.

Sickles EA, Filly FA, Callen PW. Breast cancer detection with sonography and mammography: comparison using state-of-the-art equipment. *AJR* 1983;140:843.

Staren ED. Surgical office-based ultrasound of the breast. *Am Surg* 1995;61:619.

Chapter 9

COLPOSCOPY

Created in 1925, the colposcope has slowly gained its now pivotal role in the assessment of abnormal cervical cytology. Colposcopy and exfoliative cytology complement each other by improving the diagnostic accuracy of each. Based on a simple stereoscopic operating microscope with magnifications of from 4 to 40×, the colposcope allows the clinician to identify normal landmarks, find changes suggestive of underlying abnormality, and select sites for biopsy that will yield the most information. As a simple office-based screening tool, colposcopy can be invaluable.

To allow comparison and standardization, the performance of colposcopy must follow a series of unchanging steps and use a consistent terminology. Most of the standards for the performance and documentation of colposcopy have come from the American Society for Colposcopy and Cervical Pathology and the International Federation of Cervical Pathology and Colposcopy. These groups, along with the American College of Obstetricians and Gynecologists, have sought to ensure that the maximal reliability and benefit is attained any time colposcopy is performed.

Equipment

- Colposcope with light source (Fig. 9.1)
- Endocervical speculum
- Biopsy forceps (e.g., Tischler, Kevorkian)
- Endocervical curette
- Large-tipped cotton swabs, cotton balls, or small gauze sponges
- Examination gloves
- Vaginal speculum
- Tenaculum (optional)
- Acetic acid (3–5%) (white vinegar)
- Monsel's solution (ferric subsulfate)
- Lugol's (5%) solution (supersaturated iodine; optional)
- Sputum or urine cups (to hold solutions)
- Uterine sound (optional)

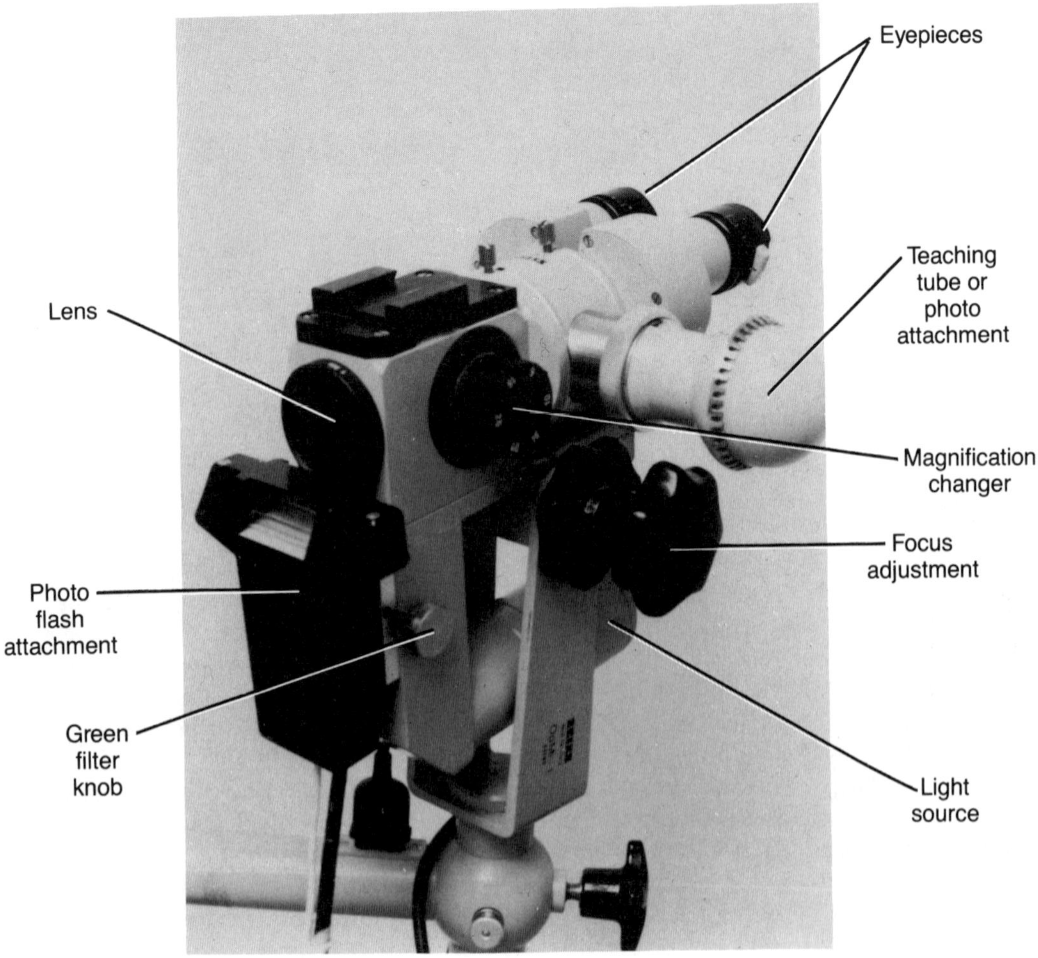

FIGURE 9.1.
Colposcope. Many different types of colposcopes are available with different features. (Reproduced with permission from Jones HW, Wentz AC, Burnett LS. Novak's Textbook of Gynecology. *11th ed. Baltimore: Williams & Wilkins, 1988:659.)*

- Sterile gloves (optional)
- Video or photographic equipment attached to the hysteroscope as desired (optional)

Training/Credentialing

No special credentialing needed; office procedure only. Self-learning packages are available from many sources, including a new computer-based interactive program from the American College of Obstetricians and Gynecologists. Free-standing courses and tutorials in conjunction with other meetings are also available. Some form of tutorial or learning package is advisable.

Coding

57452	Colposcopy (Vaginoscopy); (separate procedure)
57454	with biopsy(s) of the cervix and/or endocervical curettage

57460	with loop electrode excision procedure of the cervix
57500	Biopsy of cervix only, single or multiple
57505	Endocervical curettage (not done as part of a dilatation and curettage)

Technique

Because of the many small items, solutions, and support material needed to smoothly perform colposcopy, some advance planning is necessary. If colposcopy is to be a regular part of a clinician's practice, the advance preparation of a tray or kit containing most of the equipment needed will greatly simplify set-up. Such a kit also reduces the chances that a key piece of equipment will be missing when it is needed.

Any instrument that will enter the endocervical canal or will be used for biopsy should be sterilized before use. The use of sterile gloves is not required as long as the portions of instruments that will come in contact with the patient are handled in such a way that they remain sterile.

The most widespread application of colposcopy is for the evaluation of abnormal cervical cytologic findings (Fig. 9.2). Other common indications for colposcopy are shown in Table 9.1. The indications for colposcopy and the information expected to result from the procedure should be discussed with the patient in advance. If biopsy specimens are to be taken or local anesthetics used, informed consent should be obtained before colposcopy is done (see Chapter 2, Informed Consent). If there is a possibility that the patient could be pregnant, a pregnancy test should be performed.

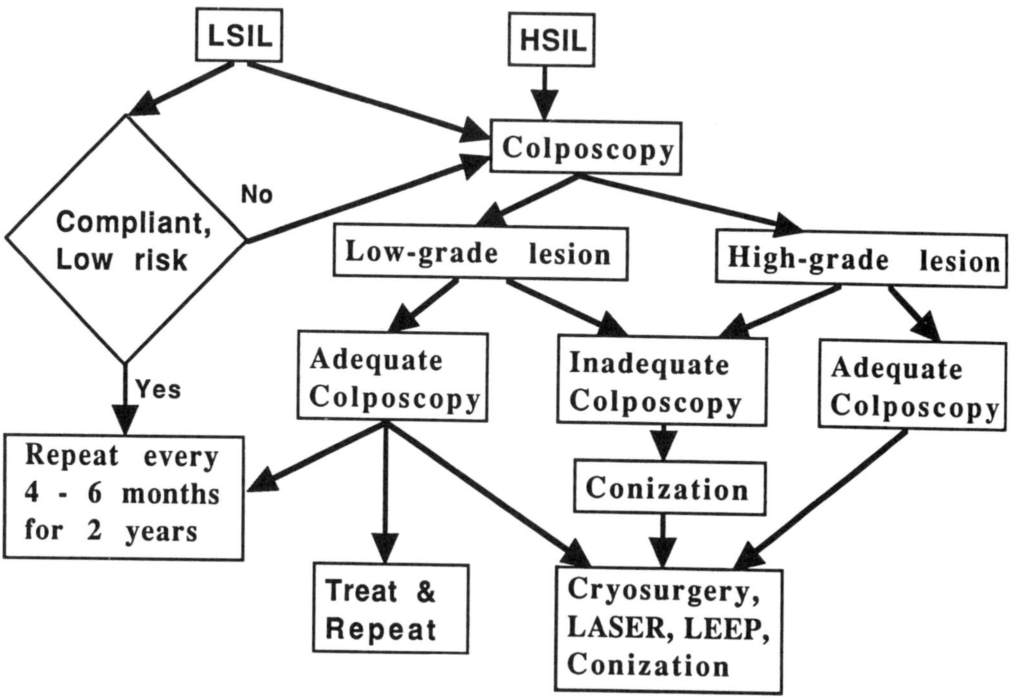

FIGURE 9.2.
Colposcopy plays a pivotal role in the evaluation and management of abnormal cervical cytology. LEEP, loop electrosurgical excision procedure. (Reproduced with permission from Smith RP. Gynecology in Primary Care. *Baltimore: Williams & Wilkins, 1997:313.)*

TABLE 9.1. Common Indications for Colposcopy

Abnormal cervical cytology (atypia, cancer, dysplasia, koilocytosis)
Cervical lesions (palpable or visible)
Condyloma (current or past) (relative indication)
Human immunodeficiency virus (HIV) infection
Intrauterine diethylstilbestrol (DES) exposure
Surveillance or follow-up

The patient should be placed in the dorsal lithotomy position and made as comfortable as possible. A bimanual examination may be considered to evaluate the location and mobility of the cervix, the length of the vagina, and the presence of any palpable lesions. If such a bimanual examination is performed, care must be used to limit the amount of lubricant used because the lubricant (and glove powder) can adversely affect cytologic studies. If the examination has recently been performed, this step may be skipped.

By using the largest warmed but unlubricated speculum the patient can comfortably accommodate, the cervix should be brought into view. Colposcopy requires a wider field of exposure than does routine screening or cytologic examinations. A wide-bladed Graves' speculum is more comfortable than a smaller speculum, which may require frequent repositioning. Patients who have redundant or lax vaginal walls may present a particular challenge to obtaining a clear view of the cervix. When this occurs, a condom or the finger of a large glove may be placed over the blades of the speculum and the tip removed. The barrel formed by the condom or glove finger and the blades of the speculum will hold the vaginal tissue safely and comfortably out of the field of view. With the cervix satisfactorily in view, the thumb screws of the speculum should be set to allow security and maximal access.

Next, the cervix and the vaginal fornices should be grossly inspected for lesions. At this time, excessive secretions may be gently blotted away, cultures may be obtained, or a repeat Papanicolaou smear may be taken. Excessive cervical mucus may be removed by using a saline moistened swab. Each of these steps may produce irritation or bleeding and should be done only when clearly indicated.

The colposcope may be moved into position either before or after the application of acetic acid, although many have suggested that initial screening be done before any agent is applied. The instrument should be positioned to provide an unobstructed view of the cervix; its position and height should be comfortable for both the patient and the examiner. With the focus of the colposcope at the middle of its range, the position of the entire instrument should be adjusted so that the cervix is in focus. This allows further fine adjustments to be made by using only the instrument's focusing mechanism and not by repositioning the instrument itself.

Acetic acid (3–5%) should be liberally applied to the cervix. This is easily accomplished by using large cotton-tipped applicators (such as those used in anoscopy or colonoscopy), cotton balls, or small gauze sponges. A cold or stinging sensation may be experienced, and the patient should be warned of this before the application. Acetic acid causes the columnar epithelial cells to swell and opacifies metaplastic and dysplastic cells. The changes brought on by the application of acetic acid are only temporary, requiring periodic reapplication approximately every 5 minutes. Gross lesions exposed by the application of the acetic acid should be noted for careful scrutiny.

Inspection of the cervix begins using the lowest magnification, with additional magnification added later if needed. The transformation zone (the area between the existing squamocolumnar junction and the original squamocolumnar junction) should be identified and inspected in its entirety. If necessary, the cervix may be manipulated using an acetic acid-soaked applicator stick, a cervical hook (similar to a skin hook retractor), or an endocervical speculum. If these are used, care must be exercised to avoid trauma. Any areas of white change, vascular abnormality, or mosaicism should be inspected under greater magnification. Vascular patterns may be made more visible by the interposition of a green filter in front of the colposcope's light source. This will make the normally red vessels appear black against the pale background of the epithelium.

Biopsy specimens of all abnormal areas should be obtained. Abnormal areas may be stained with Lugol's solution to enhance this identification, but this is rarely necessary. Lugol's solution is more useful when the transformation zone must be outlined before conization (see Chapter 20, LEEP and LLETZ Conizations). Any acetowhite area, areas of thickening, abnormal vascular pattern, or mosaicism should be sampled by using one of several different types of biopsy forceps available (Fig. 9.3). When multiple abnormalities are present, biopsies of the most severe areas take precedence. Whenever possible, the biopsy specimen should include the edge or border of the lesion. Even in the face of frank malignancy, a biopsy specimen taken from the center of the lesion may show only terminal changes or necrosis, making histologic diagnosis impossible. Biopsy specimens should be placed in a buffered formalin solution for transport to the pathology laboratory.

Curettage of the endocervical canal must be included in colposcopic examination to exclude the possibility of endocervical lesions above the limits of visibility. The endocervical curettage helps to identify lesions that are located beyond the transformation zone. Endocervical curettage is especially helpful as a first stage in the evaluation

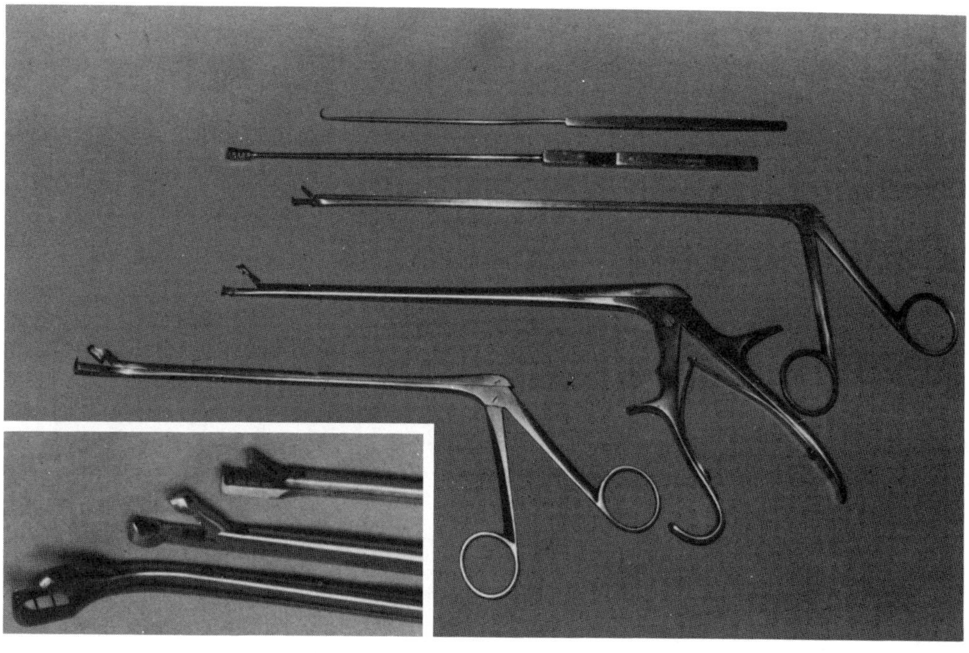

FIGURE 9.3.

Cervical biopsy instruments. The larger jaw may be used to get a deep bit of stroma to prove the presence of invasive cancer. The small hook is useful in stabilizing the cervix or tenting up the vaginal walls for a biopsy. (Reproduced with permission from Jones HW, Wentz AC, Burnett LS. Novak's Textbook of Gynecology. *11th ed. Baltimore: Williams & Wilkins, 1988:664.)*

of atypical glandular cells and should be performed under direct vision to avoid inadvertent contamination with ectocervical material. The procedure should not be performed during either known or expected pregnancy.

To perform endocervical curettage, the curette is passed into the endocervical canal to the level of the inner os. This point may be identified by a modest increase in resistance to further advancement and a slight puckering of the cervix as the canal is advanced with the curette. If neither resistance nor puckering indicates the location of the inner os, the curette should not be advanced more that about 2 cm from the external os. The entire endocervical canal should be sampled in all directions. This generally requires two or more passes with the curette; care should be taken to rotate the face of the curette toward all areas. As with any other histologic specimen, tissue obtained should be placed in a buffered formalin solution. Some laboratories prefer that these samples be placed on lens paper, Telfa, or other carrier before being placed in fixative. This should be left to the preferences of the local laboratory. Tissue that remains trapped in the opening of the curette may be freed by using the sharp tip of a broken wooden applicator stick.

If bleeding from a biopsy site persists or is heavy, Monsel's solution may be applied. Monsel's solution should only be applied after all specimens have been obtained. Because Monsel's solution can delay healing, it should be used sparingly. Once bleeding has been controlled, excessive blood, clots, and Monsel's solution should be removed by gentle swabbing. The colposcope may be moved out of the way and the speculum removed, taking care to inspect the walls of the vagina for lesions or other pathologic abnormalities as the speculum is retracted.

The location and character of all lesions and the transformation zone itself should be noted, and a drawing detailing the location of these features and the location from which biopsy specimens were obtained should be placed in the patient's chart (Fig. 9.4). The terms used and impressions rendered should be consistent.

Normal Findings

The cervix should appear smooth, pink, and glistening. The transformation zone should be fully visible and regular. There should be no abnormal vascular patterns or acetowhite areas. Typical findings and the terms used to describe them are shown in Table 9.2.

Selected Abnormal Findings

Colposcopic examinations that fail to visualize the squamocolumnar junction or the limits of any lesions present (inadequate studies) occur in roughly 15 to 20% of premenopausal women. In these patients, additional studies such as repeated cytologic samples or conization will be based on the patient's history and previous cytologic abnormality.

When abnormalities are present, an attempt to grade the lesion should be made. Criteria that aid in this determination are intercapillary distance, denseness of the white epithelium, sharpness of borders with the surrounding epithelium, and irregularity of surface contour. Flat, dense white lesions with sharp borders and widely spaced capillaries are the least ominous. Atypical vessels (Fig. 9.5) and a mosaic pattern to the surface (Fig. 9.6) suggest an abnormality from which a biopsy specimen should be obtained. Normal variants, such as nabothian cysts, may have vascular changes (Fig. 9.7), but these generally show branching and lack the close spacing, sharp angles, and tortuous spirals (hairpins) that characterize malignant and premalignant changes.

Colposcopy Record
Ambulatory Care Services
OB-GYN CLINIC

ADDRESSOGRAPH (Name, Hospital Number)

TELEPHONE #:

HUSBAND'S FIRST NAME:

AGE	PAR.	RACE	DATE

VISIT: 1st ☐ 2nd ☐ 3rd ☐ Other ☐

REASON FOR REFERRAL: ____________________

REFERRAL AGENCY, TELEPHONE #: ____________________

*BASIC INFORMATION TO BE FILLED OUT BY **NURSING PERSONNEL ON FIRST VISIT**

	YES	NO		YES	NO		YES	NO
LMP	☐	☐	HERPES	☐	☐	GC	☐	☐
PREGNANT / EDC	☐	☐	CONDYLOMATA	☐	☐	PREVIOUS CRYO	☐	☐
POSTMENOPAUSAL	☐	☐	DES EXPOSURE	☐	☐	PREVIOUS CONE	☐	☐
BIRTH CONTROL	☐	☐						
PRIOR LASER	☐	☐						

SIGNIFICANT MEDICAL HISTORY ____________________

BIMANUAL EXAM ____________________

EVERY VISIT

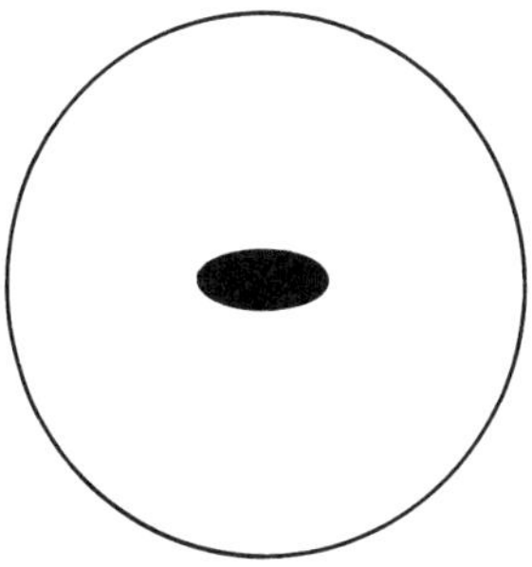

GRADE T- Z
1 ☐
2 ☐
3 ☐

☐ PAP
☐ ECC
☐ CERVICAL Bx
☐ ENDOMETRIAL Bx
☐ VULVAR/VAGINAL Bx
☐ KOH/SALINE
☐ C & S
☐ PHOTO
☐ VAGINAL pH
☐ DRY SMEAR AND STAIN
☐ OTHER

IMPRESSION ____________________

TREATMENT PLAN ____________________

____________________ RTC____________________

FIGURE 9.4.
The findings made at colposcopy should be recorded in a consistent manner using standard nomenclature. The inclusion of a drawing provides a visual record that makes follow-up examinations easier.

TABLE 9.2. Colposcopic Terminology as Adopted by the American Society for Colposcopy and Cervical Pathology

I. **Normal Colposcopic Findings**
   A. **Original Squamous Epithelium** is a smooth, pink, and featureless epithelium originally established on the cervix and vagina. There are no remnants of columnar epithelium identified, such as mucus-secreting epithelium, cleft openings, or nabothian cysts.
   B. **Columnar Epithelium** is a single-layer mucus-producing tall epithelium that extends between the endometrium cranially and either the original squamous epithelium or the metaplastic epithelium caudally. Area covered with columnar epithelium has irregular surface with long stromal papillae and deep clefts. In the colposcope after acetic acid test it has a typical grape-like structure. Columnar epithelium may be present in the endocervix, on the portio, or even in the vagina.
   C. **Transformation Zone** is the area between original squamous epithelium and columnar epithelium in which metaplastic epithelium in varying degrees of maturity is identified. Components of a normal transformation zone may be islands of columnar epithelium surrounded by metaplastic squamous epithelium, "gland openings," and nabothian cysts. In normal transformation zones, there are no colposcopic findings suggestive of cervical neoplasia.

II. **Abnormal Colposcopic Findings**
   A. **Atypical Transformation Zone** A transformation zone in which there are colposcopic findings suggestive of cervical neoplasia.
      1. *White epithelium*—a focal abnormal colposcopic pattern seen after acetic acid test. The white epithelium is a transient phenomenon that is seen in the area of increased nuclear density.
      2. *Punctation*—a focal abnormal colposcopic pattern in which the capillaries appear as a stippled pattern.
      3. *Mosaic*—a focal abnormal colposcopic lesion in which the tissue has a mosaic pattern. The fields of mosaic are separated by reddish borders.
      4. *Hyperkeratosis*—a focal colposcopic pattern in which hyperkeratosis or parakeratosis is present and appears as an elevated whitened plaque. This whitened plaque is identified before the application of acetic acid. At times, leukoplakia may be identified outside the transformation zone.
      5. *Abnormal blood vessels*—a focal abnormal colposcopic pattern in which the blood vessel pattern appears not as punctation, mosaic, or delicately branching vessels but rather as irregular vessels with abrupt courses appearing as commas, corkscrew capillaries, or spaghetti-like forms.
   B. **Suspect Frank Invasive Cancer** Colposcopically obvious invasive cancer that is not evident on clinical examination.

III. **Unsatisfactory Colposcopic Findings** Cases in which the squamocolumnar junction cannot be visualized.

IV. **Other Colposcopic Findings**
   A. **Vaginocervicitis** is a diffuse colposcopic pattern of hyperemia in which the blood vessels may appear in a diffuse stippled pattern similar to the vascular pattern in punctation.
   B. **True Erosion** is an area denuded of epithelium, usually by trauma.
   C. **Atrophic Epithelium** is an estrogen-deprived squamous epithelium in which the vascular pattern is more readily identified because of the relative thinness of the overlying squamous epithelium.
   D. **Condyloma and Papilloma** are exophytic lesions that might be inside or outside of the transformation zone.

FIGURE 9.6.
Colpophotograph of cervix in a 23-year-old woman whose Papanicolaou test result was consistent with carcinoma in situ. There is a large atypical transformation zone characterized by mosaic structure and punctation. Directed biopsy of the abnormality showed carcinoma in situ. (Reproduced with permission from Glass RH. Office Gynecology. *4th ed. Baltimore: Williams & Wilkins, 1993:141.)*

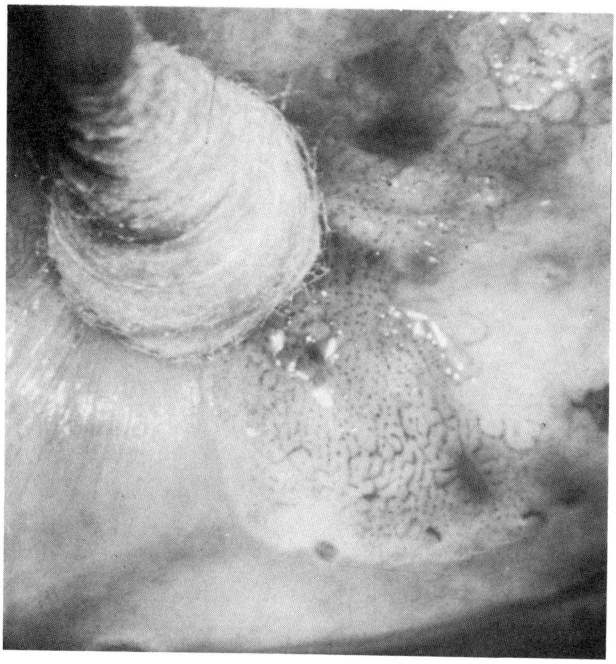

FIGURE 9.5.
Colpophotograph of the posterior cervix in a 32-year-old gravida III, para III whose Papanicolaou test result was consistent with carcinoma in situ. A highly atypical transformation zone characterized by punctation and mosaic is present. In this photograph, the cotton-tipped applicator is lifting the posterior lip of the cervix to demonstrate punctation. The borders of the lesion are sharp and the area is white. The lesion was graded as a carcinoma in situ; this classification was proven on biopsy. (Reproduced with permission from Glass RH. Office Gynecology. *4th ed. Baltimore: Williams & Wilkins, 1993: 139.)*

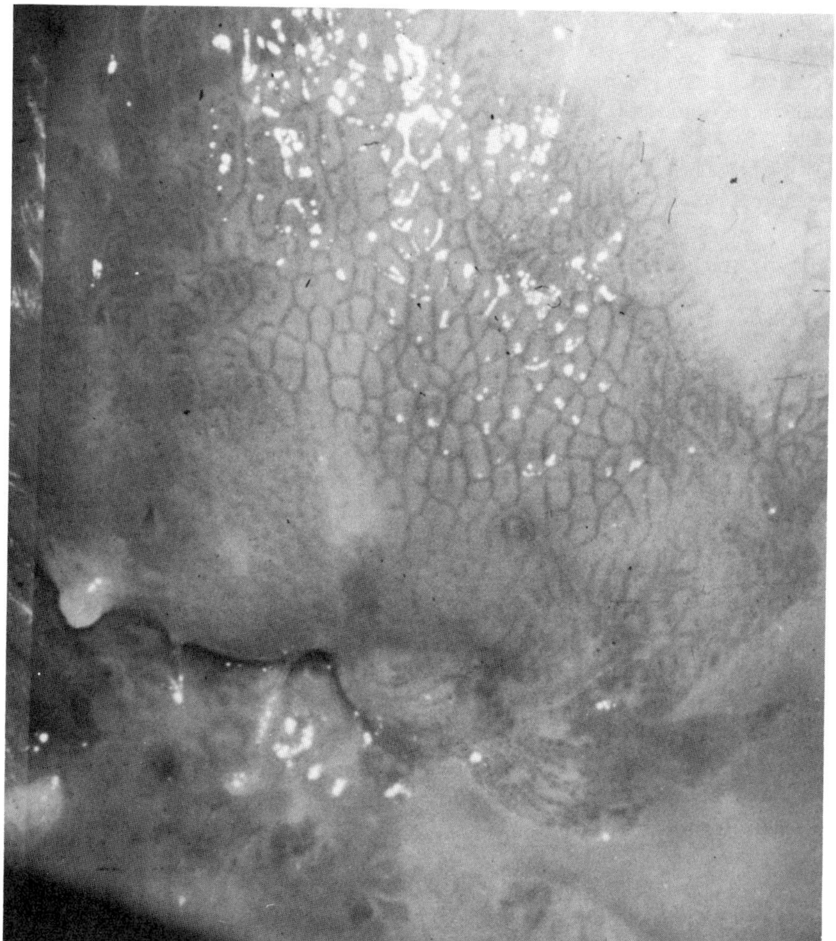

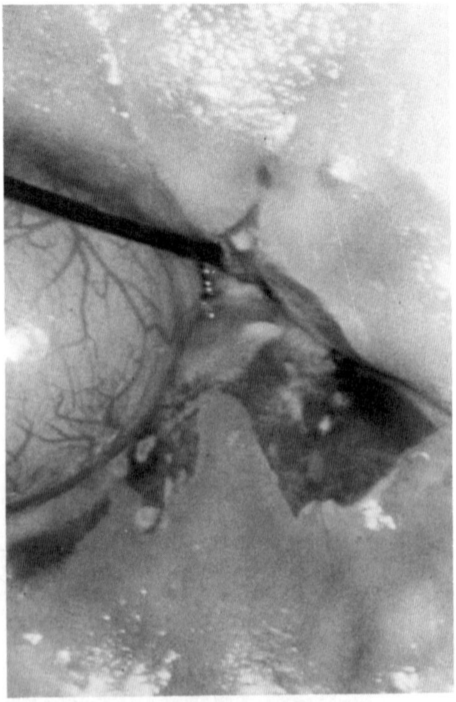

FIGURE 9.7.
Colpophotograph of the cervix in a 35-year-old woman showing a large nabothian cyst along the left-hand border of the figure. The cervical os is in the center; the string of an intrauterine device is passing anteriorly. Note the regular branching vessels overlying the nabothian cyst. Normal vessels have a regular direction. It is important to recognize and appreciate the normal blood vessel pattern in order to compare normal against abnormal vessels; the latter are associated with carcinoma. (Reproduced with permission from Glass RH. Office Gynecology. *4th ed. Baltimore: Williams & Wilkins, 1993:144.)*

Acetowhite areas (Fig. 9.8) must be differentiated from malignant change and the papillary changes of human papilloma virus infection (Fig. 9.9).

Special Notes

For a colposcopy to be considered "adequate," the entire transformation zone must be visualized. The full extent of any lesion present must also be visible for the study to be considered adequate. If the colposcopy is inadequate, diagnostic conization is required.

The following are other considerations to keep in mind. Random or "four-quadrant" blind biopsies are not adequate to rule out invasive cancer. It is less threatening to patients if the terms "vinegar" or "cleansing solution" are used rather than "acetic acid." The discomfort of cervical biopsy may be lessened by having the patient cough at the moment the biopsy is performed. The patient should be advised to expect an increased vaginal discharge if biopsy specimens were taken and Monsel's solution was used. Because of the focal length and magnification offered by the colposcope, the instrument may also be used to evaluate lesions on the vaginal wall, vulva, or other parts of the surface of the body.

If acetic acid is used on the vulva, a weaker concentration results in less burning and discomfort. Because of the relatively thicker epithelium of the vulva, the acetic acid must be left in contact with the tissues for a longer period (even if the stronger solution is chosen). This is most easily accomplished by soaking a gauze sponge and allowing it to remain in contact with the skin for several minutes. This process may be started while other preparations are under way, thereby reducing the overall time required for the evaluation.

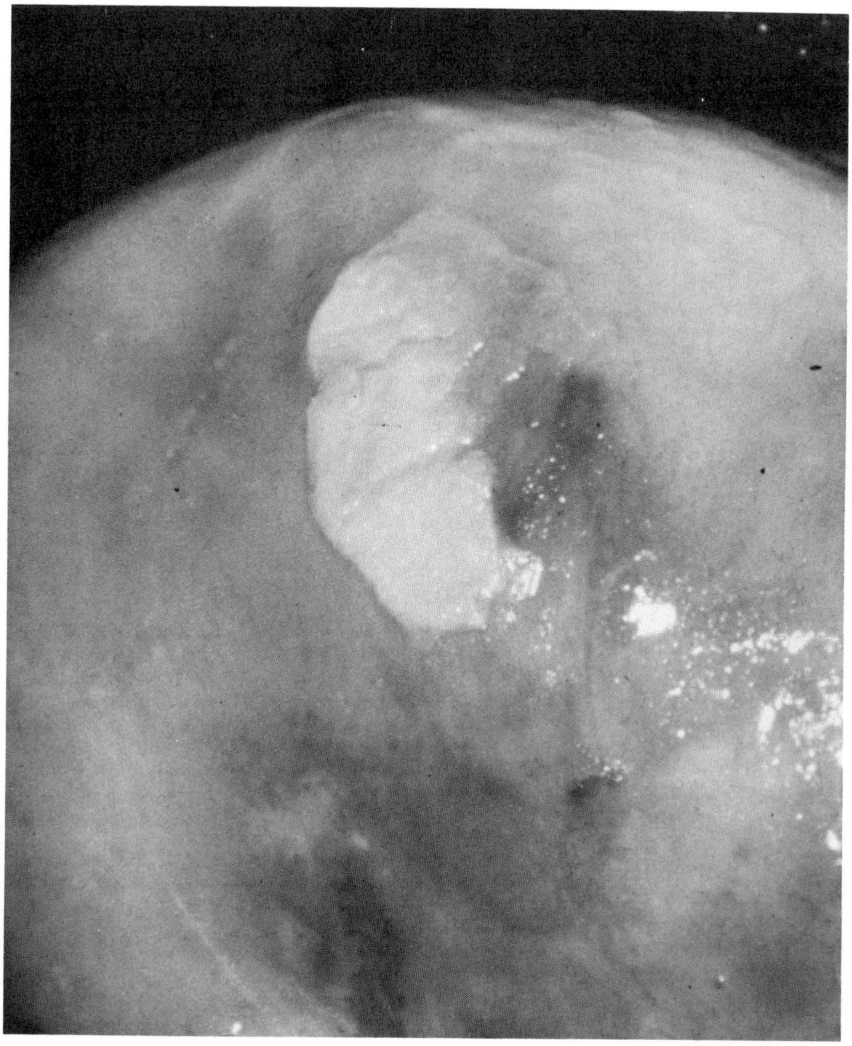

FIGURE 9.8.
Colpophotograph (original magnification, x12) of the anterior lip of the cervix in a 31-year-old gravida IV, para IV. A grossly visible white lesion was seen on the anterior cervical lip. The patient's Papanicolaou test result was normal. Directed biopsy showed hyperkeratosis and no nuclear atypia. (Reproduced with permission from Glass RH. Office Gynecology. *4th ed. Baltimore: Williams & Wilkins, 1993:143.)*

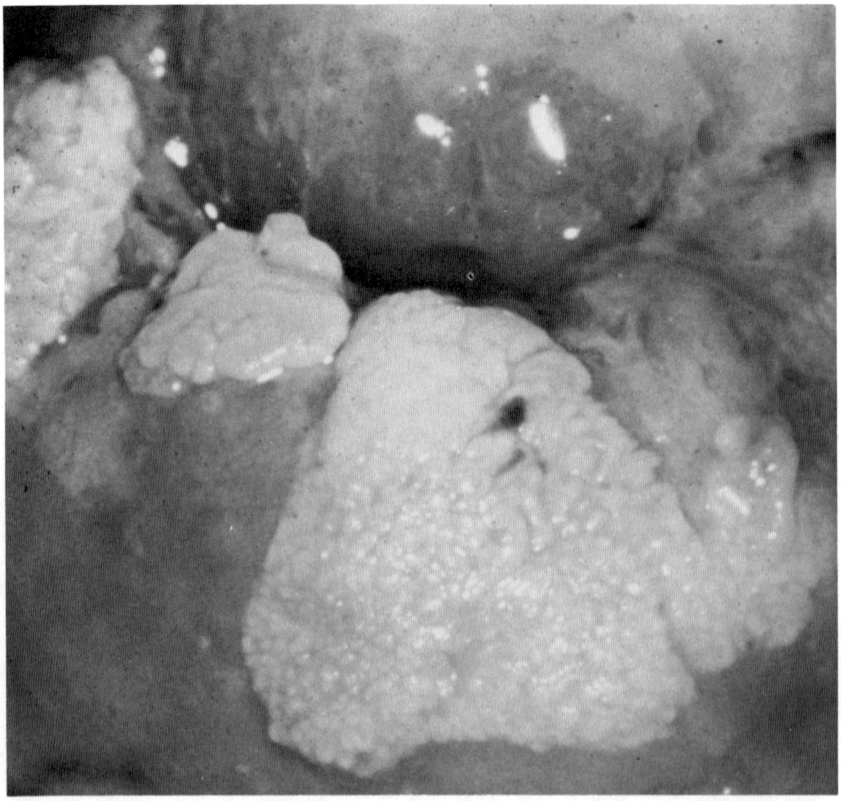

FIGURE 9.9.
Colpophotograph of posterior lip of the cervix in a 21-year-old woman who was 26 weeks pregnant. Several grossly visible, raised, white lesions were seen on the posterior lip. Colposcopically, these lesions showed irregular surface contour with an occasional double-branching vessel. The impression of condylomata acuminata was confirmed by directed biopsy. (Reproduced with permission from Glass RH. Office Gynecology. *4th ed. Baltimore: Williams & Wilkins, 1993:146.)*

Suggested Readings

Ang MS, Kaufman RH, Adam E, et al. Colposcopically directed biopsy and loop excision of the transformation zone. Comparison of histologic findings. *J Reprod Med* 1995;40:167.

Burke L, Antonioli DA, Ducatman BS. *Colposcopy: Text and Atlas.* East Norwalk, Conn: Appleton & Lange, 1991.

Craine BL, Craine ER. Digital imaging colposcopy: basic concepts and applications. *Obstet Gynecol* 1993;82:869.

Cristoforoni PM, Gerbaldo D, Perino A, et al. Computerized colposcopy: results of a pilot study and analysis of its clinical relevance. *Obstet Gynecol* 1995;85:1011.

Curry SL, Pfenniger JL, Sarma S. Colposcopy: when? why? how? *Patient Care* 1994;15:167.

Davis GD. Colposcopic examination of the vagina. *Obstet Gynecol Clin North Am* 1993;20:217.

Dunton CJ, Sedlacek TV. *Comprehensive Review of Colposcopy.* Washington, DC:

American College of Obstetricians and Gynecologists and American Society for Colposcopy and Cervical Pathology, 1996.
Johnson BA. The colposcopic examination. *Am Fam Phys* 1996;53:2473.
Kitchener HC, Cruickshank ME, Farmery E. The 1993 British Society for Colposcopy and Cervical Pathology/National Coordinating Network United Kingdom Colposcopy Survey. Comparison with 1988 and the response to introduction of guidelines. *Br J Obstet Gynaecol* 1995;102:549.
Lonky NM, Mann WJ, Massad LS, et al. Ability of visual tests to predict underlying cervical neoplasia. Colposcopy and speculoscopy. *J Reprod Med* 1995;40:530.
Luesley D. Advances in colposcopy and management of cervical intraepithelial neoplasia. *Curr Opin Obstet Gynecol* 1992;4:102.
Mayeaux EJ Jr, Harper MB, Abreo F, et al. A comparison of the reliability of repeat cervical smears and colposcopy in patients with abnormal cervical cytology. *J Fam Pract* 1995;40:57.
Reed TP, Saade G. Microcolposcopy. When and how to do it. *J Reprod Med* 1993; 38:725.
Reid R. Biology and colposcopic features of human papillomavirus-associated cervical disease. *Obstet Gynecol Clin North Am* 1993;20:123.
Richart R, Pringle P. A state of the art guide to colposcopes and accessories. *Contemp Obstet Gynecol* 1988;30:107.
Rickert VI, Kozlowski KJ, Warren AM, et al. Adolescents and colposcopy: the use of different procedures to reduce anxiety. *Am J Obstet Gynecol* 1994;170:504.
Shafi MI, Dunn JA, Chenoy R, et al. Digital imaging colposcopy, image analysis and quantification of the colposcopic image. *Br J Obstet Gynaecol* 1994;101:234.
Shier RM. The colposcopy unit. Instrumentation, colposcopic technique, recording of findings, and terminology. *Obstet Gynecol Clin North Am* 1993;20:47.
Stafl A, Wilbanks GD. An international terminology of colposcopy: report of the nomenclature committee of the International Federation of Cervical Pathology and Colposcopy. *Obstet Gynecol* 1991;77:313.
Townsend DE. Colposcopy, cryosurgery, carbon dioxide laser, and loop electrosurgical excision procedure (LEEP). In: Glass RH, ed. *Office Gynecology.* 4th ed. Baltimore: Williams & Wilkins, 1992:133.
Wright VC. Understanding the colposcope. Optics, light path, magnification, and field of view. *Obstet Gynecol Clin North Am* 1993;20:31.

Chapter 10

DIAPHRAGM FITTING

The diaphragm remains an important reversible contraceptive method for the well-motivated patient who wants an alternative to hormonal contraception. The effectiveness of the diaphragm in preventing pregnancy and reducing upper genital tract infection is predicated on the proper selection of size and type and careful instructions to the patient to ensure correct positioning of the device when in use.

Equipment

- Examination gloves and lubricant
- Set of fitting rings or diaphragms in sizes 65 to 90 mm
- Examples of each of the three spring types (arching, coil, and flat) for use in patient education (optional)
- Diaphragm introducer (for instruction; optional)

Training/Credentialing

No special credentialing needed; office procedure only.

Coding

57170	Diaphragm or cervical cap fitting with instructions (includes procedure only)

Technique

Diaphragm fitting begins with a bimanual vaginal examination with the patient in the dorsal lithotomy position. The finger or fingers of the examining hand are advanced into the vagina until they touch the posterior fornix, just posterior to the cervix (Fig. 10.1). The point on the examining hand just below the pubic symphysis is noted by placing the thumb of the same hand on the spot or by estimation. The hand is withdrawn, and the distance from under the symphysis to posterior fornix is measured. A fitting ring with this diameter is selected from a range of sizes (Fig. 10.2), and the size is confirmed by measuring the ring against the marked fingers. The most common size

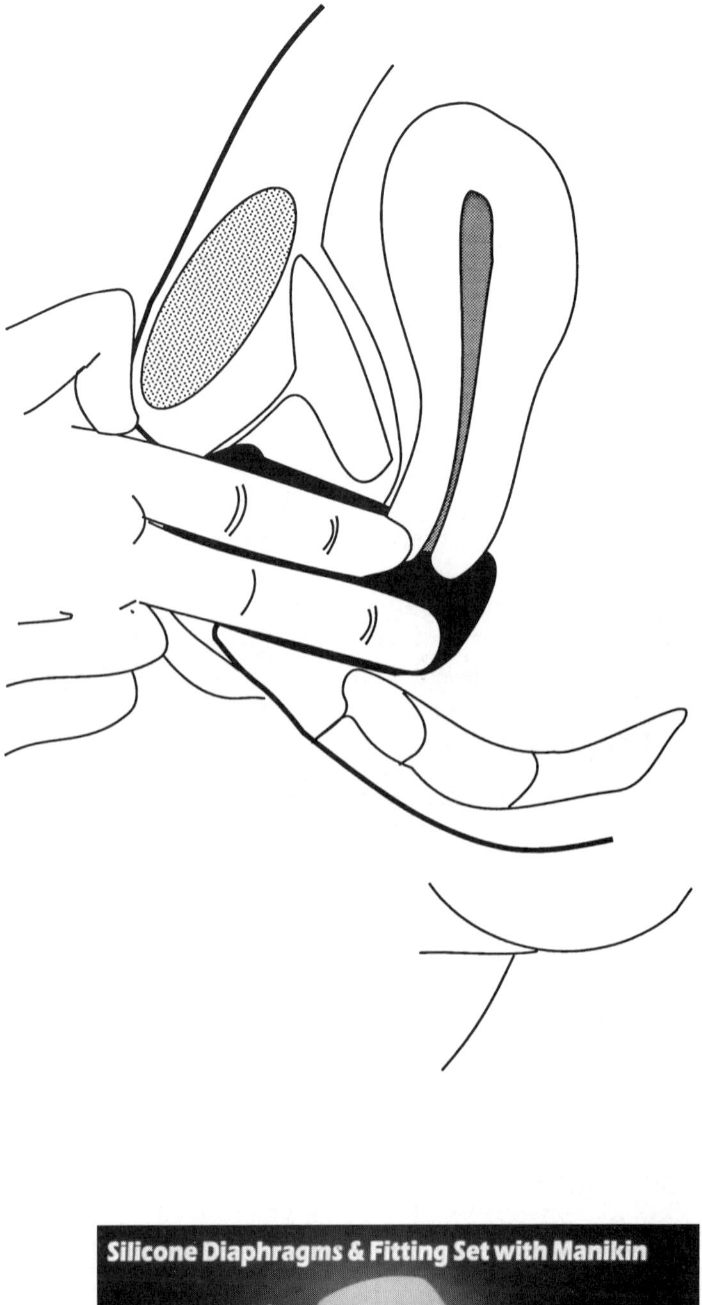

FIGURE 10.1.
The size of the diaphragm is estimated by measuring the distance from the pubic symphysis to the posterior fornix (behind the cervix).

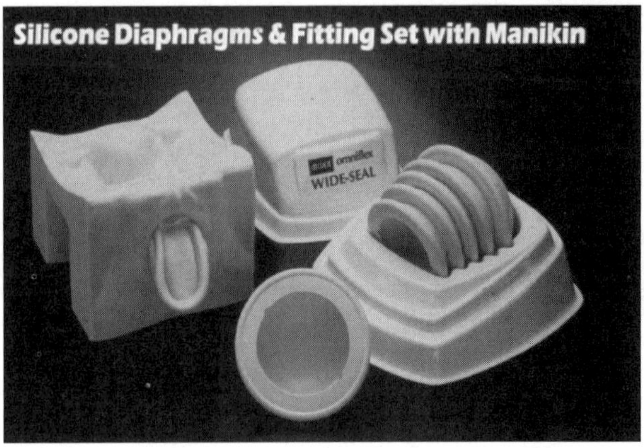

FIGURE 10.2.
Fitting ring sets, examples of various types of diaphragms, and pelvic models for practicing diaphragm fitting are available from many suppliers. (Courtesy of Milex Products, Chicago, IL.)

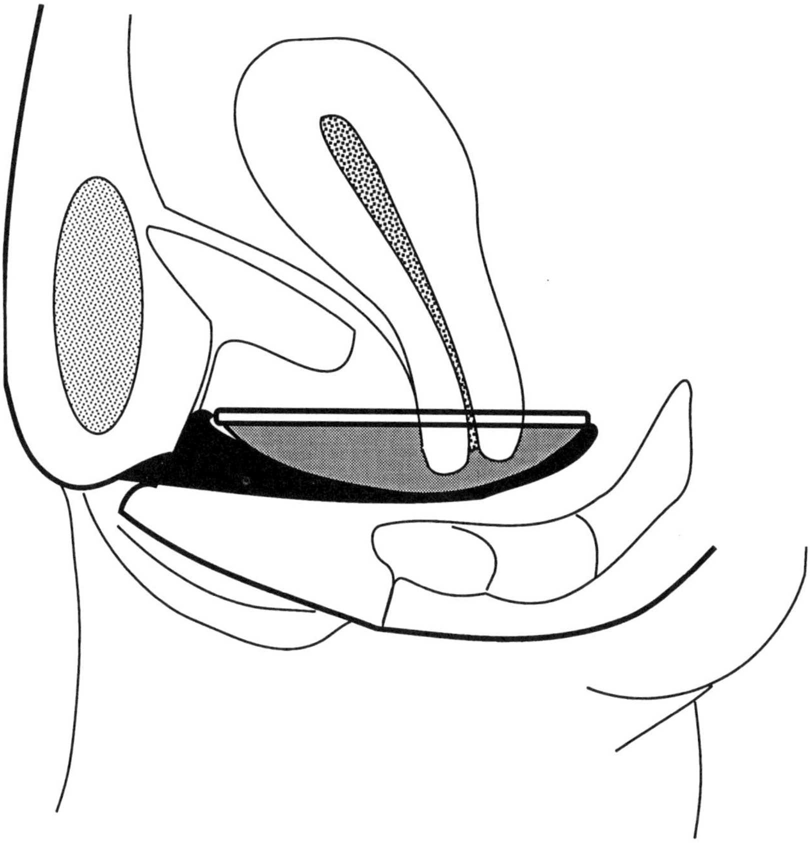

FIGURE 10.3.
The correctly fitting diaphragm should sit comfortably behind the symphsis and in the posterior vaginal fornix; the cervix should be covered and in contact with the spermicidal cream or jelly that has been applied to the dome.

used is 75 mm, although any size in the full range of 50 to 105 mm may be needed depending on the depth of the patient's vagina.

The selected ring is then lubricated and folded by compressing the sides between the fingers of one hand. The folded ring is gently inserted into the vagina and is guided to the posterior fornix by the tips of the fingers. Once the ring has been placed in the posterior fornix, behind the cervix, the opposite side should be gently placed behind the symphysis anteriorly (Fig. 10.3). The ring should fit snugly but allow a finger to pass easily between it and the vaginal wall in all directions. The examiner's hand is withdrawn and the patient is asked about her ability to perceive the diaphragm. A well-fitting diaphragm should be unnoticed or be noticed only with concentration or effort. The patient should be asked to perform a Valsalva maneuver, cough, or move about to check for comfort and to ensure against displacement with normal activities.

If there is undue pressure or if the patient is aware of the presence of the diaphragm, a smaller size or different type of spring should be chosen. If the diaphragm is displaced by normal activity, a larger size or arching spring should be tested.

Once the size has been determined, the fitting ring should be removed by sliding a finger between the ring and the symphysis anteriorly, displacing the ring downward, and withdrawing the ring with the hooked finger. The fitting ring should be disinfected

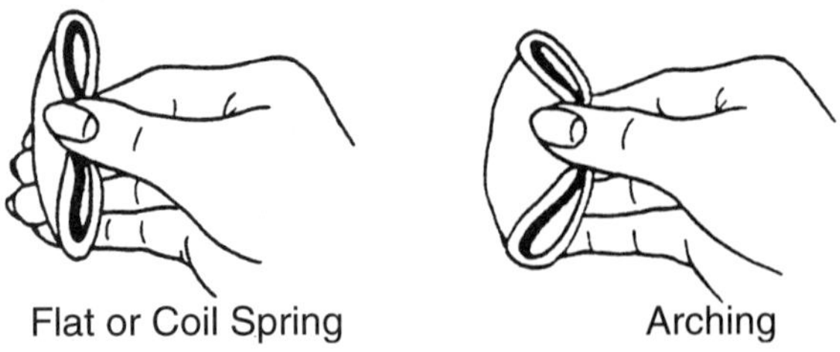

FIGURE 10.4.
When compressed, the rim of flat or coil spring diaphragms stays in one plane while arching spring types form an arch that helps to anchor the diaphragm behind the symphysis.

TABLE 10.1. Characteristics of Three Types of Diaphragms

SPRING TYPE	SHAPE WHEN COMPRESSED	USE WITH INTRODUCER	ADVANTAGES
Arching	Arch	Not needed	Firm rim, good when pelvic support is poor
Coil	Flat (will curve to fit body)	Optional	Soft, best with good support and the cervix in midplane or anterior position
Flat	Flat	Optional	Soft, remains in flat plane, best for women with narrow pubic angle or shallow retropubic space

according to the manufacturer's directions. Disinfection generally consists of cleansing with soap and water. Some clinicians prefer to sterilize the fitting rings with cold or gas before reuse.

Diaphragm springs come in several different types. The type of spring used in the construction of the diaphragm determines its behavior when compressed by the fingers or the lateral vaginal walls (Fig. 10.4). The type of spring chosen for the individual patient is often a matter of preference, although some broad guidelines are possible (Table 10.1) . Parous patients, those with early pelvic relaxation, and those with a broad pubic arch will do best with the arching type spring; patients with a narrow, poorly defined arch will do better with a flat spring. Most patients can successfully use any of the three types and may try different styles as desired. The coil and flat spring types may be used with an inserter (a rod with notches at the tip and along the shaft into which the compressed diaphragm fits). The diaphragm is lubricated, and the assembly is inserted into the apex of the vagina. A slight twisting motion dislodges the diaphragm from the inserter, leaving it in place.

The patient should be offered the opportunity to insert the diaphragm or fitting ring herself so that correct placement may be assured. If the patient feels confident about her ability or wishes more privacy, she may experiment with the diaphragm at home and return later (with the diaphragm in place) for evaluation. It is generally wise for the patient to practice insertion and removal several times before she plans to use it. Careful instruction and patient compliance are a must if the patient is to be satisfied with her choice of contraceptive methods.

Instructions for Patient Use

Diaphragms (a rubber dome with a springy ring) are used with a contraceptive jelly or creams to provide contraception by both barrier and spermicidal actions. To use, a teaspoon of spermicidal jelly or cream is applied to the cervical (concave) side and rim of the diaphragm, providing a spermicidal barrier to fertilization. The diaphragm is inserted into the vagina, beyond the cervix and behind the symphysis. In this position, the diaphragm covers the anterior vaginal wall and cervix, providing a mechanical barrier to sperm passage and positions the spermicide against the cervix to optimize its effect. The proper positioning of the diaphragm should be verified each time it is used. If the cervix may be felt through the dome of the diaphragm, the positioning is correct. The diaphragm must be inserted before intercourse begins and must be left in place for 6–8 hours after intercourse. It is then removed, washed, and stored. Should additional intercourse be desired before the 6–8 hours have lapsed, additional spermicide is applied to the vaginal side of the diaphragm (without dislodging it) and the waiting time to removal is restarted. Postcoital douching is not recommended.

The fit of a diaphragm may change with substantial change in weight, vaginal birth, or pelvic surgery. The diaphragm should be the largest that can be comfortably inserted, worn, and removed.

Special Notes

Diaphragms should not be fitted in the presence of known pelvic infection, clinically significant pelvic relaxation (large cystocele, rectocele, enterocele, or uterine prolapse), or sooner than 6 weeks after delivery. A history of recurrent urinary tract infections is a relative contraindication to the use of a diaphragm.

Although newer diaphragms are made from silicone, most are still made of latex and may produce allergic reactions in susceptible persons.

The optimal diaphragm size may change with substantial increase in weight (10–15 or more pounds), vaginal birth, or pelvic surgery. If there is any doubt, a check of the size of the device or refitting is indicated.

Some women who use the diaphragm for contraception insert the device each evening before bed and leave it in place until the following evening, when it is removed, washed, remedicated with contraceptive jelly, and reinserted. This obviates the need to insert the diaphragm during the act of intercourse. This approach should be discouraged because of the potentially prolonged interval from insertion to coitus (increasing contraceptive failure) and the possibility of vaginal or urinary tract infections, or pressure damage to the vaginal wall. The toxic shock syndrome has been reported in women who have worn a diaphragm for more than 24 hours.

Suggested Readings

Faundes A, Elias C, Coggins C. Spermicides and barrier contraception. *Curr Opin Obstet Gynecol* 1994;6:552.

Gillespie L. The diaphragm: an accomplice in recurrent urinary tract infections. *Urology* 1984;24:25.

Heaton CJ, Smith MA. The diaphragm. *Am Fam Phys* 1989;39:231.

Jaffe R. Toxic shock syndrome associated with diaphragm use. *N Engl J Med* 1981; 305:1585.

Tagg PI. The diaphragm: barrier contraception has a new social role. *Nurse Pract* 1995;20:36.

Chapter 11

CONTRACEPTIVE ROD INSERTION

Long-acting levonorgestrel implantable contraceptive rods (Norplant) provide highly effective contraception for as long as 5 years of use. With appropriate counseling and patient selection, these contraceptive rods can provide compliance-free, reliable, reversible contraception. Insertion of these devices is accomplished quickly under local anesthesia using a technique that is easy to master. The ease with which the technique is learned belies the importance that correct insertion plays in patient satisfaction and eventual removal.

Equipment

- Implantable contraceptive rod kit (contains one fenestrated sterile drape and two regular drapes, syringe, two needles, forceps, scalpel, 10-gauge trocar, six contraceptive rods, skin closure tapes, three packs of gauze sponges, stretch roller bandage, and a patient information booklet)
- Sterile gloves
- Skin preparation materials (alcohol, iodine- or hexachlorophene-based antibacterial solution [e.g., Betadine, Hibiclens])
- 1% Xylocaine without epinephrine (or similar)
- Plastic skin template to assist with placement angles (optional)
- Additional gauze sponges (optional)

Training/Credentialing

No special credentialing is needed, but specialized training is available and advisable. These training sessions provide evidence of training for the provider's records. Training may be arranged through the Norplant Procedure Instruction Program at 800–922-0877.

Coding

11975 Insertion, implantable contraceptive capsules

11977 Removal with reinsertion, implantable contraceptive capsules

Technique

PATIENT SELECTION AND COUNSELING

Although it is not in the scope of this book to extensively review the factors involved in selecting patients for this or any other contraceptive method, a brief mention of some aspects of this process is germane to overall satisfaction and long-term use. The best insertion technique and correct placement of the contraceptive rods will be wasted if the patient has not been selected and counseled regarding the use of the system.

Candidates for implantable contraceptive rods are patients who desire long-term but potentially reversible contraception. Patients who have contraindications to other methods or have significant concerns about compliance may also be considered. As with other hormonal contraceptive agents, several conditions represent relative or absolute contraindications to the use of implantable contraceptive rods (Table 11.1). In addition, patients who are unwilling or unable to tolerate the probability of menstrual irregularity during the first several months of use should choose another method. Patients should be counseled about the need for normal periodic health evaluations and the necessity of an additional procedure to remove the contraceptive system at 5 years, if conception is desired, or at any other time that a change is desired.

Because insertion of implantable contraceptive rods involves the use of a local anesthetic and a skin incision, most practitioners obtain written informed consent before beginning the procedure (see Chapter 2, Informed Consent).

INSERTION TECHNIQUE

The patient should be positioned supine on the examining table. Although either upper arm may be used for insertion, the nondominant arm is usually selected. The arm should be rested comfortably, abducted from the body at a 90° angle, with the elbow similarly flexed (Fig. 11.1). The planned site of insertion should be inspected to ensure that no lesions or other concerns might interfere with the planned insertion. A plastic template may be used to mark the fan-shaped placement planned for the contraceptive rods, but this step is optional. If a template is used, a surgical marking pen or other de-

Table 11.1. Contraindications to Use of Implantable Contraceptive Rods

Active thrombophlebitis
Acute liver disease
Known or suspected breast cancer
Benign or malignant liver tumors
Morbid obesity
Known or suspected pregnancy
Thromboembolic disease

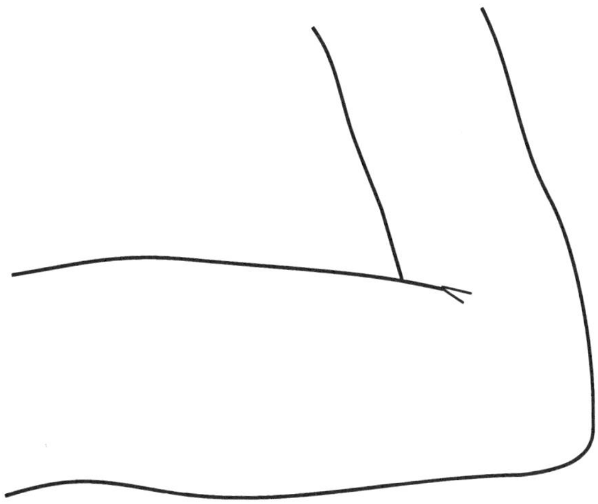

FIGURE 11.1.
The upper arm on the side chosen for insertion of contraceptive capsules should be rested comfortably at a right angle to the body, with the elbow similarly flexed.

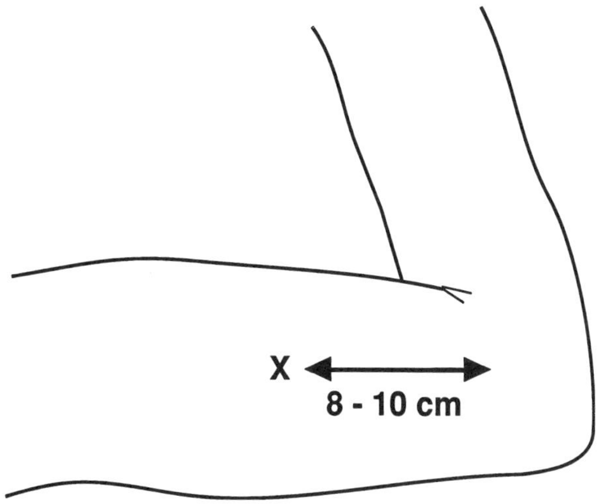

FIGURE 11.2.
The site of contraceptive capsule insertion should be approximately 8–10 cm above the crease of the elbow.

vice should be chosen that will not wash off during skin preparation. The skin of the upper arm should be cleansed with antiseptic solution as for minor surgery.

The contraceptive rod kit should then be opened. The contents of the kit are not sterile. They are, however, packaged so that they may be opened onto a sterile field. As a result, an assistant must be present to open supplies onto the sterile field or to make them available to the person performing the procedure. With the kit opened and the material laid out for ease of identification and access, sterile gloves may be donned. Sterile drapes (if desired) may now be placed around the patient's arm to provide a sterile field in which to work. A syringe and large-bore needle should next be made available so that a suitable local anesthetic may be drawn up. The local anesthetic chosen should not contain epinephrine because this drug may result in superficial tissue necrosis. In preparation for injection, a 22-gauge (1½-inch) needle is substituted for the needle used to draw up the anesthetic agent.

If not already marked, a point on the inner aspect of the upper arm roughly 8–10 cm from the crease of the elbow is identified and marked with gentle pressure from a finger nail (Fig. 11.2). This will temporarily mark the point chosen for insertion and provide pressure-induced anesthesia for the initial needle penetration as local infiltration is begun. With a minimal amount of anesthetic agent, a small skin weal is raised at the

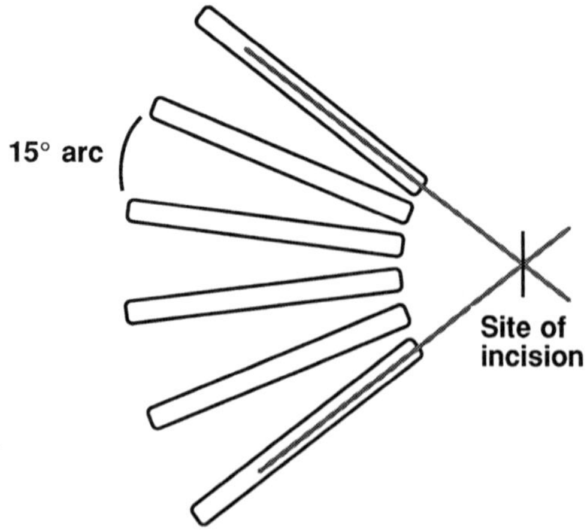

FIGURE 11.3.
When properly positioned, the implantable contraceptive system rods should be placed with the long axis of the fan parallel to the axis of the arm and separated at an angle of approximately 15°. The incision for insertion should be located at the central point of the fan as shown.

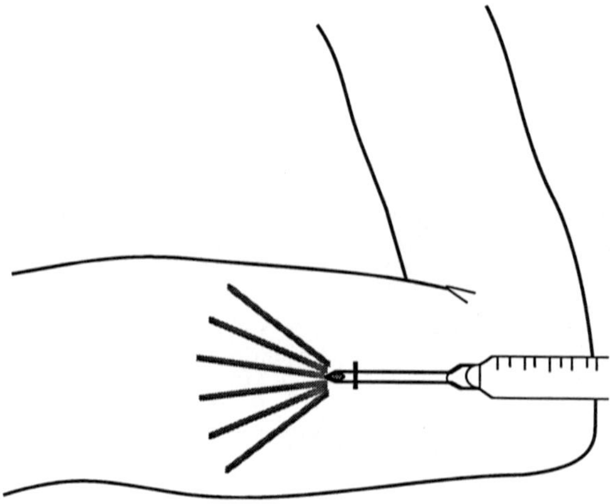

FIGURE 11.4.
Infiltration of local anesthetic should follow the track proposed for the contraceptive rods.

site marked with the finger nail (roughly where the base of the fan of contraceptive rods would meet if extended [Fig. 11.3]). The rough bounds of the fan-shaped distribution planned for the insertion of the rods should be envisioned if it has not already been marked on the skin. The needle is then advanced along one side of this fan-shaped area, remaining just under the dermis until the needle is advanced to its full length (3–4 cm) (Fig. 11.4). Anesthetic is injected into this track as the needle is withdrawn. Less than 1 mL of agent should be deposited in this track. The needle is then readvanced along the opposite boundary, raising a second track. This provides a partial field block that lessens the discomfort of subsequent injection. The proposed tracks of the remaining four rods are injected in sequence using the same technique of needle advancement and injection during withdrawal. The formation of six subdermal channels makes placement of the inserting trocar and rods much easier. Less than 5 mL of the anesthetic should be used.

As the local anesthetic sets, the scalpel, inserting trocar, and contraceptive capsules should be opened onto the sterile field. The contraceptive rods must be counted to ensure that all six are present and none has remained in the packaging material.

A shallow, 2-mm transverse incision is made at the point of the initial skin weal. This incision should penetrate only the dermis. Next, the inserting trocar should be inspected. Care must be taken to note the position of the bevel and the two incised marks used to facilitate capsule placement (Fig. 11.5). These two marks are central to

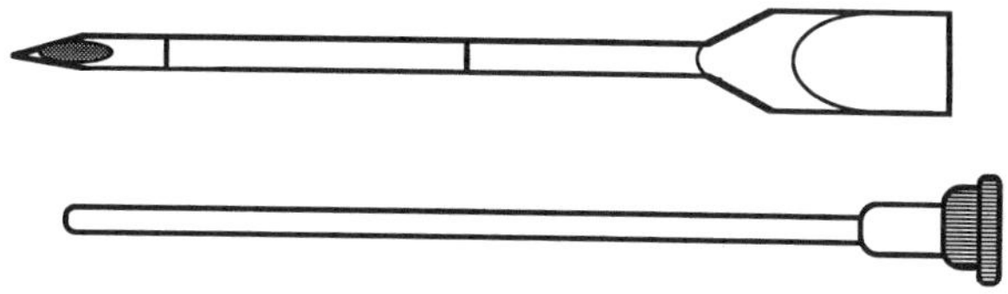

FIGURE 11.5.
The trocar used to place contraceptive capsules under the skin has two marks along its shaft. These are used to indicate the maximal depth of trocar insertion before capsule placement and the maximal amount to which the trocar should be withdrawn when moving from one capsule site to another. The trocar also has an obturator that should be in place any time the trocar is advanced through tissue.

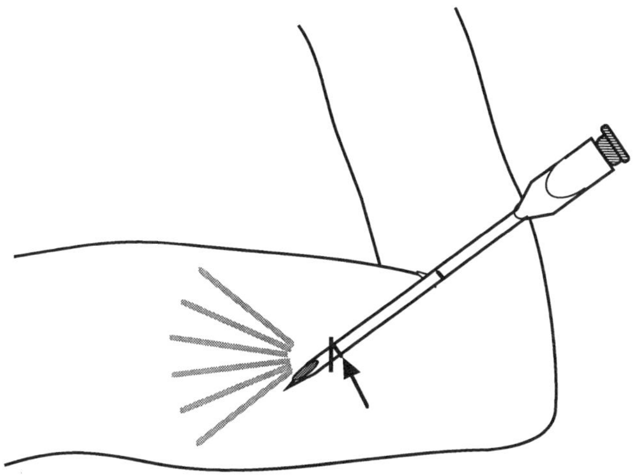

FIGURE 11.6.
The trocar should be inserted into the skin incision with the bevel upward and should advance only to the first mark.

the correct placement of the contraceptive capsules. With the obturator in place and the bevel facing upward, the trocar is placed at a shallow angle into the skin incision (Fig. 11.6). The trocar is advanced along one of the anesthetized tracks at either extreme of the fan-shaped area. The trocar is advanced until the proximal barrel mark is at or just outside of the skin incision (Fig. 11.7). The trocar must remain just below the dermis for the entire length of its insertion. Advancing the trocar in this plane requires a moderate amount of force, which is reduced somewhat by the correct placement of the local anesthetic solution. Placement may be facilitated by a gentle up-and-down or side-to-side motion as the trocar is advanced.

With the trocar held in place, the obturator is removed and a contraceptive rod is inserted into the hub (Fig. 11.8). (The capsule may be handled directly with the gloved fingers if the gloves are free of powder.) The capsule is advanced into the hub and positioned at the tip of the trocar by gently replacing the obturator just enough that resistance is felt (Fig. 11.9). If the trocar is in the correct position below the dermis, the tip of the contraceptive rod may be seen to nudge the skin at the tip of the trocar.

The contraceptive capsule is now in its final position and is ready to be left behind in the tissue. This is accomplished by holding the obturator motionless as the trocar is withdrawn to its distal mark (Fig. 11.10). It is vital to understand that the implantable contraceptive rods are left behind in the tissue as the trocar is withdrawn, not inserted by the trocar. An effort to insert the obturator to push the capsule out

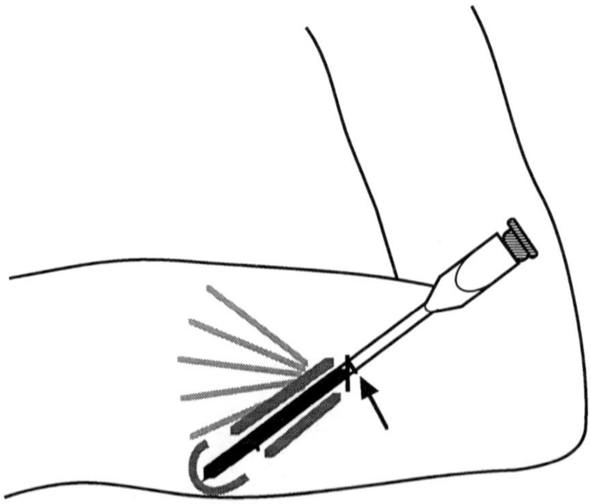

FIGURE 11.7.
The trocar should visibly tent the skin as it is advanced.

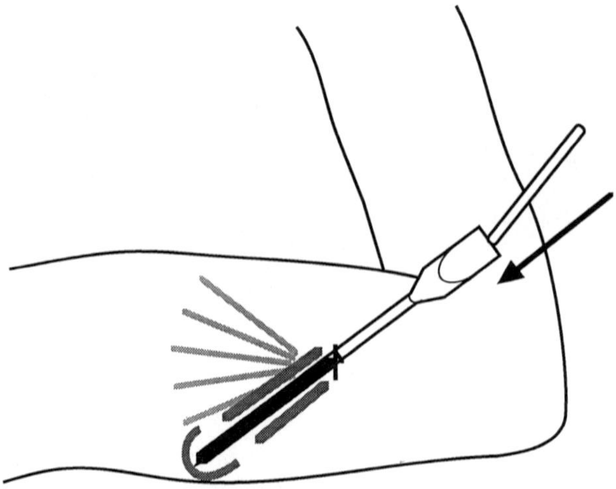

FIGURE 11.8.
With the trocar stabilized in position, the contraceptive capsule is inserted into the needle.

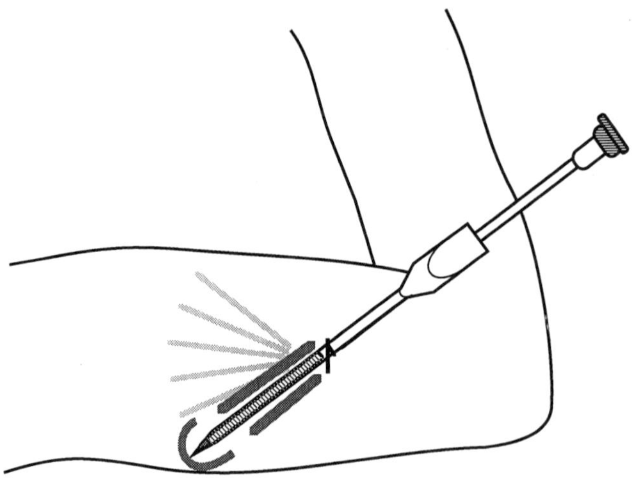

FIGURE 11.9.
The obturator is advanced sufficiently to move the capsule to the tip of the trocar, but not beyond.

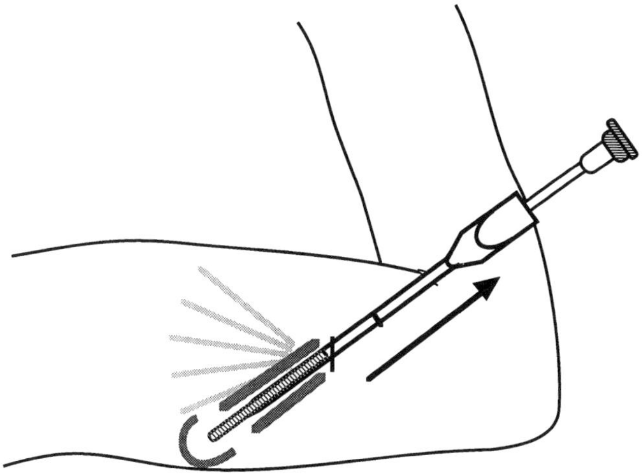

FIGURE 11.10.
The contraceptive implant is left behind under the skin as the trocar is withdrawn over the stationary obturator.

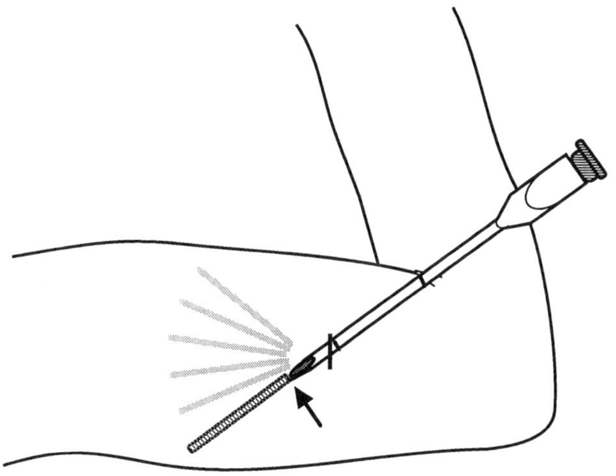

FIGURE 11.11.
The contraceptive implant must drop free of the tip of the trocar before the trocar is angled toward the next insertion tract.

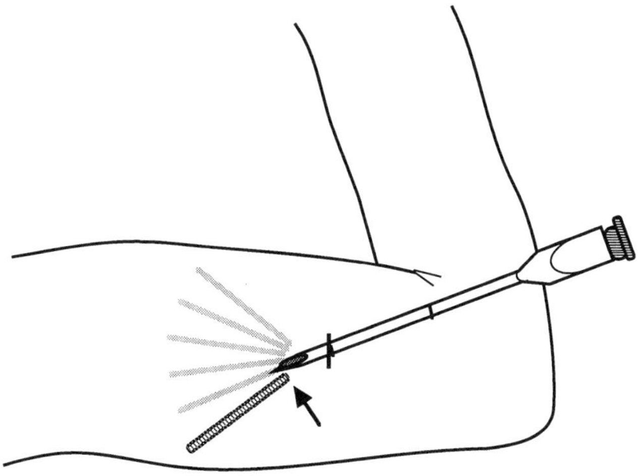

FIGURE 11.12.
Without removal of the trocar beyond the first mark, the trocar is angled toward the next insertion tract and advanced.

results in improper placement, possible capsule damage, and a more complicated removal. If the trocar and obturator are lifted upward away from the arm, placing the skin on traction, the capsule may be seen to emerge from the tip of the trocar as it is backed out of the insertion track. With careful observation, the capsule may also be seen to drop clear of the tip of the trocar just before the distal barrel mark reaches the skin opening. The trocar should not be withdrawn past this point until the sixth capsule has been placed. Deposition of the capsule clear of the tip of the trocar may also be confirmed by direct palpation (Fig. 11.11).

Once it has been confirmed that the last capsule is clear of the tip, the trocar can be safely advanced along the next track, approximately 15° from the last track (Fig. 11.12), until the proximal barrel mark is reached. To minimize the possibility of displacing the previous capsule, it may be stabilized and protected by a finger as the trocar is advanced. The obturator is removed, and the capsule is placed into the lumen and left in place as the trocar is withdrawn. This sequence of placement is repeated until all six contraceptive capsules have been placed. The trocar may then be removed.

The capsules should be palpated to insure that all six have been placed and none is closer than 5 mm to the skin incision. Placement closer than this is associated with a greater risk for expulsion or infection. Skin closure tape is placed to reapproximate the edges of the wound. A bandage may be placed as desired.

An appropriate note, including either a description or drawing of the location of the contraceptive implants, should be placed in the patient's medical record. Rods that are known to be in an atypical location (e.g., closer than normal to an adjacent rod, closer or further from the incision site, or displaced into a "U" or "S" shape) should also be noted. Such a drawing or notation can be invaluable when the capsules are to be removed.

Normal Findings

Patients should be advised that moderate bruising of the insertion site is normal and is not a cause for alarm. Bruising may be minimized by applying ice for a few hours after the procedure. After the local anesthetic wears off, a mild analgesic agent or heat relieves any discomfort experienced. The skin closure tapes may be removed in 5 to 7 days if they have not already been lost.

Special Notes

Although implantable contraceptive rods may be inserted at any point during the menstrual cycle, it is preferable to insert them during the first 7 days of the cycle to minimize menstrual irregularity and to avoid the possibility of ovulation before effective levels of contraceptive hormone have been established.

The Norplant Foundation can provide information and contraceptive kits for needy patients under certain circumstances. The address is: The Norplant Foundation, PO Box 25223, Alexandria, VA 22314; the telephone number is 703-706-5933 or 800-760-9030.

Infection at the site of insertion is rare. If infection does occur, one or more of the capsules must be removed while local treatment is undertaken.

If desired, a new set of implantable contraceptive rods may be inserted immediately after the removal of the previous set by either facing the fan of capsules in the opposite direction through the same incision or by using a new site on the opposite arm.

Suggested Readings

Alvarez-Sanchez F, Brache V, Faundes A. Recent experience with and future directions of contraceptive implants and injectable contraceptives. *Curr Opin Obstet Gynecol* 1993;5:805.

Darney PD, Klaisle CM, Walker DM, et al. The importance of proper insertion of Norplant contraceptive implants. *J Fam Pract* 1992;34:545.

Nelson AL. Neutralizing pH of lidocaine reduces pain during Norplant system insertion procedure. *Contraception* 1995;51:299.

Wehrle KE. The Norplant system: easy to insert, easy to remove. *Nurse Pract* 1994;19:47.

Chapter 12

CONTRACEPTIVE ROD REMOVAL

To reverse the action of long-acting levonorgestrel implantable contraceptive rods (Norplant), the rods must be removed through a minor surgical procedure. This procedure may be done in the office setting using only local anesthesia. Several techniques allow the contraceptive rods to be removed quickly, with a minimum of tissue trauma; however, careful, correct placement is the most important factor in ensuring an uneventful removal (see Chapter 11, Contraceptive Rod Insertion).

Equipment

- Sterile gloves
- Scalpel (#11 blade and holder, blade only, or disposable type)
- Two small hemostats (one straight and one curved), those with fine tips are preferred
- 2-mm vasectomy clamp (Norgrasp; optional)
- One fenestrated sterile drape and two regular drapes (optional)
- Additional gauze sponges
- Skin preparation materials (alcohol, iodine- or hexachlorophene-based antibacterial solution [e.g., Betadine, Hibiclens])
- 1% Xylocaine without epinephrine (or similar)
- 18-gauge half-inch and 22-gauge (1½-inch) needles for local anesthetic infiltration
- Skin closure tapes
- Stretch roller bandage (optional)

Training/Credentialing

No special credentialing is needed, but specialized training is available and advisable. These training sessions provide evidence of training for the provider's records.

Training may be arranged through the Norplant Procedure Instruction Program at 800-922-0877.

Coding

11976	Removal, implantable contraceptive capsules
11977	Removal with reinsertion, implantable contraceptive capsules

Technique

The removal of implantable contraceptive rods requires only slightly more time than the insertion process. Unlike for insertion, standardized kits containing the required equipment are not generally available. The tools needed may be easily assembled when needed or may be combined into a user-specific tray or kit that may be put up and sterilized for future use.

Because removal of implantable contraceptive rods involves the use of a local anesthetic and a skin incision, most practitioners obtain written informed consent before beginning the procedure (see Chapter 2, Informed Consent).

The patient should be positioned as for insertion of implantable contraceptive rods: supine on the examining table with the upper arm rested comfortably, abducted from the body at a 90° angle, with the elbow similarly flexed (Fig. 12.1). The site of the implantable capsules should be inspected and palpated to identify each of the six rods. It is imperative that the capsules be located accurately both before and during the process of removal.

The skin of the upper arm should be cleansed with antiseptic solution as for minor surgery, and sterile drapes should be placed as desired to provide a sterile field. A suitable local anesthetic may be drawn up by using a syringe and large-bore needle. The local anesthetic chosen should not contain epinephrine because this drug may result in superficial tissue necrosis. A 22-gauge needle is substituted for the needle used to draw up the anesthetic agent and used for tissue infiltration.

The site of injection and incision for removal of contraceptive rods depends somewhat on the technique to be used. For the "finger" and "standard" techniques, the scar

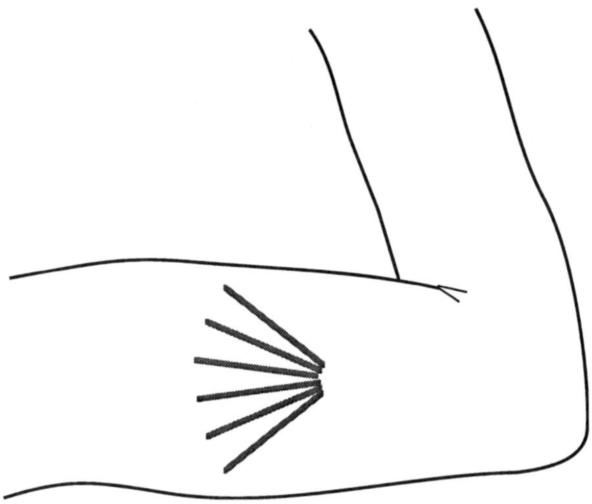

FIGURE 12.1.
The arm with the contraceptive capsules should be rested comfortably at a right angle to the body, with the elbow similarly flexed.

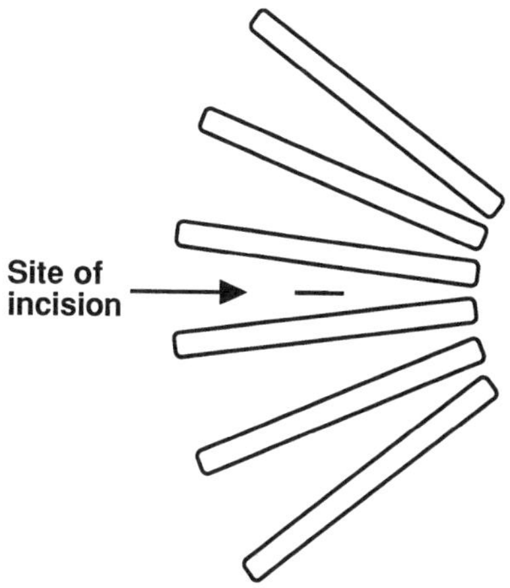

FIGURE 12.2.
For the U removal technique, the skin incision should be located parallel to the axis of the arm and capsule fan. It should be made between the third and fourth rods approximately at their midpoint.

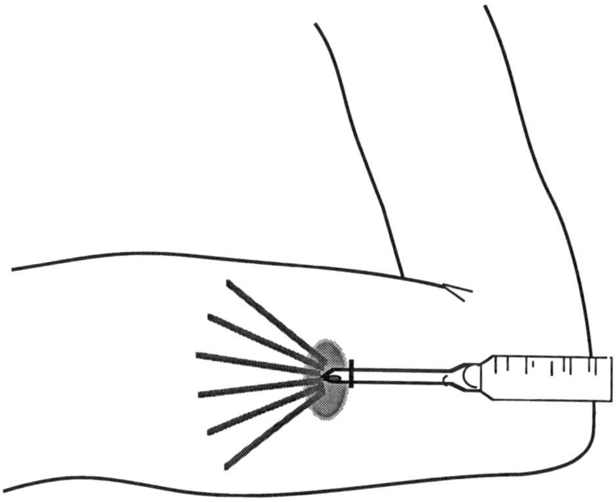

FIGURE 12.3.
The amount of local anesthetic injected should only be the amount necessary to elevate the ends of the contraceptive rods toward the skin surface.

of the original site of insertion is often reused. To be suitable for these techniques, the tips of the rods at the narrow end of the fan should be near the site of incision or easily displaced to it by finger pressure. In the "U" technique, the incision is made in a linear fashion parallel and between the third and fourth rods (Fig. 12.2). At either location, the incision should remain shallow and 3 to 4 mm in length.

Once the site of incision has been determined, a small amount of anesthetic agent is used to raise a small skin weal. For the finger and standard techniques, a total of 1 to 1.5 mL of additional anesthetic agent is injected under the proximal tips of the contraceptive rods, elevating them toward the skin surface (Fig. 12.3). The total amount of anesthetic agent should be limited so that it does not obscure identification of the rods. In the U technique, a small amount of anesthetic agent is infiltrated beneath the center of each of the rods in a similar fashion.

A shallow, 2–4-mm transverse skin incision is made at the point of the initial skin weal. This incision should penetrate only the dermis. Removal of the rods then proceeds by use of one or more of the techniques described in the following paragraphs. Although most practitioners have one technique that is preferred, a familiarity with each is advisable because it is often necessary to use more than one approach when problems with removal are encountered.

Once the contraceptive rods have been removed, they should be recounted to ensure that all six are accounted for. Because the fibrous capsule formed around the rods may be palpable for some time, the patient should be shown that all six capsules have been removed. A skin closure tape is placed to reapproximate the edges of the wound. A bandage may be placed as desired. An appropriate note, including either a description or drawing of the location of the contraceptive implants, should be placed in the patient's medical record.

DIGITAL (FINGER) TECHNIQUE

The digital removal technique begins with blunt dissection to break up adhesions around the proximal tips of the contraceptive capsules and to open the subdermal plane. The tips of a straight or curved hemostat are advanced through the skin wound, just below the dermis, then gently opened to accomplish this dissection. If the ends of one or more rods are visible at the incision, they should be grasped (individually) with a hemostat (Fig. 12.4). Care should be taken to limit this grasp to near the tip, where the rod is thickest and least likely to break or tear. A fibrous capsule formed around the rods must be removed from the tip using the tip of a needle or scalpel blade to scratch through the tissue (Fig. 12.5). A gauze sponge may also be used to bluntly remove the tissue. If a needle or scalpel is chosen, care must be used not to cut the contraceptive rod itself. Once the fibrous tissue is removed and the bare tip of the contraceptive rod is visible, the tip of the rod is regrasped with a hemostat and removed with gentle traction. Resistance to removal indicates a need to dissect additional adherent tissue.

When the proximal tips of the contraceptive rods are not visible at the incision, the distal tip of one rod should be palpated, then pushed toward the wound until the proximal is seen (Fig. 12.6). This process may be further facilitated by simultaneous traction of the skin incision in the opposite direction. The action of moving the rod and incision toward each other generally makes the tip of the contraceptive capsule visible. The tip may then be grasped, freed from the surrounding tissue, and removed as described above.

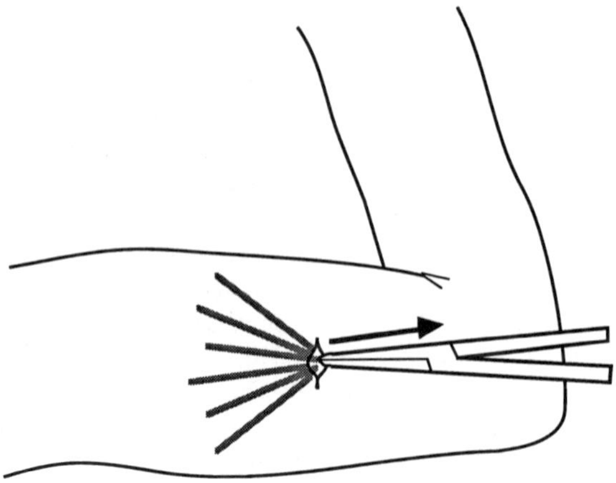

FIGURE 12.4.
If the ends of any contraceptive rods are visible in the incision, they may be grasped by their tip using a hemostat and delivered through the wound.

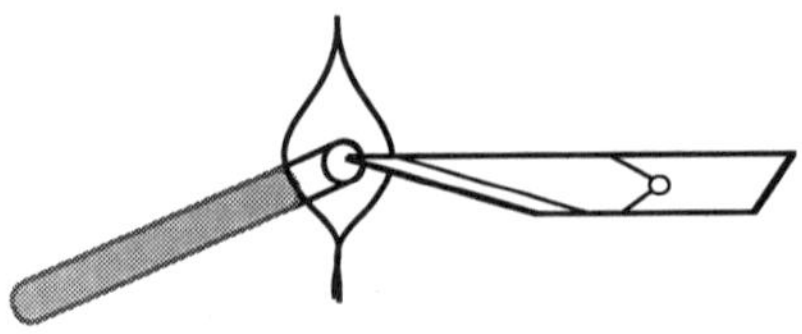

FIGURE 12.5.
The tip of a scalpel, needle, or gauze sponge may be used to dissect away the fibrous capsule encircling the contraceptive rod.

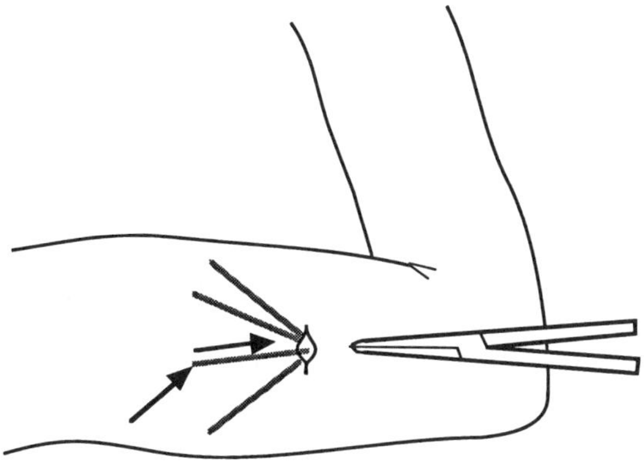

FIGURE 12.6.
Pressure on the distal end of the contraceptive capsule is often sufficient to bring the tip into the incision, from which it can be grasped and removed.

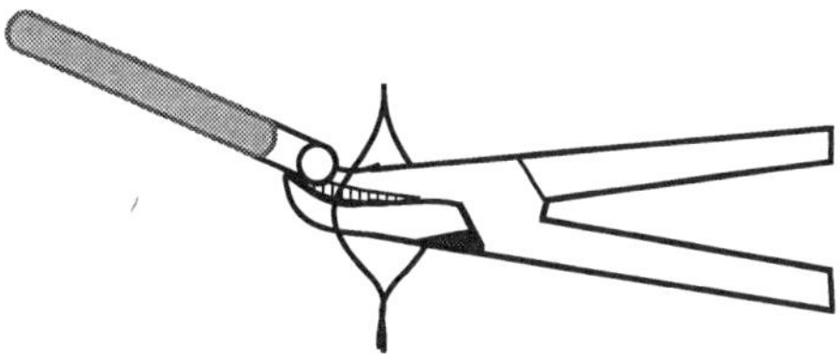

FIGURE 12.7.
A curved hemostat may be passed below the tip of the contraceptive capsule and opened, a process that allows the capsule to be grasped. A finger should be placed on the skin over the jaws of the hemostat to prevent the capsule from slipping out as the hemostat is closed.

In both the digital and standard methods, the capsules may be removed in any order; the sequence of removal is usually dictated by the location and ease of access of the individual rods. When the rods are removed in a random order, care must be taken to avoid losing track of the location of the remaining rods as the procedure progresses. Failure to do so may mean that the remaining rods will be difficult to find at the end of the procedure or that they will be inadvertently left behind.

STANDARD TECHNIQUE

In the standard technique, any capsules visible at the incision site are removed as above. The remaining capsules are removed by advancing a curved hemostat to below the proximal end of the rod (Fig. 12.7). The jaws of the hemostat are elevated and opened so that they are located on either side of the capsule. By using gentle downward pressure from a finger to prevent the capsule from slipping from the hemostat's grasp, the hemostat is closed, grabbing the tip of the contraceptive capsule. Gentle traction then delivers the capsule and the surrounding fibrous tissue to the wound, where the tissue is dissected free and the rod is removed as in the digital method.

The movement of the capsule to the incision may be facilitated by rotating the hemostat upward and back along the axis of the rod (Fig. 12.8). This results in traction on the rod toward the incision at the same time the incision itself is moved toward the rod. The rod will be bent into a "J" shape, with the curve visible below the hemostat in the opening of the wound. This portion may be cleansed of surrounding tissue, allowing removal through this point.

Some practitioners prefer to grasp the contraceptive rods with the modified vasectomy clamp. This clamp is less likely to break or damage the rods. This is a matter of personal preference.

U TECHNIQUE

The U technique allows the physician to grasp the implants anywhere along their shaft, not just near the tip. The U technique requires the use of ring-tipped forceps

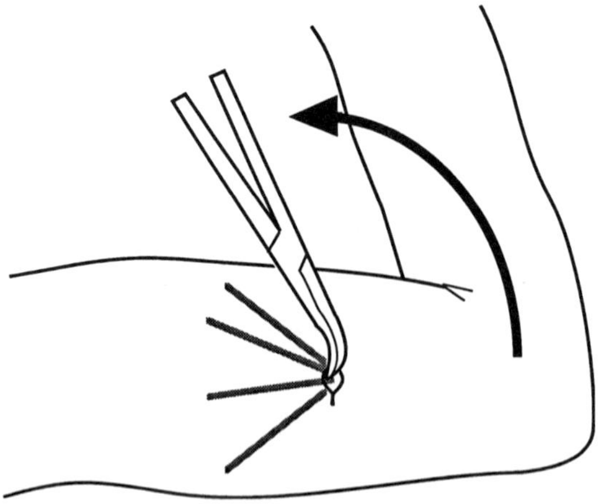

FIGURE 12.8.
By rotating the hemostat back along the axis of the rod, the tip of the capsule and the skin incision will be moved toward each other, thereby making the tip accessible.

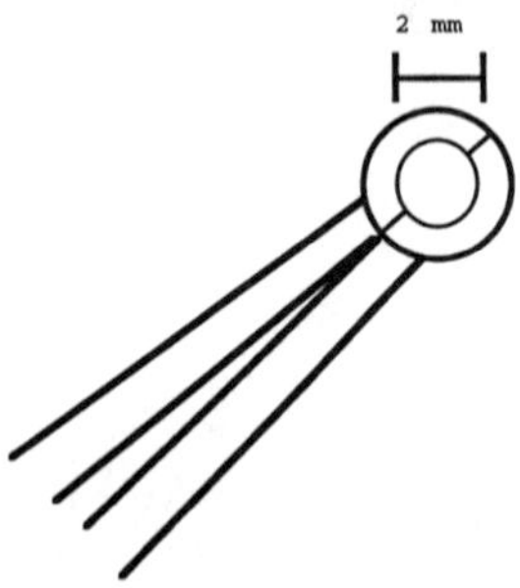

FIGURE 12.9.
The tip of the modified vasectomy clamp (Norgrasp) forms a ring with an opening that is approximately the size of the contraceptive rods; this allows a firm grasp but does not lead to the cuts or breakage that might occur with a hemostat.

with a circular or oval tip (Fig. 12.9). This instrument, called Norgrasp, is a modification of the vas deferens fixation forceps used in the no-scalpel vasectomy technique. The clamp is advanced under the contraceptive rod adjacent to the skin incision, is opened, and is closed around the rod, thereby providing a firm grasp. The rod is delivered into the wound; in so doing, the rod is bent into a U shape, giving the method its name. As in the digital and standard methods, the fibrous capsule around the rod must be carefully dissected, freeing the rod for its removal. If a needle or scalpel is used to incise the fibrous tissue surrounding the contraceptive rod, care must be taken to do so along the axis of the rod itself. This minimizes the possibility of breaking the rod when it is removed.

THE DIFFICULT REMOVAL

Missing Capsules

If it is difficult to see or feel the capsules before starting the removal process, it is unlikely that the removal will be routine or easy. When direct palpation and inspection do not clearly indicate the location of each rod, inspection may be enhanced by painting the skin surface with a povidone–iodine solution, then gently scraping away the excess solution using a straight edge (such as the side of a scalpel handle). The location of the rods may appear as light areas in the otherwise darkened field.

When one or more capsules cannot be located during the process of removal, serious consideration should be given to abandoning the search; after the arm heals for 6 weeks, the location of the missing rods can be reassessed. This allows the edema that has invariably accumulated during the attempt to dissipate, revealing the location of the missing rods. When the rods are still not apparent, they may be sought using such imaging and localization techniques as ultrasonography or fluoroscopy. Each may be performed with or without needle localization of the rods. It is imperative that during the interval from first attempt to final removal the patient is advised to use some other form of contraception if pregnancy is to be avoided.

Broken Rods

If a contraceptive capsule is broken during the removal process, care must be taken to account for all portions. As each segment is removed, it should be placed with the other pieces so that the original capsule is reconstructed. Once all segments are thought to have been recovered, an undamaged rod should be placed along side the damaged one for comparison. By checking the length on the undamaged rod against the reconstructed rod, the possibility of additional unrecovered fragments may be determined.

Further Assistance

Assistance with problems in the removal of contraceptive rods may be obtained by contacting the Norplant Consultant's Network at 800-922-0877. This group provides free consultation with an expert who is experienced in the use, insertion, and removal of contraceptive rods.

Special Notes

Videotapes illustrating removal techniques, plastic arm models that allow the learner to practice removal skills, the Norgrasp clamp, and enrollment in the Procedure Instruction Program may be obtained by contacting the Norplant Foundation at the following address: PO Box 25223, Alexandria, VA 22314; telephone number, 703-706-5933 or 800-760-9030.

If desired, another set of capsules may be inserted immediately after the removal of the previous set by facing the fan of capsules in the opposite direction through the same incision or by using a new site on the opposite arm.

Suggested Readings

Berg WA, Hamper UM. Norplant implants: sonographic identification and localization for removal. *AJR* 1995;164:419.

Cecil H, Reed D, Holtz J. Norplant removal facilitated by use of ultrasound for localization. *J Fam Pract* 1995;40:182.

Glauser SJ, Scharling ES, Stovall TG, et al. Ultrasonography: usefulness in localization of the Norplant contraceptive implant system. *J Ultrasound Med* 1995;14:411.

Kirk EP, Field CS. Difficult Norplant removal facilitated by fluoroscopy. *Am J Obstet Gynecol* 1993;169:748.

Lang JF, Heine MW, Purdon TF. Use of needle localization for difficult Norplant removal. *Am J Obstet Gynecol* 1994;171:1161.

Monaghan JC. Norplant insertion and removal. *Patient Care* March 1992:231.

Praptohardjo R, Praptohardjo U. 'U' technique and standard technique of Norplant removal. *Adv Contracept* 1995;11:115.

Praptohardjo U, Wibowo S. The "U" technique: a new method for Norplant implants removal. *Contraception* 1993;48:526.

Reynolds RD. The 'Modified U' technique: a refined method of Norplant removal. *J Fam Pract* 1995;40:173.

Sarma SP, Hatcher R. The Emory method: a modified approach to Norplant implants removal. *Contraception* 1994;49:551.

Sarma SP, Hatcher RP. Neurovascular injury during removal of levonorgestrel implants. *Am J Obstet Gynecol* 1995;172:120.

Shihata AA, Salzetti RG, Schnepper FW, et al. Innovative technique for Norplant implants removal. *Contraception* 1995;51:83.

Shoupe D, Mishell DR. Norplant: subdermal implant system for long-term contraception. *Am J Obstet Gynecol* 1989;160:1286.

Soloman G. Vasectomy technique for Norplant removal. *J Fam Pract* 1995;40:121.

Zuber TJ, DeWitt DE, Patton DD. Skin damage associated with the Norplant contraceptive. *J Fam Pract* 1992;34:613.

Chapter 13

INTRAUTERINE CONTRACEPTIVE DEVICE INSERTION

The intrauterine contraceptive device (IUCD) remains a cost-effective contraceptive method for many women. Although best suited for parous, monogamous women who are unlikely to want future fertility, the IUCDs of today may be used by almost any patient. The device is easily inserted, but the process is still a surgical procedure that carries the possibility of substantial complication if not performed carefully and properly.

Equipment

- IUCD in sterile package (ParaGard T380A or Progestasert)
- Antiseptic solution (e.g., povidone–iodine solution)
- Vaginal speculum
- Tenaculum
- Uterine sound (optional)
- Nonsterile examination gloves
- Scissors (long)
- Sterile gloves (optional with "no touch" technique)

Training/Credentialing

No special credentialing needed; office procedure only.

Coding

58300	Insertion of intrauterine device (IUD), not including device
X4633	Charge for cost of copper IUD
X4634	Charge for cost of progesterone IUD

Technique

Before any attempt is made to insert an IUCD, the size, shape, and location of the uterus should be determined. This should be done even if the patient has recently been examined. Except in the most obese or uncooperative patients, these uterine characteristics can be determined by simple bimanual examination. When such examination cannot be done, the advisability of IUCD use should be seriously reconsidered before tests such as ultrasonography are used.

Once the position of the uterus has been determined, the cervix should be visualized with the aid of a speculum, then disinfected. In parous patients who do not have substantial uterine flexion, it is often not necessary to use a tenaculum. Because a tenaculum produces discomfort in its own right, an attempt to insert the IUCD without it is reasonable whereever possible.

The technique used to place the contraceptive device in its proper location in the uterine cavity varies slightly depending on the brand chosen. Each of the currently available types uses the same general sequence of steps: loading the IUCD into its carrier or placement device, placing the IUCD in position in the uterine cavity, withdrawal of the placement instrument leaving the IUCD behind, verification of correct placement, and trimming of the marker stings. Because of individual differences in the insertion device and thus the technique of placement, each of the two available devices will be discussed separately.

PARAGARD T380A

The IUCD must be loaded into its insertion device, which varies somewhat with the type of IUCD. In the case of ParaGard, this may be done using either sterile gloves or a "no touch" technique. With sterile gloves, the device is grasped, folded, and inserted into the distal end of the insertion tool (Fig. 13.1). The "no touch" method has the same goals, but these are reached by manipulating the IUCD through the outer package wrapper. With practice this method can be just as fast and safe, while saving the time and cost of donning sterile gloves. For the inexperienced, this approach can be frustrating and risks contamination. If there is doubt, the sterile glove method is always safer.

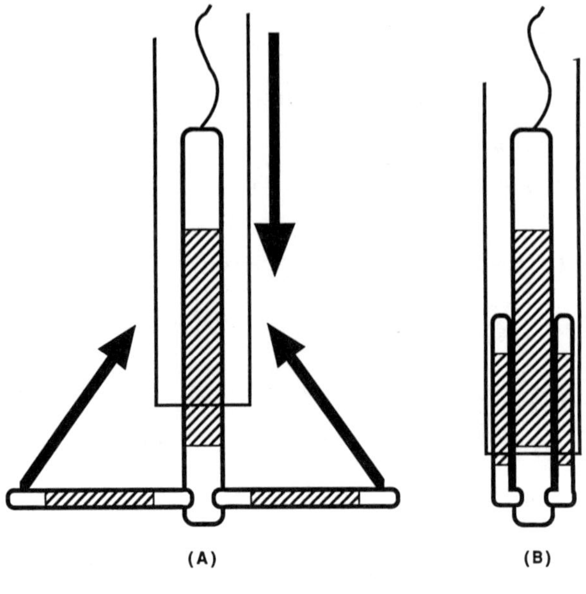

FIGURE 13.1.
*The ParaGard IUCD is grasped through the outer sterile wrap and the wings folded downward as the insertion tube is advanced (**A**). The IUCD is brought to its final position with its wings completely enclosed in the insertion tube (**B**).*

Once in place in the insertion device, the moveable flange is moved backward on the insertion tube until it corresponds to the expected or measured depth of the uterus. Next, the IUCD and inserter are placed at the disinfected external cervical os and gently advanced until resistance indicates that the fundus had been reached. With the obturator held in place, the insertion tube is withdrawn, leaving the device in the correct position. Care should be used that the obturator is not inadvertently advanced as the insertion tube is partially withdrawn. Failure to perform this in the correct way may result in the IUCD being forced into or through the wall of the uterus. The insertion tube may be slightly readvanced to ensure that the IUCD lies against the fundus; it is then withdrawn completely.

The string of the device should be trimmed at a point approximately 1–2 cm from the external os.

PROGESTASERT

The Progestasert IUCD is supplied with an integrated inserter and loading device (Fig. 13.2). The loading device (arm-cocker) allows the IUCD to be loaded into its inserter without the use of sterile gloves. To load the IUCD into the inserter, the package is opened; care should be taken to retain the sterility of the inner wrapping and to ensure that the retaining plug (Fig. 13.3, *insert*) is not disturbed. The inserter assembly is

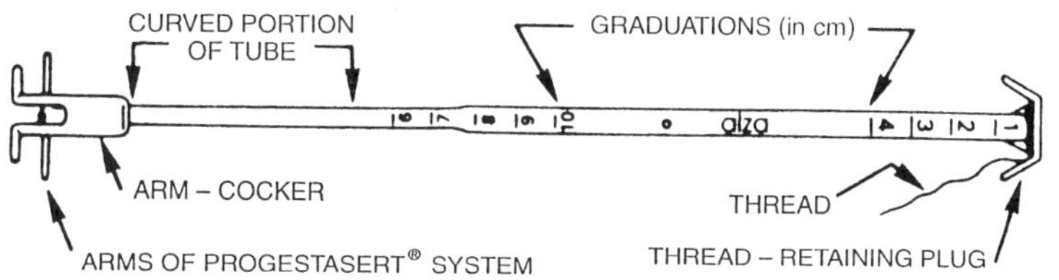

FIGURE 13.2.
The Progestasert contraceptive device is supplied with an integrated inserter and loading tool. (Courtesy of ALZA Corporation, Palo Alto, CA 94303.)

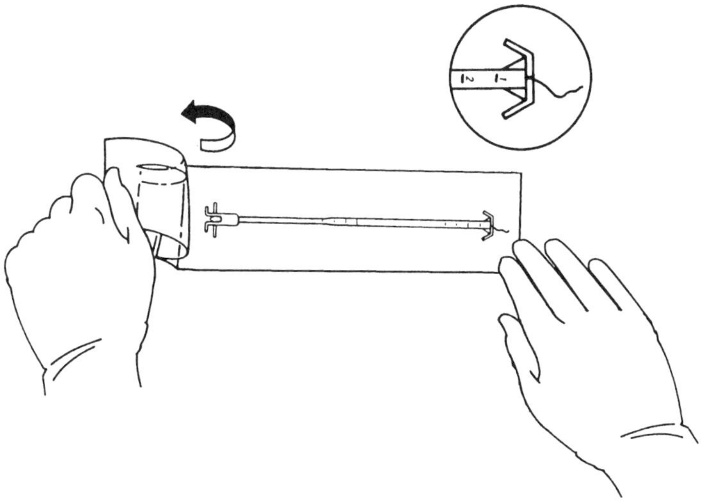

FIGURE 13.3.
When the Progestasert package is opened, the retaining plug (insert) should be left in place. (Courtesy of ALZA Corporation, Palo Alto, CA 94303.)

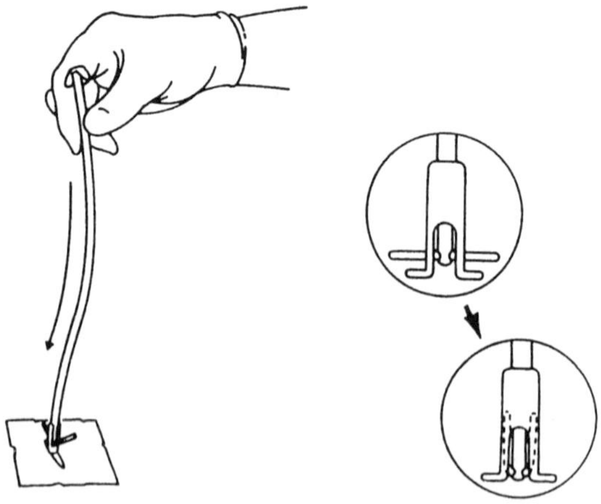

FIGURE 13.4.
With gentle pressure against a sterile surface, the arms of the IUCD will fold backward in preparation for insertion into the uterine cavity. (Courtesy of ALZA Corporation, Palo Alto, CA 94303.)

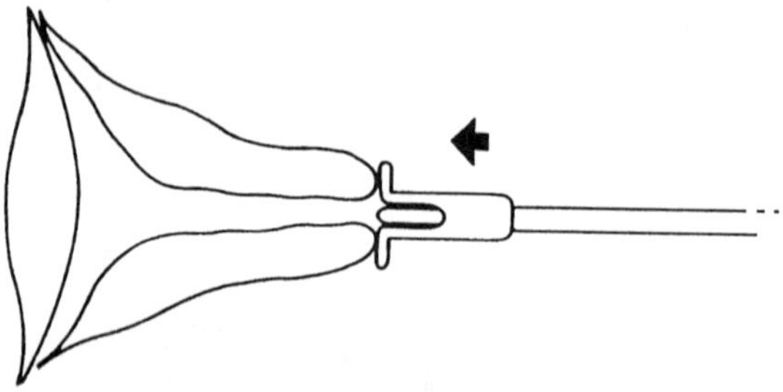

FIGURE 13.5.
The tip of the IUCD and the wings of the loading tool are placed at the external cervical os and gently advanced. (Courtesy of ALZA Corporation, Palo Alto, CA 94303.)

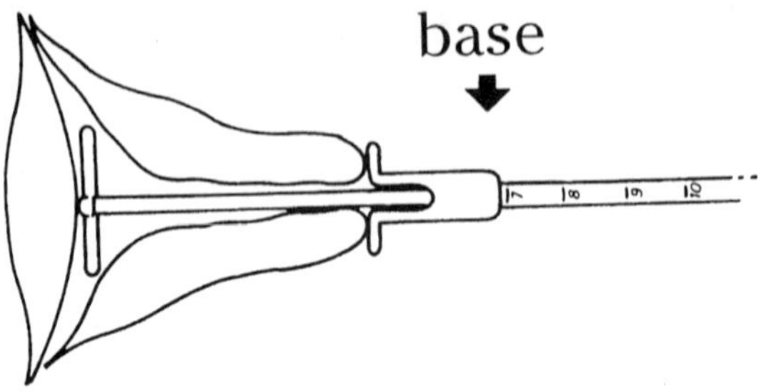

FIGURE 13.6.
The depth of the uterus may be gauged by the centimeter mark visible at the base of the loading tool. (Courtesy of ALZA Corporation, Palo Alto, CA 94303.)

picked up by the end that is opposite to the IUCD, and the face of the loading tool is placed against the sterile surface of the sterile package wrapper. When gentle downward pressure is applied on the shaft of the inserter, the arms of the IUCD fold backward into the proper position for insertion (Fig. 13.4).

To place the IUCD in the uterine cavity, the tip of the IUCD and insertion tool are placed against the disinfected cervical os (Fig. 13.5); the curve of the insertion device is directed in the same direction as any uterine flexion that may be present. Gentle pressure is exerted on the shaft of the inserter, and the tip is advanced until the fundus is reached. The depth of the uterus may be measured or verified by noting the centimeter mark at the base of the loading tool (Fig. 13.6).

Once the IUCD had been delivered to the apex of the uterine cavity, the retaining plug is removed from the inserter by squeezing the wings together and pulling backward, freeing the retaining string (Fig. 13.7). The IUCD may now be deposited clear of the insertion tool by gently removing the tool, with care taken not to snag the retaining string (Fig. 13.8). The proper positioning of the IUCD at the fundus of uterine cavity may be verified by reversing the insertion tool and measuring the length of the short string protruding from the external os. The shorter (indicator) string has a length

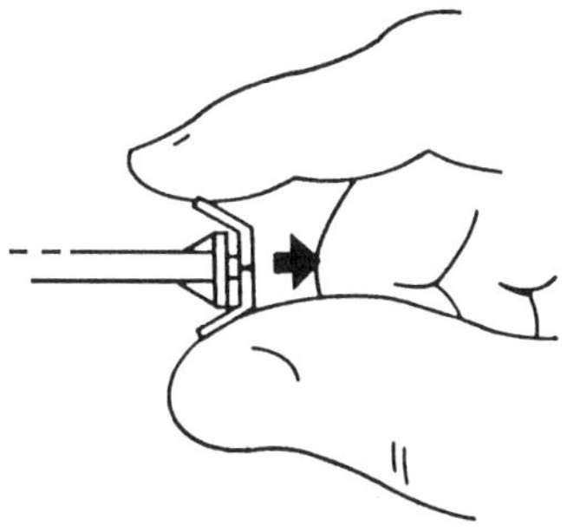

FIGURE 13.7.
The IUCD retaining plug is removed by compression and traction. (Courtesy of ALZA Corporation, Palo Alto, CA 94303.)

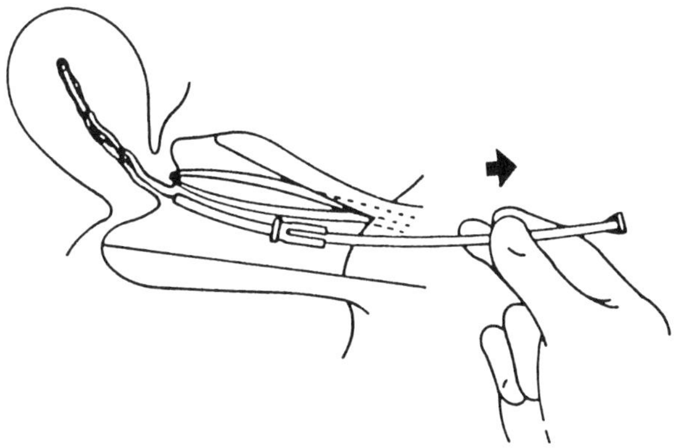

FIGURE 13.8.
Gentle traction on the insertion tool will result in the IUCD being left behind in the uterine cavity. (Courtesy of ALZA Corporation, Palo Alto, CA 94303.)

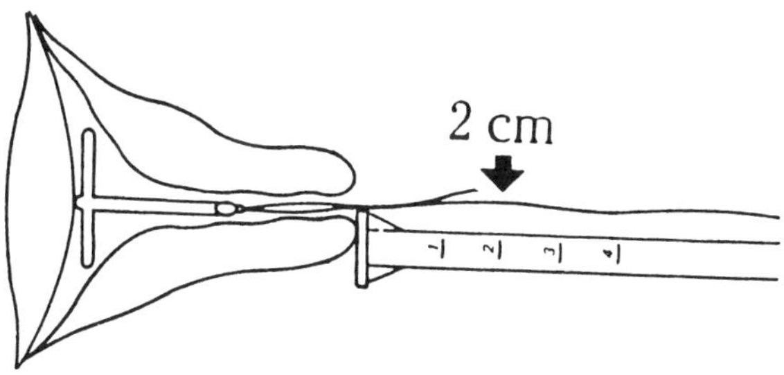

FIGURE 13.9.
For most patients, approximately 2 cm of indicator string will be visible outside the opening of the cervix. (Courtesy of ALZA Corporation, Palo Alto, CA 94303.)

of 9 cm. As a result, the length of string visible outside the cervix should equal 9 minus the depth of the uterus, as measured by uterine sound or the mark seen on the insertion device at the time of placement. In the case illustrated in Figure 13.9, 2 cm of string (9 − 7 = 2) should remain outside the cervical canal. Once this has been confirmed, the longer retaining string should be cut approximately 1 cm longer than the indicator string. This allows the position of the IUCD to be verified at any future time by measuring the shorter of the two strings.

Special Notes

Although an IUCD may be inserted during any point in a menstrual cycle (where pregnancy has been ruled out), it is preferable to insert the device at the time of regular menstruation. This offers three advantages: 1) Pregnancy is unlikely; 2) the cervical os is often slightly dilated at this time, which facilitates insertion; and 3) any bleeding caused by the insertion process will be lost in the normal menstrual process.

The discomfort of IUCD placement may be minimized by premedicating the patient with a nonsteroidal anti-inflammatory agent 30 to 60 minutes before the start of the procedure.

Table 13.1. Contraindications to Placement of IUCD

Active cervical infection
Acute sexually transmissible infection
Allergy to copper (copper IUCD only)
Dysfunctional uterine bleeding (undiagnosed)
Dysmenorrhea
Genital actinomycoses
History of ectopic pregnancy (relative)
Immediate postpartum period (less than 8 weeks)
Immunocompromise
IUCD in situ (unremoved)
Malignant condition (uterine or cervical, known or suspected)
Menorrhagia
Multiple sexual partners (relative)
Previous pelvic inflammatory disease (relative)
Known or suspected pregnancy
Uterine cavity malformation
Vaginitis
Wilson's disease (copper IUCD only)

When gentle pressure does not cause the IUCD insertion tool to advance through the cervix, a tenaculum may be used to stabilize the cervix. Traction on the tenaculum may result in some straightening of the canal, further aiding insertion. In some cases, it may be necessary to use a sterile uterine sound to identify the axis of the canal, modestly dilate the canal, or confirm the depth to the uterine cavity. Because the use of both the tenaculum and the sound potentially cause pain and increase the risk for infection, they should be used with caution.

Intrauterine contraceptive devices should not be left in the folded position inside the inserter for more than 1–2 minutes. As a result of prolonged folding, the device will not unfold properly in the uterine cavity, increasing the risk for expulsion or contraceptive failure.

Patients should be reminded to use an alternate form of contraception for the first month after IUCD placement. Ideally, this method should not be one associated with intermenstrual spotting, which could confuse the assessment of possible side effects of the IUCD. General contraindications to the use of an IUCD are shown in Table 13.1.

Suggested Readings

Anteby E, Revel A, Ben-Chetrit A, et al. Intrauterine device failure: relation to its location within the uterine cavity. *Obstet Gynecol* 1993;81:112.

Anwar M. An evaluation of IUD insertion by a non-clinical delivery system. *Adv Contracept* 1992;8:303.

Duenas JL, Albert A, Carrasco F. Intrauterine contraception in nulligravid vs parous women. *Contraception* 1996;53:23.

Farley TM, Rosenberg MJ, Rowe PJ, et al. Intrauterine devices and pelvic inflammatory disease: an international perspective. *Lancet* 1992;339:785.

Morrison C, Waszak C, Katz K, et al. Clinical outcomes of two early postpartum IUD insertion programs in Africa. *Contraception* 1996;53:17.

O'Hanley K, Huber DH. Postpartum IUDS: keys for success. *Contraception* 1992; 45:351.

Reinprayoon D. Intrauterine contraception. *Curr Opin Obstet Gynecol* 1992;4:527.

Richardson A, Paul C. A national study to monitor the safety of IUCD use. *Contraception* 1993;47:359.

Saarikoski S. Contraception during lactation. *Ann Med* 1993;25:181.

Toivonen J. Intrauterine contraceptive device and pelvic inflammatory disease. *Ann Med* 1993;25:171.

Walsh TL, Bernstein GS, Grimes DA, et al. Effect of prophylactic antibiotics on morbidity associated with IUD insertion: results of a pilot randomized controlled trial. IUD Study Group. *Contraception* 1994;50:319.

Xu JX, Reusche C, Burdan A. Immediate postplacental insertion of the intrauterine device: a review of Chinese and the world's experiences. *Adv Contracept* 1994; 10:71.

Zorlu CG, Aral K, Cobanoglu O, et al. Pelvic inflammatory disease and intrauterine devices: prophylactic antibiotics to reduce febrile complications. *Adv Contracept* 1993;9:299.

Chapter 14

INTRAUTERINE CONTRACEPTIVE DEVICE REMOVAL

Currently available intrauterine contraceptive devices (IUCDs) may be left in place for 1 to 10 years before they should be removed. For most patients, removal is quick and easy. For some, however, the removal process may be more complicated than the insertion itself. A familiarity with several removal techniques will allow the practitioner to successfully remove the IUCD in the office in almost all cases.

Equipment

- Vaginal speculum
- Tenaculum
- Uterine packing forceps or other long forceps
- IUD or "crochet" hook (optional)
- Nonsterile examination gloves
- Antiseptic solution (e.g., povidone–iodine solution) if hook or other intrauterine instrument is used

Training/Credentialing

No special credentialing needed; office procedure only.

Coding

58301 Removal of intrauterine device (IUD)

Technique

Because it is almost never known in advance which patient may require intrauterine manipulation to retrieve an IUCD, a bimanual examination should precede any at-

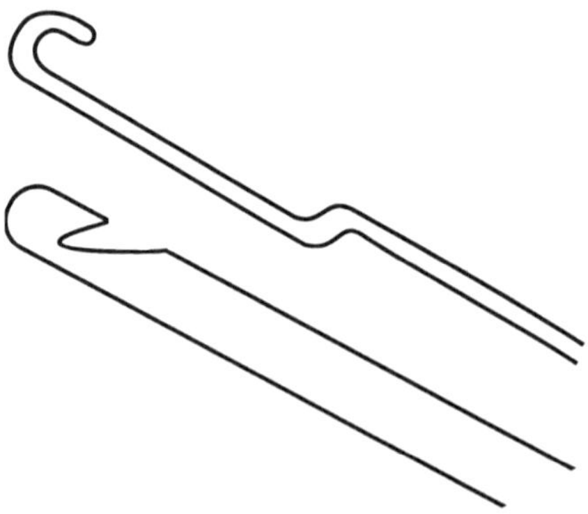

FIGURE 14.1.
Several different styles of IUCD hooks can be used to retrieve missing devices.

tempt at removal. This examination determines the size, shape, and position of the uterus, information that is vital to ensuring the safety of intrauterine manipulation.

When the IUCD string or strings are visible at the cervical os, gentle traction with a uterine packing forceps or other suitable grasping device results in the delivery of the IUCD. When the string is not apparent, gentle probing of the outer portion of the cervical canal with the forceps or a sterile crochet hook often yields the string, which may then be grasped as above. If these two maneuvers are unsuccessful in retrieving the IUCD, the cervix should be disinfected before any further attempts. The possibility of an ongoing pregnancy must also be considered.

An IUCD ("crochet") hook may be used to retrieve the missing strings of an IUCD or the device itself (Fig. 14.1). In most cases, if a hook must be used a tenaculum to stabilize the cervix is helpful. The hook is passed through the cervix to the level of the uterine fundus. Because of the larger size of the hook, passage through the cervix may be more difficult and produce more discomfort than would an endometrial biopsy. As the hook is advanced, the shaft of the device should be carefully monitored for vibrations, sounds, or the "feel" that the tip has encountered the IUCD. This information is helpful in identifying the possible location of the IUCD. Once the hook has reached the fundus (or the level of the IUCD if it is felt), the hook is slowly rotated through 180 to 360° and withdrawn. Moderate resistance to withdrawal is associated with capture of the IUCD, and persistent traction often delivers the device. Even when no resistance is felt, removal of the hook often delivers the string or strings, allowing removal of the IUCD by conventional traction. If neither the IUCD nor its string has been retrieved in several attempts, the effort should be abandoned until the presence of the IUCD in the body has been confirmed and removal through hysteroscopy or laparoscopy has been considered.

Special Notes

When the strings of an IUCD are not visible at the cervix, the possibility that the device had been expelled at some time in the past must be considered. Ultrasonography, plain radiography, or computed tomography may be used to identify the presence and location of a missing IUCD if it is still contained in the body.

The discomfort of IUCD removal may be minimized by premedicating the patient with a nonsteroidal anti-inflammatory agent 30 to 60 minutes before the start of the procedure.

If a pregnancy occurs and the strings of the IUCD are still visible, removal of the device by gentle traction is desirable. If the strings cannot be seen or are not located just inside the external cervical os, no further attempts at removal are necessary.

Suggested Readings

Assaf A, Gohar M, Saad S, et al. Removal of intrauterine devices with missing tails during early pregnancy. *Contraception* 1992;45:541.

Duenas JL, Albert A, Carrasco F. Intrauterine contraception in nulligravid vs parous women. *Contraception* 1996;53:23.

Ranzini AC, Wapner RJ, Davis GH. Ultrasonographically guided intrauterine contraceptive device removal before chorionic villus sampling. *Am J Obstet Gynecol* 1995;173:603.

Reinprayoon D. Intrauterine contraception. *Curr Opin Obstet Gynecol* 1992;4:527.

Sachs BP, Gregory K, McArdle C, et al. Removal of retained intrauterine contraceptive devices in pregnancy. *Am J Perinatol* 1992;9:139.

Wyatt S, Gallen IW, Nicholls A. A potential hazard of prolonged insertion of an intrauterine device. *N Engl J Med* 1994;330:1395.

Zhang J. Factors associated with copper T IUD removal for bleeding/pain: a multivariate analysis. *Contraception* 1993;48:13.

Chapter 15

CRYOSURGERY

The use of cold to produce "frost bite" can provide a convenient office method for destroying cervical, vaginal, or vulvar lesions. The equipment necessary to perform cryosurgery is common, simple to operate, and relatively inexpensive to purchase and maintain.

Equipment

- Cryosurgery unit powered by nitrous oxide
- Flat and conical cryoprobes of assorted sizes
- Water-soluble lubricant (e.g., K-Y Jelly)
- Timer (optional but recommended)
- Vaginal speculum
- Colposcope (if colposcopy has not been previously performed or the boundaries of the lesion are not visible)
- 3–5% acetic acid (white vinegar) or Lugol's (5%) solution
- Gauze pads or cotton balls
- Vaginal sidewall retractor (optional)

Training/Credentialing

No special credentialing needed; office procedure only.

Coding

57511	Cauterization of cervix; cryocautery, initial or repeat (surgical procedure only)
56501	Destruction of lesion(s), vulva; simple, any method
56515	extensive, any method
57061	Destruction of lesion(s), vagina; simple, any method
57065	extensive, any method

Technique

CRYOSURGERY OF THE CERVIX

Before cryosurgery is done, the risks, benefits, and alternatives should be explained to the patient. A history or pregnancy test should be done to determine that the patient is not pregnant. If desired, the patient may be given pretreatment analgesia either to be taken at home or in the office. Ibuprofen (800 mg) or other similar nonsteroidal anti-inflammatory agent is sufficient to reduce the cramping associated with the procedure. This drug should be taken approximately 1 hour before therapy.

Once informed consent has been obtained, the patient, undressed from the waist down, is positioned on the examination table as for a speculum examination. The cervix should be brought into view using a standard speculum. Any cultures or cytologic smears to be obtained should be taken at this stage. If a significant period has elapsed since the last colposcopic examination, colposcopy should be repeated (see Chapter 9, Colposcopy). If the extent of the lesion has not been documented or is not immediately visible, acetic acid or Lugol's solution should be applied to the cervix to delineate the area of abnormality.

A cryoprobe tip should be selected so that the freezing effect extends approximately 5 mm beyond the extent of the lesion (Fig. 15.1). Whenever possible, the probe should be flat or slightly conical to minimize the risk for extensive endocervical freezing. This should, in turn, minimize the risk for inward migration of the squamocolumnar junction. The selected tip should be attached to the cryocautery handle, following manufacturer's directions. When the tip is attached, the gas supply tank valve should be in the "off" position. Once the tip is secured, the gas supply should be turned on and the tank pressure checked to ensure an adequate supply.

A water-soluble gel or lubricant is applied to the tip of the cryoprobe. Lidocaine jelly may be substituted if desired. The tip of the probe should be placed against the cervix, covering the lesion. Care must be used that the probe is not in contact with the side walls of the vagina.

The patient is informed that the procedure is about to start and that the machine may make sounds upon activation. The unit is activated, and after approximately 5 seconds, the tip adheres to the cervix. Once the tip is adhered to the cervix, the device is maneuvered outward and further away from the vaginal sidewalls to avoid adherence of the vaginal wall to the gun. This outward movement brings along the cervix and also minimizes lateral freezing.

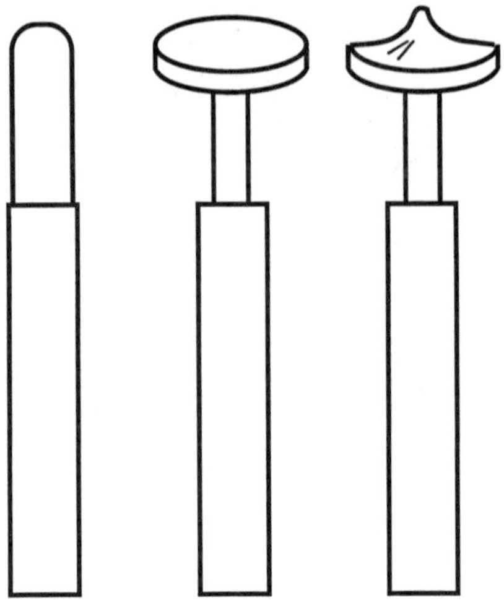

FIGURE 15.1.
Many shapes and sizes of tips are available for most cryocautery machines. The size and shape of the tip should assure complete coverage of the lesion. The tip should provide good contact to the surface of the cervix but not extend far into the endocervical canal.

Freezing should continue for 3 minutes, resulting in an iceball that extends 5 mm beyond the cervical lesion. The freezing mechanism is then deactivated to allow the lesion to thaw for 5 minutes. The probe should not be actively loosened from the cervix but allowed to defrost and detach by itself. After thawing for 5 minutes, the lesion is refrozen as above for another 3 minutes. A single 5-minute freeze may also be used, but with either method, the iceball must extend to a distance of more than 5 mm for the procedure to be effective.

After the final freeze, the patient should be told that postoperative discharge may be expected to occur for several weeks. In addition, a follow-up sequence of Papanicolaou smears should be discussed with the patient. The first smear should not be done for at least 3 months to allow for complete healing.

APPLICATIONS BEYOND THE CERVIX

The use of cold to selectively destroy lesions may be applied in other areas of the body as well as the cervix. In gynecology, this usually involves lesions of the vaginal wall or vulva, most notably condyloma acuminata. When cryosurgery is used for this purpose, the lesion should be moistened with water or a water-soluble gel. A fine tip should be chosen and attached to the cryocautery unit according to the manufacturer's directions. The tip is placed in contact with the moistened lesion and cooling is begun. Once the tip has adhered to the lesion, traction should be supplied to lift the tip (and lesion) away from the surrounding skin. The same freeze-thaw-freeze sequence used for cervical lesions should be applied to lesions located elsewhere in the genital tract.

The patient should be told that the lesion will swell during the ensuing hours, become vesicular, and slough in 3 to 5 days. Little pain should be felt after the initial sharp pain of freezing. A watery discharge from the site is common.

Normal Findings

Patients may report uterine cramping or hot flashes during the procedure or shortly thereafter. These findings are normal and will be self-limited.

Selected Abnormal Findings

Persistent pain or discharge after cryosurgery may suggest incidental freezing of the vaginal wall. Examination may be warranted depending on the individual case.

Special Notes

Patients may be given topical vaginal medications such as Triple Sulfa cream or an acidifying cream (e.g., Amino-Cerv) to reduce discharge after cryosurgery. Theoretical cervical stenosis as a result of the procedure is highly unlikely unless the procedure is done repetitively or if a probe tip that extends high into the endocervix is used.

Suggested Readings

Andersen ES, Thorup K, Larsen G. Results of cryosurgery for cervical intraepithelial neoplasia. *Gynecol Oncol* 1988;30:21–5.

Benedet JL, Miller DM, Nickerson KG, et al. The results of cryosurgical treatment of cervical intraepithelial neoplasia at one, five, and ten years. *Am J Obstet Gynecol* 1987;157:268–73.

Ferris DG. Lethal tissue temperature during cervical cryotherapy with a small flat cryoprobe. *J Fam Pract* 1994;38:153.

Gage AA. Cryosurgery in the treatment of cancer. *Surg Gynecol Obstet* 1992;174:73.

Loobuyck HA, Duncan ID. Destruction of CIN 1 and 2 with the Semm cold coagulator: 13 years' experience with a see-and-treat policy. *Br J Obstet Gynaecol* 1993;100:465.

Mathevet P, Dargent D, Roy M, et al. A randomized prospective study comparing three techniques of conization: cold knife, laser, and LEEP. *Gynecol Oncol* 1994;54:175.

Ostergard DR. Cryosurgical treatment of cervical intraepithelial neoplasia. *Obstet Gynecol* 1980;56:231–3.

Townsend DE. Cryosurgery for CIN. *Obstet Gynecol Surv* 1979;34:828.

Chapter 16

ENDOMETRIAL BIOPSY

The advent of simple, office-based endometrial sampling systems makes this procedure quick, easy, inexpensive, and safer than the traditional dilatation and curettage.

Equipment

- Disposable endometrial sampling device (e.g., Accurette, Explora, Gynocheck, Pipelle, and Z-Sampler) or reusable curette (Novak or other curette)
- Sterile single-tooth tenaculum (optional)
- Sterile uterine sound (optional)
- Sterile lacrimal duct probe (optional)
- Skin preparation materials (generally an iodine-based antibacterial solution such as Betadine)
- Buffered formalin or other histologic fixative
- Pelvic examination equipment (examination gloves, lubricant, speculum, light source)

Training/Credentialing

No special credentialing needed; office procedure only.

Coding

58100	Endometrial sampling (biopsy) with or without endocervical sampling (biopsy) without cervical dilatation, any method (separate procedure)

Technique

Several sampling devices (e.g., Accurette, Explora, Gynocheck, Pipelle, Z-Sampler, and others [Fig. 16.1]) have been shown to provide reliable tissue diagnosis in 90–100% of cases. This office diagnostic technique is valuable for evaluating patients suspected of having endometrial cancer because of irregular perimenopausal or postmenopausal bleeding. This procedure is best suited for diagnosis, not screening, because it causes

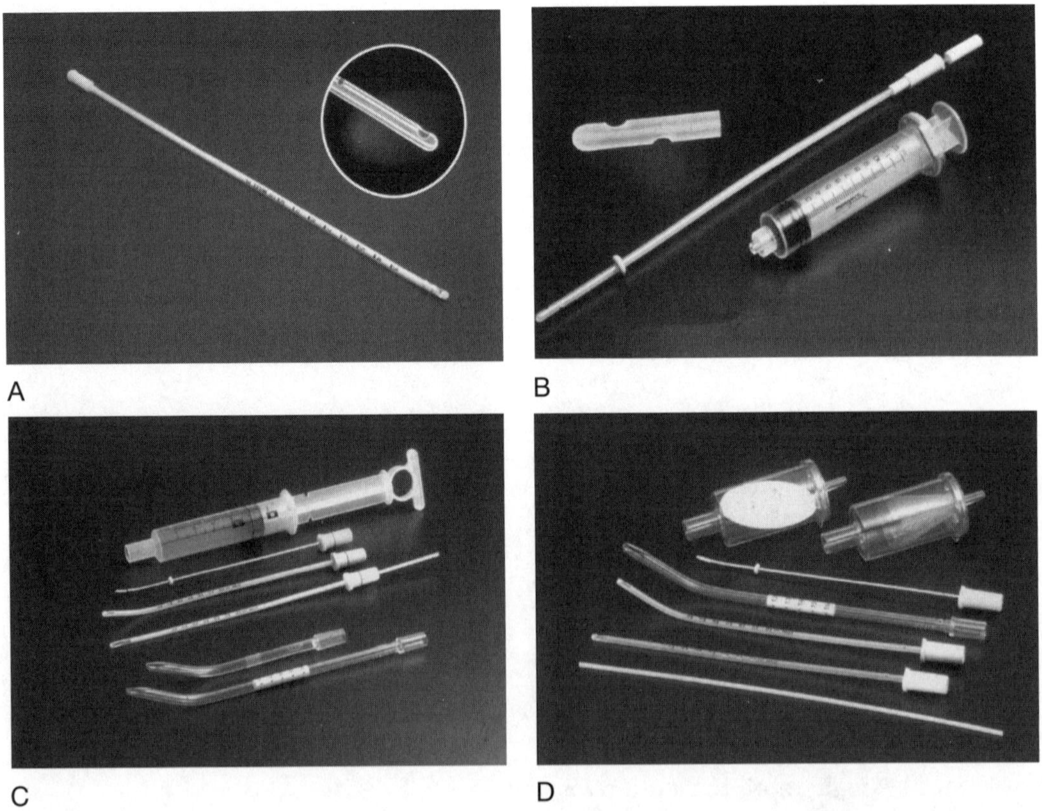

A B C D

FIGURE 16.1.
*Office endometrial sampling may be accomplished using one of several inexpensive and disposable devices. These devices include simple cannulas incorporating a piston to provide suction (**A**), those that use a syringe (**B, C**), and larger cannula and tissue collections systems designed to be used with a larger suction source (**D**). (Courtesy of Milex Products, 5915 Northwest Highway, Chicago, IL 60631.)*

some discomfort, is associated with a small but not insignificant risk for perforation or infections, and carries the cost of not only the procedure but also histologic diagnosis.

Much of the technique for currently available office endometrial biopsy methods is similar: once the cervix has been visualized, it is disinfected with a topical antiseptic (e.g., Betadine). When the patient is parous, the endometrium may be sampled without stabilizing or dilating the cervix, both of which produce mild to moderate discomfort and therefore should be avoided when possible. The sampling device is gently introduced into the uterine cavity, and the depth is noted. For suction devices such as the Pipelle or Z-Sampler, the piston is withdrawn (producing a vacuum) and the curette itself is gradually withdrawn using a spiral or twisting motion (Fig. 16.2). The procedure is complete after adequate tissue samples are placed in fixative. If additional tissue is needed, the piston may be advanced to a point just short of expelling the already obtained sample, the device again advanced into the uterine cavity, and the procedure repeated.

Open curettes, such as the Novak, or rigid suction cannula (Fig. 16.3), should be gently inserted to the apex of the uterine cavity and then withdrawn in a straight line, using light pressure against the uterine wall. Tissue obtained may be removed from the opening of the curette using the point of a broken (but still sterile) wooden, cotton-tipped applicator.

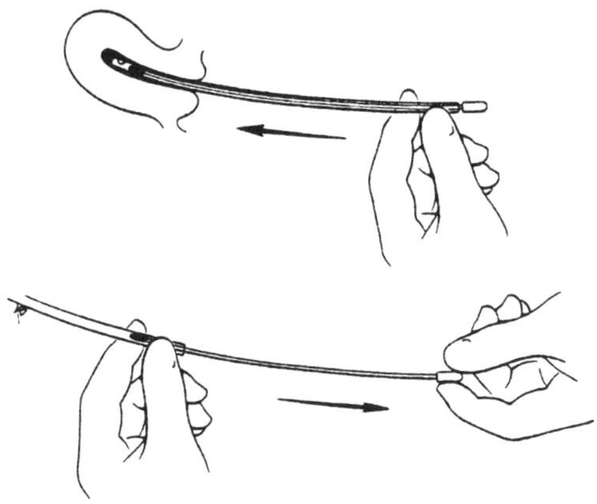

FIGURE 16.2.
Disposable suction-type sampling devices should be gently inserted into the uterus until the fundus is reached and the depth noted. The piston is then withdrawn, producing suction, and the device is withdrawn in a spiral motion. (Reproduced with permission from Beckmann RB, Ling FW, Barzansky BM, et al. Obstetrics and Gynecology. *2nd ed. Baltimore: Williams & Wilkins, 1995:26.)*

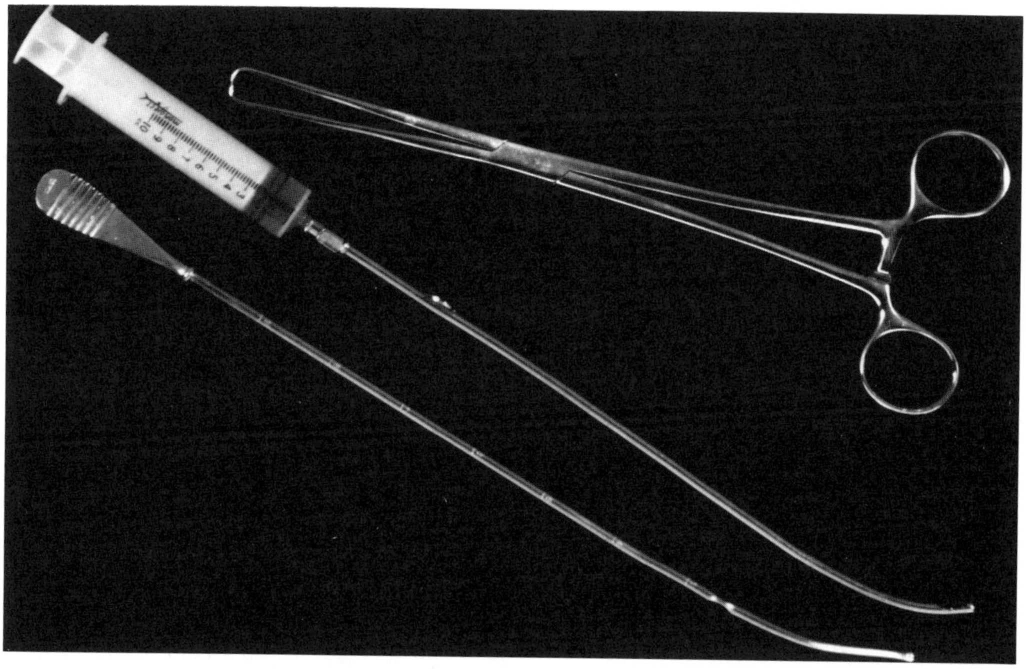

FIGURE 16.3.
Endometrial biopsy instruments. After the uterus is sounded, the thin hollow curette is inserted with the syringe during curettage. (Reproduced with permission from Jones HW, Wentz AC, Burnett LS. Novak's Textbook of Gynecology. *11th ed. Baltimore: Williams & Wilkins, 1988:746.)*

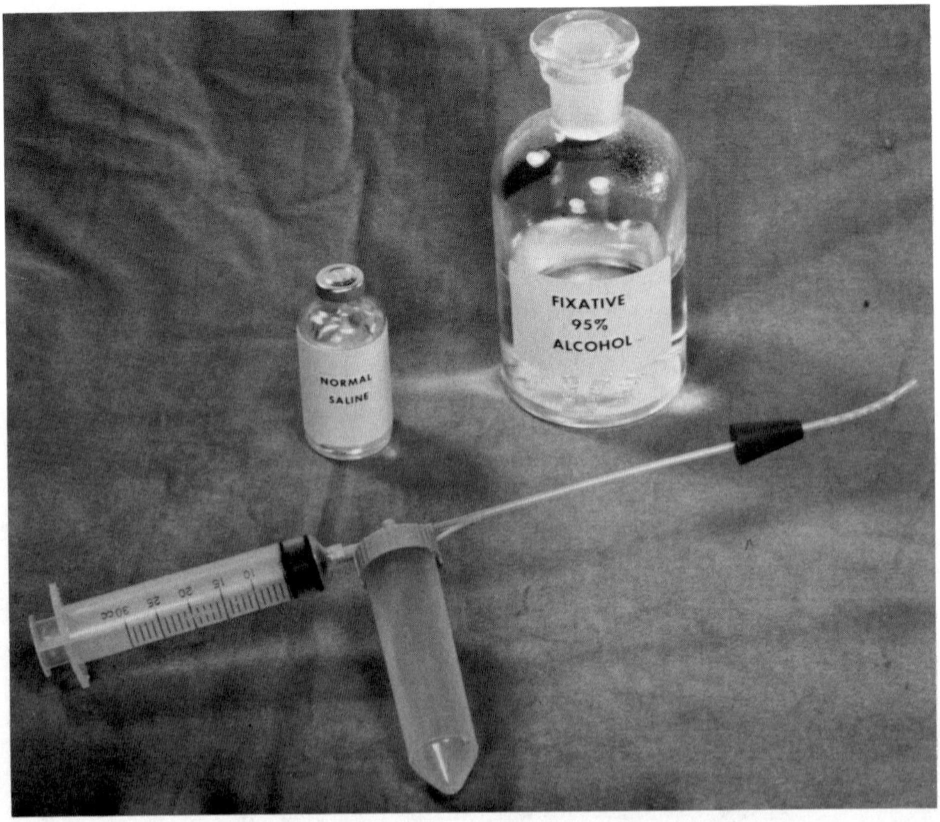

FIGURE 16.4.
Gravlee jet washer for endometrial sampling. Normal saline is lavaged through the uterine cavity through the double-bore cannula. (Reproduced with permission from Jones HW, Wentz AC, Burnett LA. Novak's Textbook of Gynecology. *11th ed. Baltimore: Williams & Wilkins, 1988:745.)*

Intrauterine cytologic specimens may be obtained in a similar manner using the Gravlee jet washer (Fig. 16.4).

Special Notes

If tissue already obtained is to be expelled before the procedure is attempted again, care must be taken to avoid contact with the fixative solution or bacterial contamination.

The discomfort of endometrial biopsy may be decreased by premedicating the patient with a single oral dose of a nonsteroidal anti-inflammatory agent given in doses usually used to treat dysmenorrhea.

Suggested Readings

Chambers JT, Chambers SK. Endometrial sampling: When? Where? Why? With what? *Clin Obstet Gynecol* 1992;35:28.

Ferry J, Farnsworth A, Webster M, et al. The efficacy of the Pipelle endometrial biopsy in detecting endometrial carcinoma. *Aust NZ J Obstet Gynaecol* 1993;33:76.

Goldchmit R, Katz Z, Blickstein I, et al. The accuracy of endometrial Pipelle sampling with and without sonographic measurement of endometrial thickness. *Obstet Gynecol* 1993;82:727.

Kaunitz AM, Masciello A, Ostrowski M, et al. Comparison of endometrial biopsy with the endometrial Pipelle and Vabra aspirator. *J Reprod Med* 1988;33:428.

Koonings PP, Moyer DL, Grimes DA. A randomized clinical trial comparing Pipelle and Tis-u-trap for endometrial biopsy. *Obstet Gynecol* 1990;75:293.

Larson DM, Broste SK. Histopathologic adequacy of office endometrial biopsies taken with the Z-sampler and Novak curette in premenopausal and postmenopausal women. *J Reprod Med* 1994;39:300.

Law J. Histological sampling of the endometrium—a comparison between formal curettage and the Pipelle sampler. *Br J Obstet Gynaecol* 1993;100:503.

Lipscomb GH, Lopatine SM, Stovall TG, et al. A randomized comparison of the Pipelle, Accurate, and Explora endometrial sampling devices. *Am J Obstet Gynecol* 1994;170:591.

Nolan TE, Smith RP, Smith MT, et al. A prospective evaluation of an endometrial suction curette. *J Gynecol Surg* 1992;8:231.

Reid PC, Brown VA, Fothergill DJ. Outpatient investigation of postmenopausal bleeding. *Br J Obstet Gynaecol* 1993;100:498.

Stovall TG, Ling FW, Morgan PL. Prospective, randomized comparison of the Pipelle endometrial sampling device with the Novak curette. *Am J Obstet Gynecol* 1991;165:1287.

Warwick A, Ferryman S, Musgrove C, et al. An evaluation of the gynocheck for endometrial sampling. *J Obstet Gynaecol* 1993;13:198.

Chapter 17

FINE-NEEDLE ASPIRATION OF THE BREAST

Fine-needle aspiration of cells from a breast mass can provide histologic confirmation of malignancy and help direct definitive therapy.

Equipment

- Skin preparation materials (alcohol, iodine- or hexachlorophene-based antibacterial solution; e.g., Betadine, Hibiclens)
- 10-mL disposable syringe
- 16- to 22-gauge needle
- Glass microscope slide and fixative (based on preference of local cytology laboratory)
- Self-adherent bandage (optional)

Training/Credentialing

No special credentialing needed; office procedure only.

Coding

88170	Fine-needle aspiration with or without preparation of smears; superficial tissue (e.g., thyroid, breast, prostate)
19100	Biopsy of breast; needle core (separate procedure)
19101	incisional

Technique

Although commercial devices are available, fine-needle aspiration may be performed using a 16- to 22-gauge needle mounted on a standard 10-mL syringe (Fig. 17.1). After skin preparation, the needle is inserted into the mass and negative pressure is applied by the syringe. Several (15 or more) short passes at varying angles are made through the

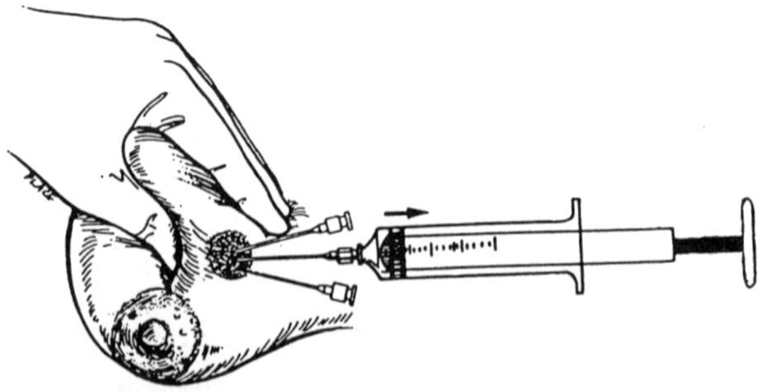

FIGURE 17.1.
Fine-needle aspiration (biopsy) using a standard 16- to 22-gauge needle and syringe. The needle is passed into the mass, suction is applied using the syringe, and multiple passes in various directions are made. Local anesthesia may be used at the discretion of the clinician. (Modified from Mitchell GW, Bassett LW. The Female Breast and Its Disorders. *Baltimore: Williams & Wilkins, 1990:186.)*

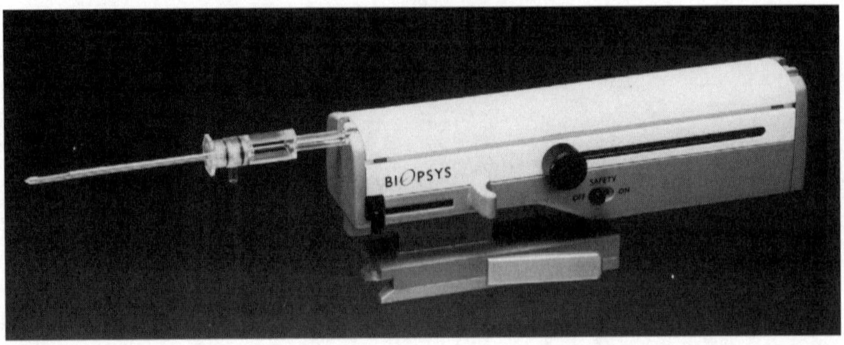

FIGURE 17.2.
Several self-contained systems are now available to obtain core biopsy specimens of breast masses. (Courtesy of Biopsys, 245 Willowsprings Drive, Encinitias, CA 92024.)

tissue to obtain cells or tissue. Negative pressure is maintained throughout these passes but is released before the needle is withdrawn from the skin. Once the needle is removed from the skin, the material collected is transferred onto a glass slide, smeared, and fixed. This sample is then examined histologically or cytologically for evidence of malignancy. Local anesthesia may be offered, but the pain of establishing the anesthesia is generally the same or worse than that associated with the procedure.

Several core biopsy instruments have recently been introduced that allow collection of histologic samples (Fig. 17.2). These instruments are similar to core biopsy needles used in other applications (e.g., percutaneous liver biopsy) but are self-contained. They include a vacuum source and collecting chamber that allow multiple samples to be obtained without removing the needle from the tissue (Fig. 17.3). Core biopsy instruments are usually best reserved for applications such as stereotactic-directed biopsy rather than blind sampling of breast masses in the office setting.

Special Notes

Fine-needle aspiration is 70–90% accurate but carries a 20% false–negative rate. Thus, if results of aspiration of a solid mass are negative, open biopsy is still required. Because of the possibility of hematoma formation or swelling after fine-needle aspiration, any desired mammography should be performed before the procedure or delayed for 4 to 6 weeks.

The smearing and fixing techniques used for fine-needle aspirates are often different

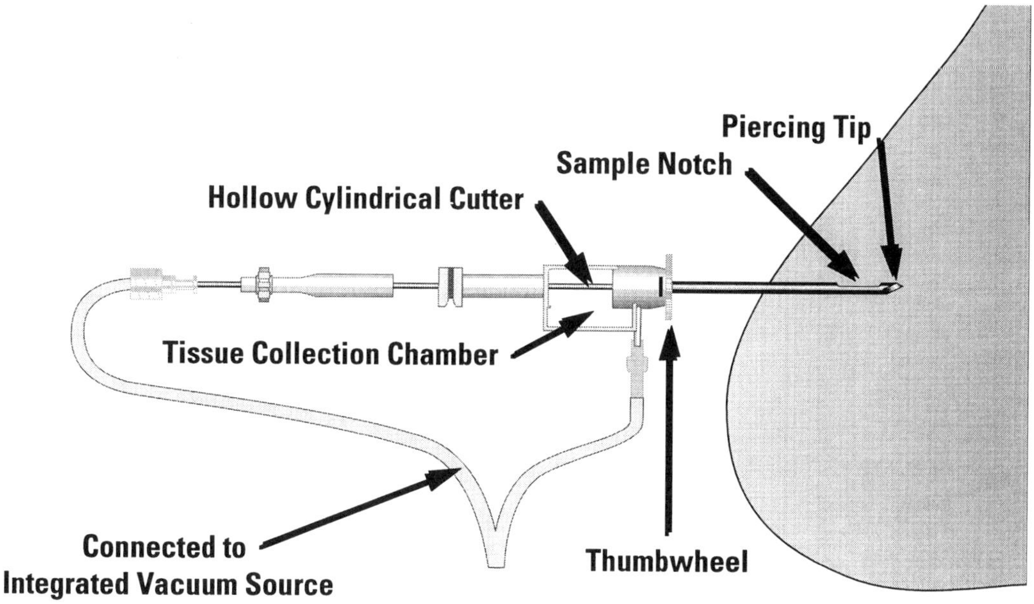

FIGURE 17.3.
Core biopsy needles have an open side into which tissue falls before being excised by a sharp cutter. In some self-contained systems, a tissue collection system and source of vacuum allow several samples to be obtained. (Courtesy of Biopsys, 245 Willowsprings Drive, Encinitias, CA 92024.)

than those used for a Papanicolaou smear and vary somewhat from laboratory to laboratory. Before this procedure is performed, it is best to determine the preferences of the persons who will be reviewing the material. In some cases, a technician may be sent to perform the smear, fix the sample, and transfer it to the laboratory.

Core biopsy (large-needle biopsy) or fluoroscopically directed stereotactic biopsy can yield larger histologic specimens with better preservation of the architecture of the tissue sampled. Many physicians believe, however, that if that degree of investigation is warranted, an excisional biopsy is more appropriate. Local custom and the preferences of the individual consultants are probably the best guide to the role of this procedure in the absence of conclusive studies.

Suggested Readings

Atamdede FI, Isaacs JH. The role of fine-needle aspiration in the diagnosis of breast lesions. *Gynecol Oncol* 1993;50:159.

Bates AT, Bates T, Hastrich DJ, et al. Delay in the diagnosis of breast cancer: the effect of the introduction of fine needle aspiration cytology to a breast clinic. *Eur J Surg Oncol* 1992;18:433.

Bauer TL, Pandelidis SM, Rhoads JE Jr. Five-year survival of 100 women with carcinoma of the breast diagnosed by screening mammography and needle-localization biopsy. *J Am Coll Surg* 1994;178:427.

Casey TT, Rodgers WH, Baxter JW, et al. Stratified diagnostic approach to fine needle aspiration of the breast. *Am J Surg* 1992;163:305.

Gordon PB, Goldenberg SL, Chan NH. Solid breast lesions: diagnosis with US-guided fine-needle aspiration biopsy. *Radiology* 1993;189:573.

Hindle WH, Hale RW. Breast evaluation and diagnosis by obstetrician-gynecologists. Survey of practice patterns. *J Reprod Med* 1992;37:857.

Marchant DJ. Diagnosis of breast disease and the role of the gynecologist. *Curr Opin Obstet Gynecol* 1993;5:67.

Mikhail RA, Nathan RC, Weiss M, et al. Stereotactic core needle biopsy of mammographic breast lesions as a viable alternative to surgical biopsy. *Ann Surg Oncol* 1994;1:363.

Nyirjesy I, Billingsley FS. Management of breast problems in gynecologic office practice using sonography and fine-needle aspiration. *Obstet Gynecol* 1992;79:699.

Phillips G, McGuire L, Clowes D. The value of ultrasound-guided fine needle aspiration in the assessment of solid breast lumps. *Aust Radiol* 1994;38:187.

Shaw de Paredes E. Evaluation of abnormal screening mammograms. *Cancer* 1994;74:342.

Teixidor HS, Wojtasek DA, Reiches EM, et al. Fine-needle aspiration of breast biopsy specimens: correlation of histologic and cytologic findings. *Radiology* 1992;184:55.

Vega A, Garijo F, Ortega E. Core needle aspiration biopsy of palpable breast masses. *Acta Oncol* 1995;34:31.

Chapter 18

HYSTEROSCOPY

Diagnostic, panoramic hysteroscopy can be performed in an office setting with minimal discomfort to the patient. As an office procedure, it is one of the most valuable ways to detect intrauterine lesions; it enables physicians to search for organic intrauterine abnormalities and select appropriate therapy on the basis of these observations. Even when no pathologic abnormality is seen, the patient may be reassured and further surgical interventions can be avoided.

The hysteroscope is a versatile instrument that can have significant benefit for both diagnosis and therapy. With appropriate patient selection, recognition of limitations in experience and skills, and adequate instrumentation and support staff, complications can be minimized. As experience with the instrument and its applications increases, indications for its use may change. It is unlikely, however, that the hysteroscope will completely replace other procedures. In the future, some investigational procedures may find applications in practice. In the meantime, office hysteroscopy is an important adjunct to other diagnostic methods.

Equipment

- Hysteroscope (flexible or rigid, 3–5-mm diameter, 0°, 12°, 30°, or 70° viewing angle)
- Insufflator (carbon dioxide, constant flow type) and light source (both compatible with the brand and type of hysteroscope chosen; other distending media may be used, but CO_2 offers the most suitable media for office use)

or

- Contact hysteroscope substituted for the above (this requires less equipment but provides a more restricted view, does not allow endoscopy, and requires more experience)
- Operating vaginal speculum (open-sided)
- Antiseptic solution (e.g., povidone–iodine solution)
- Tenaculum
- Uterine sound (optional)
- Sterile gloves

- Lidocaine (1%) without epinephrine, syringe, and 22- to 25-gauge spinal (4-inch) needle (optional)
- Video or photographic equipment attached to the hysteroscope as desired (optional)

Training/Credentialing

No special credentialing is needed if performed as office procedure only. Instruction and preceptorship are desirable in all cases and may be required for credentialing if the procedure is performed in an ambulatory surgery center or hospital operating room. Opportunities for such instruction are often available through free-standing courses or through the sponsorship of equipment manufacturers.

Coding

56350	Hysteroscopy, diagnostic (separate procedure)
56351	Hysteroscopy, surgical: with sampling (biopsy) of endometrium and/or polypectomy; with or without D & C
56355	Hysteroscopy, surgical: with removal of impacted foreign body

Technique

Contraindications to hysteroscopy are shown in Table 18.1. Because of the nature and risks of hysteroscopy, informed consent should be obtained before the procedure is begun.

The patient should be placed in the dorsal lithotomy position and made as comfortable as possible. A pelvic examination should be performed to determine the size, shape, and position of the uterus. This examination should be done even if the patient has recently been examined. The operating vaginal speculum should be placed to allow clear access to the cervix.

With the cervix in view, sterile gloves are donned and the cervix is disinfected with an appropriate antiseptic solution. If an anesthetic is to be used, a pudendal or cervical block may be placed at this time. Many patients can tolerate gentle hysteroscopy without such an anesthetic; the decision is made by the patient and practitioner.

A tenaculum may not be needed if the patient is parous and the cervical os is open, although it is generally recommended. If a tenaculum is placed, it should be attached in a transverse plane on the anterior lip of the cervix. Placing the tenaculum in this plane keeps the handles of the instrument out of the way of the hysteroscope as it is

Table 18.1. Contraindications to Office Hysteroscopy

Acute bleeding (if CO_2 is used)
Known or suspected acute pelvic infection
Known uterine or cervical cancer
Known or suspected pregnancy
Recent uterine perforation
Uncooperative patient
Vaginitis (relative)

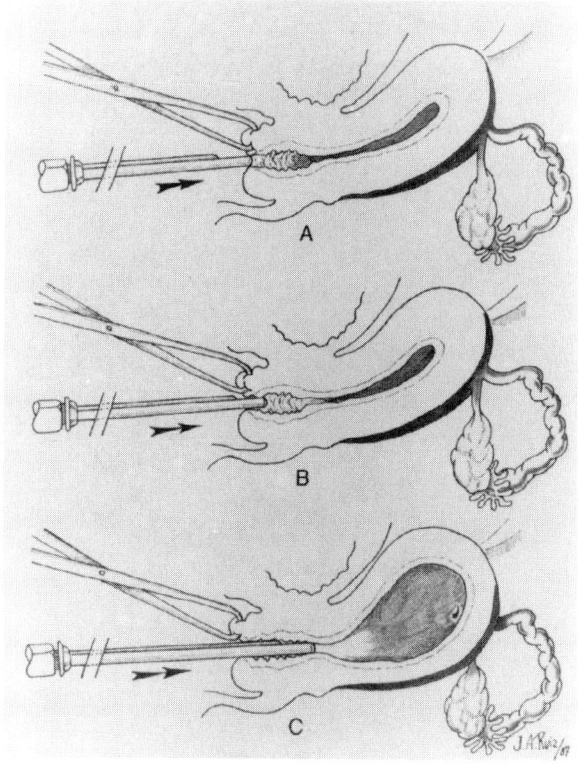

FIGURE 18.1.
*Hysteroscopy with diagnostic endoscopes (<4 mm optical density). Examination begins at external cervical os without previous cervical dilatation (**A**). The endoscope is advanced under direct vision (**B**), and after the endoscope crosses the internal cervical os, the uterine cavity is systematically examined (**C**). (Reproduced with permission from Baggish MS, Barbot J, Valle RF.* Diagnostic and Operative Hysteroscopy: A Text and Atlas. *St. Louis: Mosby-Year Book, 1989:98.)*

maneuvered to visualize the entire uterine cavity. If an anesthetic has not been used, the discomfort of the tenaculum placement may be minimized by raising an anesthetic weal or by asking the patient to cough at the moment the tenaculum is placed. A uterine sound may be used to gently dilate the cervix or provide information about the axis and depth of the uterine cavity, if needed.

The hysteroscope selected should provide the best view with the least discomfort. In general, nulliparous patients and those with a narrow cervix or small uterus are best served by the smallest hysteroscope. Patients with a large or patulous os, those with a large cavity, or those with distortion caused by fibroids or polyps may require a larger instrument. Hysteroscopes with a diameter of 5 to 10 mm are required for surgical procedures but are best suited to the ambulatory surgery setting rather than office hysteroscopy. Flexible hysteroscopes are more expensive but provide the ability to maneuver around significant distortions in the uterine cavity or follow the curvature of a flexed uterus.

With the hysteroscope appropriately connected to the insufflator and light source, the tip of the hysteroscope is brought in contact with the external cervical os and insufflation is begun. A rate of 30 mL per minute is generally appropriate. The hysteroscope may then be advanced along the endocervical canal under direct vision (Fig. 18.1). Advancement should only be done when a clear view ahead is available and resistance to advancement is minimal. When the body of the uterus is entered, carbon dioxide flow rates may have to be increased to 40 or 50 mL per minute to provide adequate distension of the cavity. Intrauterine pressure should never be allowed to exceed 100 torr (mm Hg).

The entire uterine cavity should be systematically inspected. The front, back, and lateral walls of the endometrial cavity in the body of the uterus are inspected in order, often in a circular manner. The tubal ostia should be identified and the fundus of the uterus inspected. If the endocervical canal was not evaluated at the beginning of the procedure, it should be inspected as the hysteroscope is withdrawn.

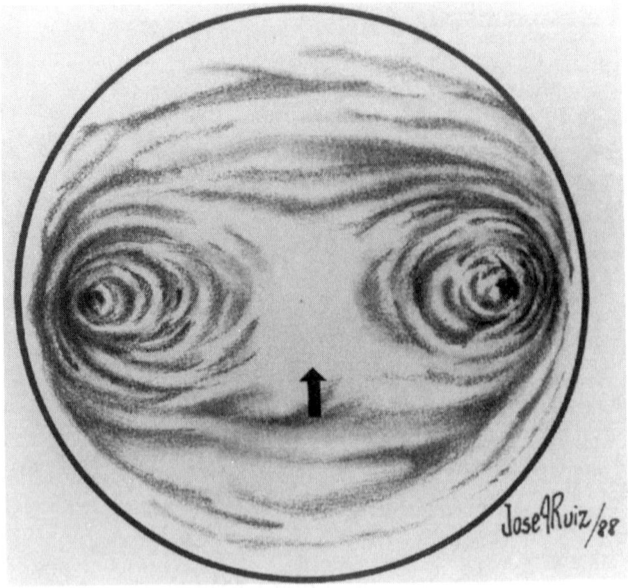

FIGURE 18.2.
When the fundus of the uterine cavity is approached, one or both tubal ostia may be visible; a slightly blanched segment of endometrium connects them and crosses the fundus. This lighter area is sometimes mistaken for a small septum or indentation. (Reproduced with permission from Baggish MS, Barbot J, Valle RF. Diagnostic and Operative Hysteroscopy: A Text and Atlas. *St. Louis: Mosby-Year Book, 1989:20.)*

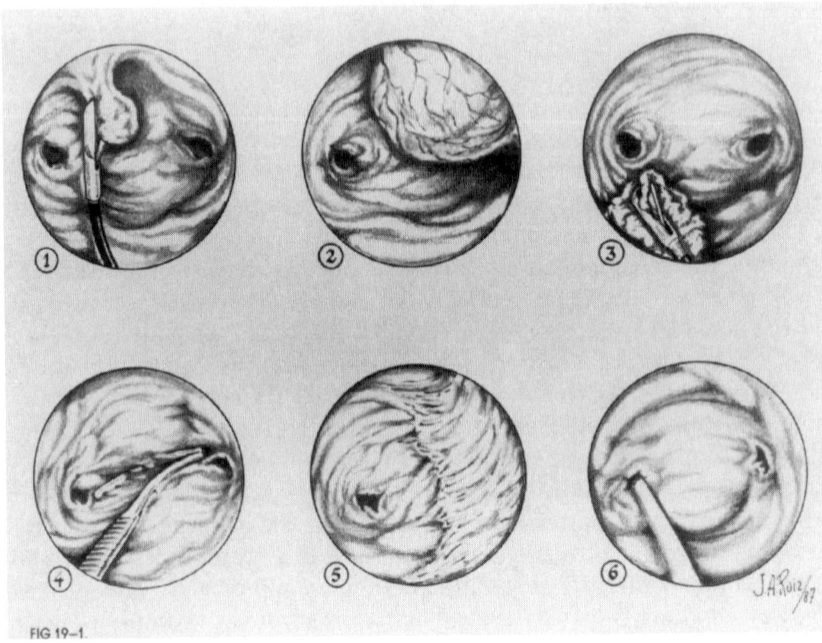

FIGURE 18.3.
A range of common hysteroscopic findings are shown: ***1,*** *pedunculated endometrial polyp (the narrow pedicle is being transected);* ***2,*** *sessile submucous leiomyoma;* ***3,*** *hysteroscopic biopsy of focal endometrial lesion;* ***4,*** *misplaced, partially embedded intrauterine contraceptive device;* ***5,*** *partial occlusion of the uterine cavity by a thick adhesion (only right tubal opening is seen); and* ***6,*** *tubal cannulation. (Reproduced with permission from Baggish MS, Barbot J, Valle RF.* Diagnostic and Operative Hysteroscopy: A Text and Atlas. *St. Louis: Mosby-Year Book, 1989:158.)*

Once the uterine cavity has been completely inspected and any biopsies or other surgical procedures have been accomplished, the hysteroscope, tenaculum (if used), and speculum should be removed. The patient may be allowed to sit upright, although the possibility of syncope should be considered. Unilateral or bilateral shoulder pain is common if CO_2 is used.

The hysteroscope should be cleansed according to the manufacturer's recommendations and should then be stored. A notation, written or dictated, should be placed in the patient's record documenting the procedure and findings.

Normal Findings

The healthy endometrium should appear pink, with a fine network of capillaries visible below the surface. The surface may range from smooth to somewhat lush in appearance as the menstrual cycle progresses. The endometrium will bleed easily if touched or traumatized, and a groove may be seen where the hysteroscopy has rested. The view within the uterine cavity should suggest a cave, with the lining receding into darkness until the fundus is approached. The tubal ostia with a slightly blanched, smooth fundus may be seen (Fig. 18.2).

Because of the magnification inherent in the optics of hysteroscopy, objects appear much larger that they really are. As a result, small areas of lush endometrium may appear to be heaped up or polypoid. True polypoid growths have a narrow base and are restricted to one or a few select areas of the uterine cavity.

Selected Abnormal Findings

Many abnormalities may be encountered, documented, and, in some cases, treated through hysteroscopy (Fig. 18.3). In general, any asymmetric thickening, change in color, or contour of the endometrium should suggest an abnormality that warrants further evaluation. A full discussion of the range of possible findings is beyond the scope of this book. Excellent discussions of such findings, along with photographic atlases, are identified in the suggested reading list.

Special Notes

Hysteroscopy is most easily performed during the early follicular phase when the endometrium is thinnest.

The discomfort of hysteroscopy may be minimized by premedicating the patient with a nonsteroidal anti-inflammatory agent 30–60 minutes before the procedure is begun.

The hysteroscope may be used to perform vaginoscopy in young girls or infants. When used in this way, distending media is generally not required or indicated.

Infection rarely develops after hysteroscopy, and prophylactic antibiotics are not recommended unless indicated by such factors as valvular heart disease.

Suggested Readings

American College of Obstetricians and Gynecologists. *Hysteroscopy.* ACOG technical bulletin 191. Washington, DC: ACOG; 1994.

Apgar BS, DeWitt D. Diagnostic hysteroscopy. *Am Fam Phys* 1992;46(5 Suppl):19S.

Baggish MS, Barbot J, Valle RF. *Diagnostic and Operative Hysteroscopy: A Text and Atlas.* St. Louis: Mosby-Year Book, 1989.

Gambone JC, Munro MG. Office sonography and office hysteroscopy. *Curr Opin Obstet Gynecol* 1993;5:733.

Gimpelson RJ. Office hysteroscopy. *Clin Obstet Gynecol* 1992;35:270.

Gimpelson RJ, Rappold HO. A comparative study between panoramic hysteroscopy with directed biopsies and dilatation and curettage. *Am J Obstet Gynecol* 1988;158:489.

Lindemann HJ. The future of hysteroscopy. *Obstet Gynecol Clin North Am* 1995;22:617.

Lindemann HJ. The use of CO_2 in the uterine cavity for hysteroscopy. *Int J Fertil* 1972;17:221.

March CM. Hysteroscopy. *J Reprod Med* 1992;37:293.

Mencaglia L, Perino A, Hamou J. Hysteroscopy in premenopausal and postmenopausal women with abnormal uterine bleeding. *J Reprod Med* 1987;32:577.

Shapiro BS. Instrumentation in hysteroscopy. *Obstet Gynecol Clin North Am* 1988;15:13.

Siegler AM. Office hysteroscopy. *Obstet Gynecol Clin North Am* 1995;22:457.

Siegler AM, Kemmann E. Hysteroscopy. *Obstet Gynecol Surv* 1975;30:567.

Siegler AM, Valle RF. Therapeutic hysteroscopic procedures. *Fertil Steril* 1988;50:685.

Taylor PJ. Hysteroscopy: where have we been, where are we going? *J Reprod Med* 1993;38:757.

Wheeler JM, DeCherney AH. Office hysteroscopy. *Obstet Gynecol Clin North Am* 1988;15:29.

Chapter 19

LASER ABLATION

Lasers deliver an intense, but very localized, transfer of energy to tissue. Lasers are used in many gynecologic procedures for cutting and coagulation. Photodynamic therapy is used clinically for malignant conditions and dysplastic lesions of the lower genital tract and may be used for endometrial ablation. Improvements in control and delivery systems have increased user friendliness and have reduced costs so that office or ambulatory surgery settings may be able to justify the expense of this equipment. Laser surgical systems carry unique risks along with their capabilities. For this reason, familiarity with their special properties is imperative if these tools are to be correctly chosen and used.

Equipment

- Office laser unit (generally a CO_2 laser)
- Dedicated smoke evacuation unit with virus particle filter
- Protective goggles for patient, provider, and others in the room
- Colposcope (preferably with attachment to allow the laser to be directed through the colposcope [Fig. 19.1])
- Colposcopy supplies (acetic acid, gauze pads or cotton balls, etc.; see Chapter 9, Colposcopy)
- Wet towels (water or saline)
- Wooden tongue depressor
- Nonreflective speculum (for intravaginal and cervical applications)
- When the laser is used on the cervix or upper vagina, a laser speculum with integrated smoke evacuation is desirable
- Micro ruler (for cervical ablations)
- Nonreflective retractors, probes, or cervical specula as required
- Local anesthetic (if desired) based on location and planned procedure

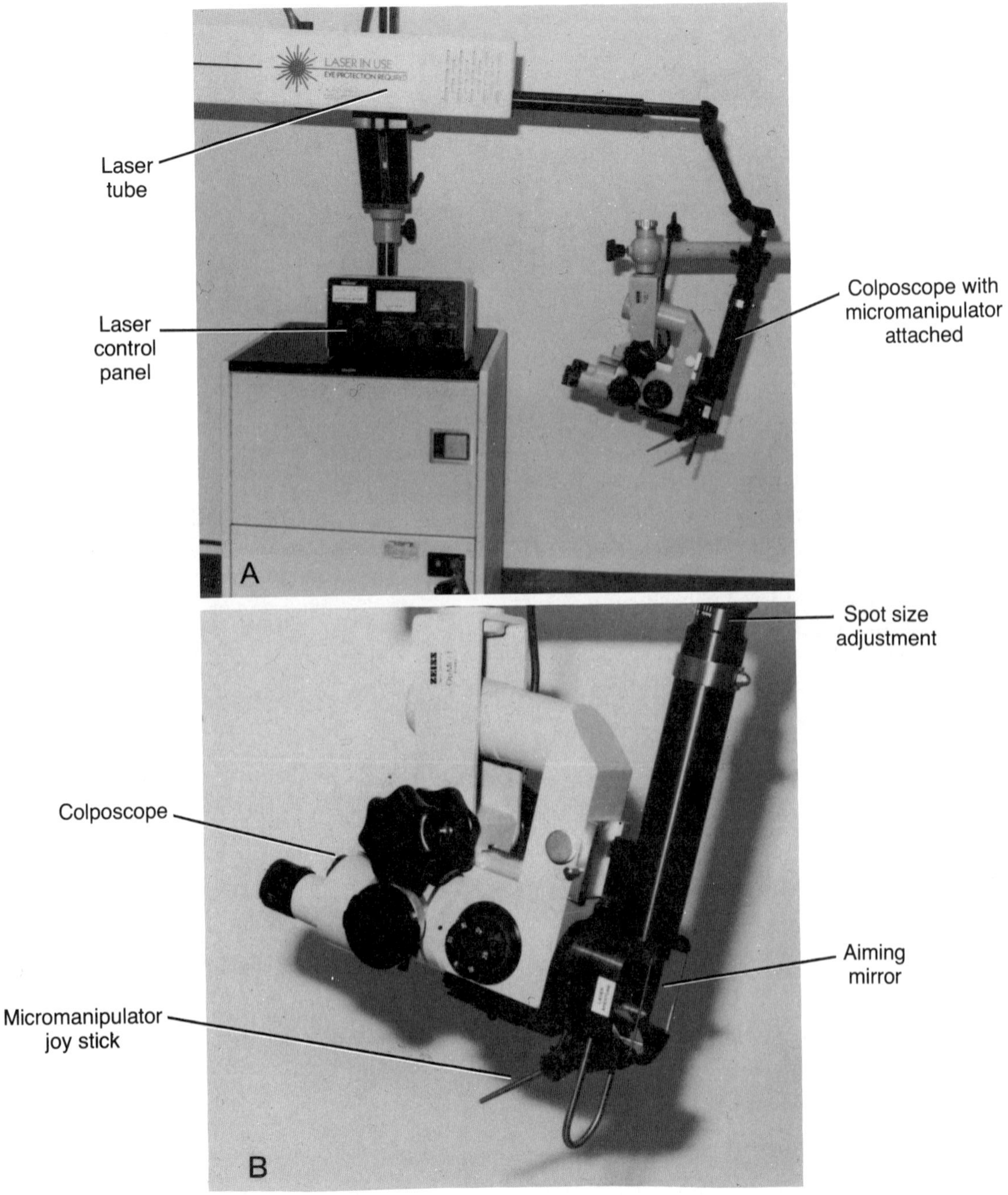

FIGURE 19.1.
***A.** Carbon dioxide laser attached to the colposcope for cervical therapy.* ***B.** The micromanipular attachment is shown in detail. (Reproduced with permission from Jones HW, Wentz AC, Burnett LS.* Novak's Textbook of Gynecology. *11th ed. Baltimore: Williams & Wilkins, 1988:669.)*

Training/Credentialing

Most hospitals and ambulatory surgery units have specific credentialing procedures. These generally include evidence of course or didactic work on the physics of lasers and the interaction of light and tissues. Evidence of proctored experience is also required. When performed in the office setting, these minimum training requirement are not required but should be strongly considered.

Coding

56501	Destruction of lesion(s), vulva; simple, any method
56515	extensive, any method
57061	Destruction of vaginal lesion(s); simple, any method
57065	extensive, any method
57513	Cauterization of cervix, laser ablation
57520	Conization of cervix, with or without fulguration, with or without dilation and curettage, with or without repair; cold knife or laser

Technique

The main lasers used in gynecology are CO_2, neodymium-yttrium aluminum garnet (Nd:YAG), and potassium tatanyl-phosphate-doubled Nd:YAG. Pulsed Ho:YAG laser looks promising, as do diode lasers. Holmium-yttrium aluminum garnet and diode lasers will be soon available commercially. Because of cost and other considerations, the CO_2 type is the most commonly used in the office setting and is the only type considered here.

PHYSICS AND SAFETY ISSUES

Lasers as Energy Sources

Although it is outside the scope of this book to extensively discuss the physics of medical lasers, it is critical that the user of these devices be familiar with the aspects of laser operation that bear directly on technique and safe application of this method. The main strengths of medical lasers (the ability to deliver intense energy at a distance) are the very aspects that raise the possibility of risk.

Laser light differs from ordinary light in a few ways: it is monochromatic (one wave length) and coherent (all of the light is in phase and tightly collimated). Laser light is generally equated with high intensity, but this is neither unique to light generated by lasers nor an automatic attribute. When the light emitted from a laser is tightly focused, it can produce local energy levels that exceed 20,000 W/cm^2. This power density may be generated by lasers whose energy consumption is similar to that of a refrigerator light bulb. This is accomplished not by brute force but by the effects of tight focus and the consistency of the coherent beam.

The effects that laser light will have on tissue are a function of the light and the tissue itself (Table 19.1). Characteristics of the light affect the amount of energy that is contained in the beam and thus is potentially available to perform work. Characteristics of the tissue determine the degree to which this energy may be absorbed, dissipated, or scattered. For example, the transfer of energy may be altered by changing either part of this equation; light intensity may be increased, the duration of exposure may be changed, or the tissue may be made more receptive. Un-

Table 19.1. Factors Affecting Light–Tissue Interactions

Properties of the light
Duration of exposure
Power density (W/cm^2)
Wavelength
Properties of the tissue
Absorption coefficient
Density
Scatter
Thermal conductivity

derstanding this interaction is vital to choosing an appropriate device and technique for the task at hand.

In general, when the task calls for coagulation of tissue or hemostasis, energy must be delivered at a lower level over a relatively longer period. For this purpose, intensity levels are reduced, and spot size (related to focus) is increased to yield a lower power density (W/cm^2). When cutting is required, energy transfer must be greater and more rapid, which leads to the formation of steam in tissues and results in their disruption. Here, high-power densities are achieved with greater beam intensity and a narrow, well-focused spot. In gynecologic applications, vaporization power densities vary from 350 W/cm^2 for the fleshy, poorly vascularized tissue of condyloma of the vulva or vagina to 2500 W/cm^2 for the dense vascular tissue of the cervix.

Safety Issues

When light is used to transfer energy to tissues, it does so at a distance from the device (e.g., hand piece, laparoscope, colposcope). This has some advantages but also results in a disconnection between apparent cause and effect. Unless the density of the laser beam decreases dramatically (which it generally does not), the light energy it contains can cause damage even after traveling a considerable distance or being reflected several times. For this reason, great care must be taken that the effects of laser light are limited to only those places intended. Nonreflective surfaces should be used where possible, "back stops" to absorb light transmitted beyond the tissue of interest must be used, and protective eye wear must be used by all persons in the area (including the patient). When the CO_2 laser is used (which emits light in the infrared wavelength), wet towels should be placed around the area to be treated to absorb and dissipate any stray light.

Because of the intensity of the energies used in laser ablation, steam is produced, molecules are disrupted, and combustion of materials (cellular or otherwise) is common. As a result, flammable materials should not be used in the presence of laser energy. Such materials include flammable anesthetic agents, skin preparation solutions, and paper or cloth drapes (unless wet with water).

The combustion of carbon-based molecules in tissue results in smoke and the liberation of particulate matter. In this vigorous process, material is ejected from the light-tissue interface at speed that exceeds the speed of sound. (This is why a buzzing sound is heard when laser vaporization is underway.) Because of the liberation of smoke and the possible aerosolization of intact cells or virus particles the issue of smoke evacuation and containment must be considered. Although no studies have documented transmission of such viruses as human papilloma virus or human immunodeficiency virus by this route, prudence dictates caution. A dedicated smoke evacuation system with virus particle filter should be used in every procedure.

Table 19.2. Approximate Power Densities Achieved on the Basis of Spot Size and Power Output

	POWER DENSITY, W/CM²			
	EFFECTIVE SPOT SIZE			
POWER, W	0.5 mm	1.0 mm	1.5 mm	2.0 mm
10	4000	1000	450	250
20	8000	2000	875	500
30	12,000	3000	1350	750
40	16,000	4000	1775	1000
50	20,000	5000	2250	1250

VAPORIZATION TECHNIQUES

Preparation

Patient preparation must include the usual preoperative discussions about the procedure planned, expected outcomes, possible complications, and accepted alternate therapies available. Informed consent should be obtained (see Chapter 2, Informed Consent). On the basis of the location and character of the lesion to be treated, the patient should be positioned to allow unimpeded access to the site. This position must be as comfortable as possible to ensure a minimum of patient movement during what may be a prolonged procedure.

The laser system must be activated and tested before use. Although systems vary, all systems require that the light output level be set and that the beam be focused. The final spot density, which determines the energy delivered to the tissue, is a function of both output and focus, as shown in Table 19.2. Focusing of the beam and active testing of the system may be assisted using a wooden tongue depressor. To do this, the laser is aimed (using the red aiming beam) at the middle portion of one end of the tongue depressor and the laser is fired briefly. A point of char appears on the wood. The size of this char and the speed with which it appears indicate the degree of focus and magnitude of power being delivered.

The operating mode of the laser system must be selected. Most currently available machines have three modes: continuous mode, in which the output of the laser lasts as long as the system is activated by the control switch; pulsed mode, in which the laser light is emitted for a predetermined duration and then ceases even if the control switch remains activated; and repeat pulse mode, in which a series of short pulses is emitted for as long as the control switch is pressed. The continuous mode is well suited to the destruction of wide areas of tissue. The pulse mode controls the energy into small aliquots that are shorter than the operator could produce manually. The repeat pulse mode is a hybrid in which pulses are emitted in rapid succession and that allows the control of the pulse mode with the speed of treatment offered by the continuous mode. Regardless of the mode chosen, the foot switch that activates the system must be placed for easy but secure use.

The final step in preparation is exposure of the operative site. On the basis of the site of proposed laser therapy, this may be as simple as uncovering the perineum or as complex as ensuring a complete view of the cervix using a nonreflective speculum. In all cases, the view of the operative site must be unimpeded and all adjacent areas protected with the use of towels wet with water or saline. Any instruments to be used near the site of laser treatment must be nonreflective. Finally, the smoke evacuation system must be in place and working.

Specific Applications

Vulva and Vagina. Vulvar or vaginal lesions, such as intraepithelial neoplasia or condyloma, lend themselves well to laser-based therapy. Laser ablation of vulvar lesions requires anesthesia. If extensive areas are to be ablated, general anesthesia is appropriate. Local anesthesia is acceptable for smaller lesions, but the administration of the anesthetic, typically xylocaine (1%, as much as 20 mL) is uncomfortable and causes a distinct burning sensation.

A slightly defocused beam may be used to deliver superficial coagulation of tissue over a wide area, whereas a narrow, high-intensity beam may be used to vaporize and remove warts. Because of the nature of the vulvar and vaginal tissues, lower output levels and spot densities may be used for many applications. When vaporization is indicated, it should be performed only to a depth of 3 mm. Begin ablation at the lowest area of the surgical field and work toward the top. Vaporize using small circular motions of the wrist. As char forms, wipe it away from the treated tissue with a gauze or cotton swab soaked with acetic acid solution.

Postoperative management for patients with vulvar lesions include sitz baths four times a day using a sea water solution; blow drying of the perineum with a hair dryer at low setting; cleansing of the perineum with diluted betadine solution, 1:4 strength; and analgesia administered for approximately 5–7 days when nerve endings regenerate. The area should heal in 4–6 weeks.

Cervical Applications. Because the goal of most laser ablation treatments of the cervix is to destroy or resect tissue, either for a local lesion or as a conization, cervical laser treatment customarily requires a higher spot density. When moderately large areas are to be treated, many physicians prefer to outline the area with a series of spot lesions placed at the boundaries of treatment. Outlining the lesion beforehand reduces the problem of distorted anatomy, which sometimes occurs once laser vaporization begins. This is most easily accomplished by setting the laser system to an intermittent or time-limited pulse. These settings allow the light to be delivered in a predetermined (short) duration that is well suited to making small dot-like lesions. Once the area to be treated has been outlined with this method, the laser may be reset to the continuous mode.

Mentally visualize the cervix divided into four quadrants, with vaporization to be completed in one quadrant before moving on to the next. Vaporization should start in one of the lower quadrants by moving the joy stick in vertical, horizontal, and diagonal directions within the quadrant to be vaporized. Rapid movement of the beam minimizes a build-up of heat in the tissue, resulting in less uterine cramping and a shorter operative time. In addition, the heat conduction to surrounding tissue is reduced, thereby reducing scarring. Beginning in a lower quadrant also prevents blood from running down into the operative field. Should uterine cramping occur, direct the laser to a different quadrant of the cervix and continue vaporization in that area as outlined above. Alternatively, the procedure can be temporarily halted to allow the heat to dissipate.

Vaporize the cervical lesion as well as the entire transformation zone to a depth of at least 6 mm to ensure thorough treatment of the lesion, including any that extends into a cervical crypt. Extend the depth of treatment higher in the central area than in the periphery. This is necessary because of the anatomy of the cervix . Using a micro ruler, measure the depth of ablation both along the lateral walls and in the central area of treatment. Depths of 6–8 mm along the lateral margins and 8–12 mm in the central region of treatment are appropriate.

After the procedure, the patient should be instructed to follow the precautions used in other forms of conization: take a mild analgesic as necessary; refrain from douching, using tampons, and sexual intercourse for approximately 3 weeks; and call if any significant bleeding greater than spotting occurs. The need for close surveillance for follow-up of abnormal Papanicolaou smears must also be stressed.

Special Notes

The output of a CO_2 laser is in the invisible infrared range. The red spot seen when using these devices is the result of a separate helium-neon laser (like the laser pointer used in lectures) that is provided solely for the purpose of aiming the device. Without this aiming beam, the interaction between site and laser will be unknown and uncontrolled. It is also true that the actual beam that produces the desired results is not the light that we can perceive, making impossible any independent assessment of risk from direct, reflected, or other casual exposure.

For the most part, the energy chosen for a given application should be the highest that may be safely handled and applied for the shortest time possible. This results in the least amount of collateral tissue damage and must be balanced against the potentially greater depth of penetration caused by even brief exposure.

Bleeding that is encountered during laser ablation may be stopped by defocusing the laser beam (increasing spot size and thereby reducing spot intensity) and applying this beam to the bleeding site. Some authors recommend injecting pitressin, 1.5% solution, into the cervical stroma either before or after surgery. This is used to reduce the size of the vessel lumens to produce improved hemostasis. Hemostatic sutures may be necessary. Delayed bleeding may be handled by packing (vaginal or cervical cases) or by applying hemostatic agents (see Chapter 4, Hemostasis).

Suggested Readings

Baggish M. A comparison between laser excisional conization and laser vaporization for the treatment of cervical intraepithelial neoplasia. *Am J Obstet Gynecol* 1986;155:39.

Baggish M. High-power-density, carbon dioxide laser therapy for early cervical neoplasia. *Am J Obstet Gynecol* 1980;136:117.

Bhatta N, Isaacson K, Bhatta KM, et al. Comparative study of different laser systems. *Fert Steril* 1994;61:581.

Ferenczy A, Bergeron C, Richart RM. Human papillomavirus DNA in the laser-generated plume of smoke and its consequences to the surgeon. *Obstet Gynecol* 1990;75:114.

Gibson KF, Kernohan WG. Lasers in medicine—a review. *J Med Engr Technol* 1993;17:51.

Helkjaer PE, Schultz H, Eriksen PS, et al. Thermal artifacts and inter-gynecologist variation of laser cone biopsies of the cervix. *Obstet Gynecol* 1993;82:435.

Luesley D. Misuse of lasers in gynaecology. *Br J Obstet Gynaecol* 1994;101:847.

Partington CK, Turner MJ, Soutter WP, et al. Laser vaporization versus laser excision conization in the treatment of cervical intraepithelial neoplasm. *Obstet Gynecol* 1989;73:775.

Riva JM, Sedlacek TV, Cunnane MF, et al. Extended carbon dioxide laser vaporization in the treatment of subclinical papillomavirus infection of the lower genital tract. *Obstet Gynecol* 1989;73:25.

Stafl A, Wilkinson EJ, Mattingly RF. Laser treatment of cervical and vaginal neoplasia. *Am J Obstet Gynecol* 1977;128:128.

Chapter 20

LEEP AND LLETZ CONIZATIONS

The availability of inexpensive electrosurgical units and a growing body of experience with their use in conization has moved the procedure from the hospital operating room to the office or ambulatory care setting. For selected patients, these procedures may provide diagnosis or therapy in a more convenient, less expensive, and less threatening environment. Despite the growing perception that these procedures are "routine," they are still surgical procedures and as such require care and attention to technique to ensure safety and an appropriate outcome.

Equipment

- Electrosurgical generator that includes the following features: output capability of at least 50 watts in both coagulation and cutting modes; variety of wave form outputs (pure cut, blended current, and coagulation current); patient grounding pad monitor; and isolated circuitry
- Loop electrodes (various sizes, reusable or disposable types)
- Ball electrode for fulguration
- Patient return electrode
- Speculum (either plastic or metal coated with a nonconductive material), with adapter for use with a smoke evacuator
- Smoke evacuator with odor and viral filter
- Colposcope
- 3–5% acetic acid (white vinegar) or Lugol's (5%) solution
- Gauze pads or cotton balls
- Ring forceps
- Monsel's paste (ferric subsulfate solution evaporated to the consistency of paste)
- Kevorkian endocervical curette or similar curette
- Histology fixative (10% formalin) in containers

- Syringe with 25- or 27-gauge, 1½-inch needle for anesthetic injection
- Lidocaine, 1 or 2% with or without epinephrine, 1:100,000
- 12-inch needle holder
- 2-0 suture material (or similar)
- Vaginal pack (optional)
- Vaginal sidewall retractor (optional)

Training/Credentialing

Appropriate supervised experience with colposcopy and loop electrosurgical excision procedure (LEEP) should be undertaken before this technique is used. No specific credentialing is required.

Coding

57460	Colposcopy with loop electrosurgical excision(s) of the cervix (LEEP)
57500	Biopsy (cervical), single or multiple, or local excision of lesion, with or without fulguration (separate procedure)
57505	Endocervical curettage (not done as part of a dilation and curettage)
57520	Conization of cervix, loop electrode excision
99070	Supplies and materials

Technique

Before the patient arrives at the office for the procedure, she should be sent patient education information on abnormal Papanicolaou smears and LEEP. The patient may take as much as 800 mg of ibuprofen or similar nonsteroidal anti-inflammatory agent approximately 1 hour before the procedure.

Once informed consent has been obtained, the patient, undressed from the waist down, should be positioned on the examination table as for a speculum examination. Attach the return electrode (grounding pad) to the patient's thigh with the long edge directed toward the hip. This is then connected to the electrosurgical generator.

The cervix should be visualized using a nonconductive speculum with smoke evacuator attachment. The speculum may be attached to the smoke evacuation system at this point or just before the start of the excision. If any cultures or cytologic smears are to be obtained, they should be taken at this stage. If a long period has elapsed since the last colposcopic examination, colposcopy should be repeated (see Chapter 9, Colposcopy). Acetic acid or Lugol's solution should be applied to the cervix to delineate the area of abnormality.

Local anesthetic should be injected submucosally into the cervix at the 3, 6, 9, and 12 o'clock positions. These injections should be approximately 3 to 5 mm deep. While the anesthetic takes effect, the appropriate loop should be selected on the basis of the size of the lesion to be treated. Lesions confined to the portio are most often treated with a round loop, 2 cm in width and 0.8 cm deep. For a nulliparous, small cervix, a loop 1.5 cm wide and 0.7 cm deep should be used. For lesions extending into the endocervix, a square loop electrode, 1 cm × 1 cm, can be used. This electrode can be combined with an ectocervical loop to create a "top hat" procedure.

The power setting for the electrosurgical generator depends on the manufacturer of the generator and the diameter of the loop. The 2 × 0.8 cm loop requires 35–45 W of power, whereas the 1 × 1 cm loop requires 20–30 W. A blended current should be used. The specific technique used varies somewhat with the type of lesion to be treated.

SMALL ECTOCERVICAL LESIONS

For small ectocervical lesions, a loop size of 1.5 to 2 cm width and 0.8 cm depth works best. Hold the loop several millimeters lateral to the edge of the lesion and simulate passing the loop over the lesion to ensure that no obstacles are present. Next, activate the loop by switching on the electrosurgical generator in the "cut" mode. This is usually accomplished by using a switch on the hand piece, although some units may use a foot switch instead. Press the loop perpendicular into the tissue to a depth of 5 to 8 mm and drag the loop laterally across and through the endocervix. The loop should be pulled to a point several millimeters past the lesions or beyond the transformation zone, whichever is further (Fig. 20.1). The resulting specimen should be dome-shaped with the endocervical canal visible in the middle (Fig. 20.2). The loop should not be pressed more than 4 or 5 mm deep at the lateral borders of the cervix because of the arterial blood supply to the cervix entering at the 3 o'clock and 9 o'clock positions.

LARGE ECTOCERVICAL LESIONS

If the lesion is too large to be removed in a single pass, first remove the central portion of the lesion using a 2-cm-wide loop as described above. Make additional passes using

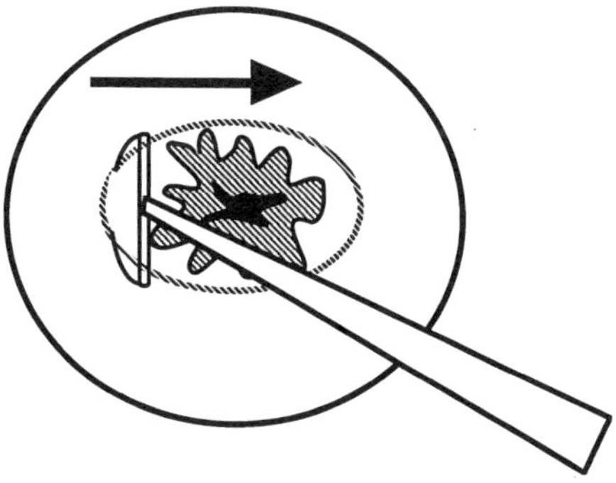

FIGURE 20.1.
For small superficial ectocervical lesions, the loop electrode may be used in a single pass to remove the lesion.

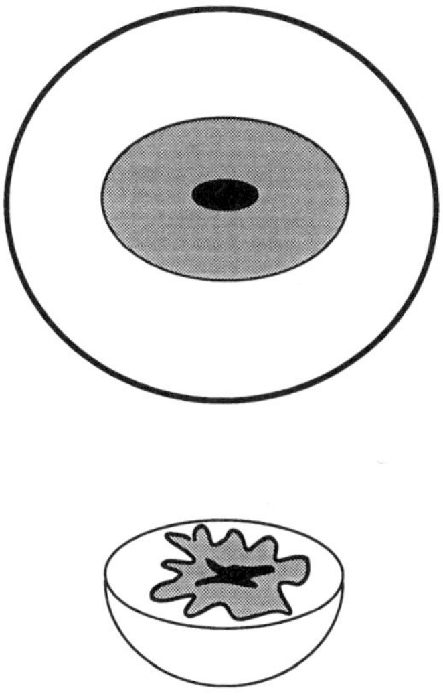

FIGURE 20.2.
When the procedure is correctly performed, the specimen removed has a dome-shaped contour and completely contains the lesion identified by colposcopy.

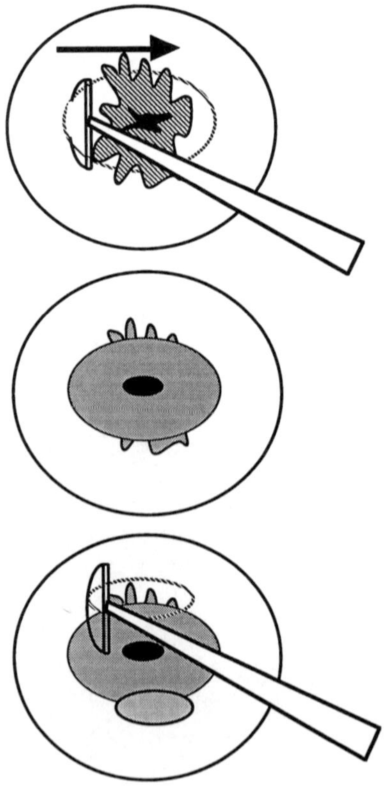

FIGURE 20.3.
Large lesions may require two or more passes to ensure complete removal. The size and shape of each pass may be adjusted on the basis of the lesion present.

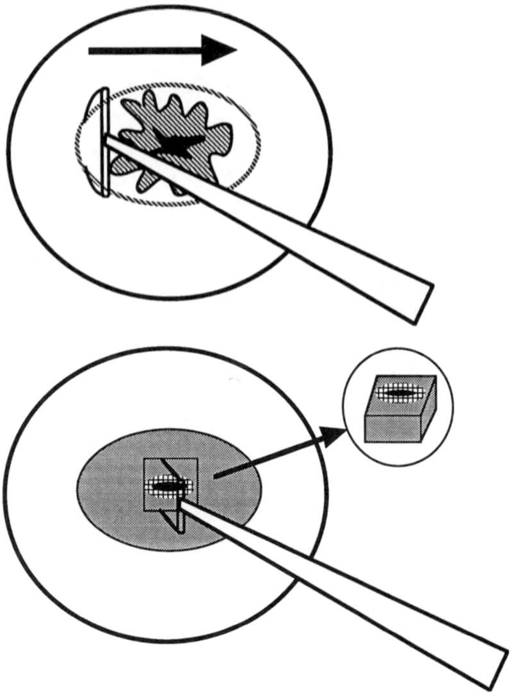

FIGURE 20.4.
When the lesion of concern involves the endocervical canal, a separate pass, either before or after the removal of the exocervix, is required. This extra pass is usually done using either a small-loop or, most commonly, rectangular electrode. The resultant square specimen (insert) should contain the endocervical margin of the lesion.

the same loop to remove remaining lesion and the transformation zone (Fig. 20.3). After LEEP has been performed, some physicians use endocervical curettage to sample the cervix above the excised tissue.

LESIONS INVOLVING THE ENDOCERVICAL CANAL

When the lesion to be excised extends into the outer portion of the endocervical canal, a two-step procedure using both a 2-cm loop and a 1-cm rectangular loop can be used. The procedure begins by excising the endocervical portion using the 1-cm rectangular electrode. This removes a deep rectangular portion that should include the upper parts of the lesion. The ectocervical portion is then excised using the techniques described above. Some physicians prefer to remove the ectocervical portion of the specimen first, then excise the endocervical portion as described above (Fig. 20.4). The sequence used is discretionary. Endocervical and exocervical portions should be sent for histologic evaluation in separate containers.

HEMOSTASIS

If a blended current is used, bleeding from the base of the excision site is generally minimal. If necessary, fulguration of bleeders using the ball electrode with the "coagulation" setting may be performed. When a 5-mm ball is used, power settings of 40 to 55 W are used. Monsel's solution may also be applied if needed. The use of either of these methods delays healing somewhat and thus should be used only when necessary.

PATIENT FOLLOW-UP

The patient should be instructed to avoid vaginal intercourse, use of tampons, or douching for 2 to 3 weeks. She should also be instructed to contact the physician if bleeding equals or exceeds a normal period or lasts more than 2 weeks from the time of the procedure. The patient should contact the physician if vaginal discharge becomes foul smelling or if fever develops.

Selected Abnormal Findings

Stalling of loop passage may occur because of movement that is too rapid, cutting power that is set too low, or excessive carbon build-up on the electrode. If stalling occurs, passing the electrode from the opposite side may be of benefit.

Special Notes

Tagging the surgical specimen with a suture at the 12 o'clock position helps the pathologist orient the specimen. Inadvertent burns to the vaginal sidewall can occur but are rare. Care must be taken to avoid any inadvertent contact between the electrode, tissues, or instruments when the electrosurgical unit has been triggered.

Cervical infection can be treated with either doxycycline or metronidazole. Cervical incompetence and stenosis are unlikely.

Suggested Readings

Ferris DG, Hainer BL, Pfenninger JL, et al. Electrosurgical loop excision of the cervical transformation zone: the experience of family physicians. *J Fam Pract* 1995; 41:337.

Gold M, Dunton CJ, Murray J, et al. Loop electrocautery excisional procedure: therapeutic effectiveness as an ablation and a conization equivalent. *Gynecol Oncol* 1996;1:241.

Mathevet P, Dargent D, Roy M, et al. A randomized prospective study comparing three techniques of conization: cold knife, laser, and LEEP. *Gynecol Oncol* 1994; 54:175.

Monk A, Pushkin SF, Nelson AL, et al. Conservative management of options for patients with dysplasia involving endocervical margins of cervical cone biopsy specimens. *Am J Obstet Gynecol* 1996;174:1695.

Muntz HG. Can cervical adenocarcinoma in situ be safely managed by conization alone? *Gynecol Oncol* 1996;61:301.

Prendiville W, Cullimore NS. Large loop excision of the transformation zone (LLETZ): a new method of management for women with cervical intraepithelial neoplasia. *Br J Obstet Gynaecol* 1989;96:1054.

Widrich T, Kennedy AW, Myers TM, et al. Adenocarcinoma in situ of the uterine cervix: management and outcome. *Gynecol Oncol* 1996;61:304.

Chapter 21

PESSARY FITTING

Pessaries can provide mechanical support for the pelvic organs.

Equipment

- Pelvic examination equipment (examination gloves, lubricant, speculum, light source)
- Examples of appropriate pessaries in a variety of sizes (generally the "average size" and at least one size larger and smaller)

Training/Credentialing

No special credentialing needed; office procedure only.

Coding

57160	Fitting and insertion of pessary or other intravaginal support device (procedure only)

Technique

Available in various types and sizes (Fig. 21.1), pessaries are worn in the vagina to replace missing structural support and to diffuse the forces of descent over a wide area. To varying degrees, the pessary occludes the vagina and holds the pelvic organs in a relatively normal position. Pessaries offer an excellent alternative to surgical repair, but the use of a pessary requires the patient's cooperation and involvement. Patients who are unable or unwilling to manage the periodic insertion and removal of the device are poor candidates for their use.

Before a pessary is fitted, the anatomic defects must be carefully assessed and the patient's symptoms must be determined. The presence or absence of normal pelvic support will help to determine the type of pessary best suited for the patient at hand. The most commonly used forms of pessary for pelvic relaxation are the ring (or donut), the ball, and the cube. The type chosen for a given patient is determined by the anatomic defect and the symptoms the patient is experiencing. The indications for various types of commonly used pessaries are shown in Table 21.1. For occasional use, a large tampon may serve the same purpose.

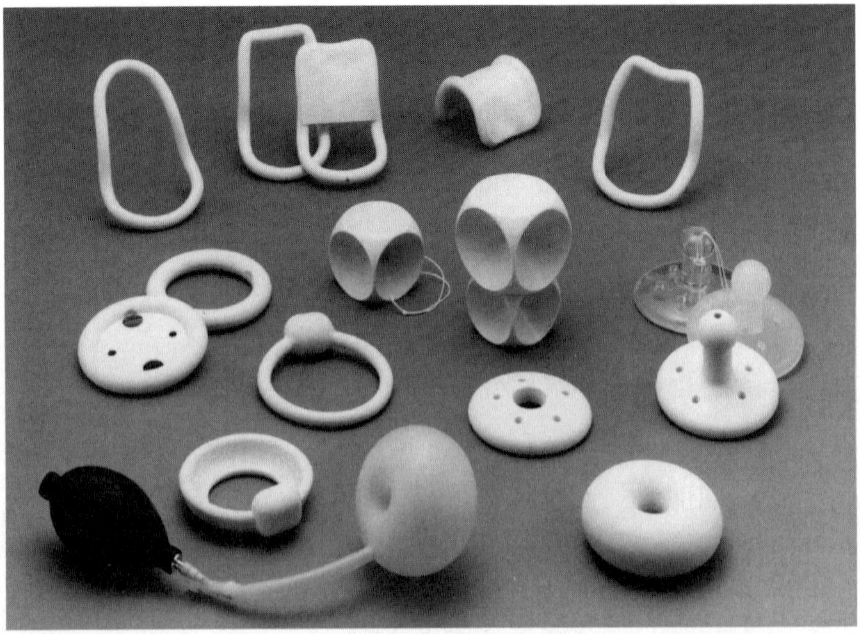

FIGURE 21.1.
Pessaries are available in many sizes and shapes. Because each type serves slightly different purposes, care must be exercised in selecting the specific type and size needed by each patient. (Courtesy of Milex Products, 5915 Northwest Highway, Chicago, IL 60631.)

TABLE 21.1. Indications for Common Pessaries

INDICATION	TYPE OF PESSARY
Malposition	Lever type (Hodge)
Prolapse	
Uterine	Gellhorn, ring, doughnut, cube
Vaginal	Doughnut, cube, ball, (Gehrung)
Cystocele / Rectocele	Gehrung
Incompetent cervix	Lever, ring
Incontinence	Doughnut, lever, ring-incontinence
Preoperative	Based on defect
Drug delivery	Experimental ring (17β-estradiol, medroxyprogesterone)

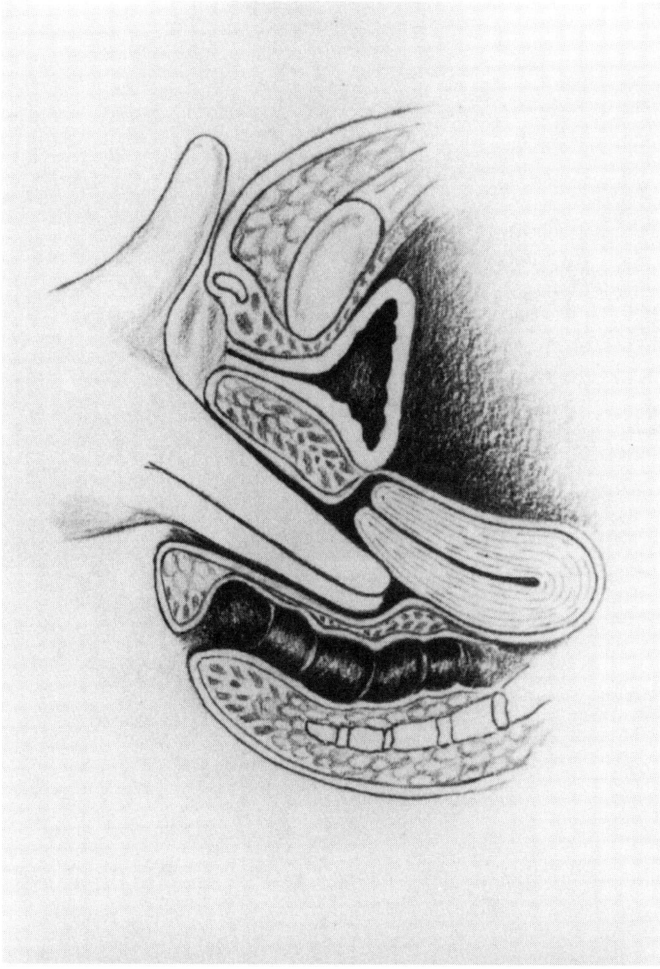

FIGURE 21.2.
The process of fitting a pessary begins with a thorough examination of the pelvic organs and their support. The vaginal depth and breadth are assessed to make a preliminary determination of the type and size of pessary to be fitted. (Courtesy of Milex Products, 5915 Northwest Highway, Chicago, IL 60631.)

Pessaries are fitted and placed in the vagina in much the same way as is a contraceptive diaphragm: the depth of the vagina and the integrity of the supporting structures of the vagina are gauged as a part of the pelvic examination (Fig. 21.2). The size of pessary to be fitted is based on the findings of the pelvic examination (Fig. 21.3). The pessary is lubricated with a water-soluble lubricant, folded or compressed, and inserted into the vagina. The pessary is then adjusted according to the type of device so that it is in the proper position: Ring and lever pessaries should sit behind the cervix (when present) and rest in the retropubic notch (Fig. 21.4); the Gellhorn pessary should be contained entirely within the vagina, with the plate resting above the levator plane (Fig. 21.5); the Gehrung pessary must bridge the cervix, with the limbs resting on the levator muscles on each side (Fig. 21.6); and the ball or cube pessaries should occupy and occlude the upper vagina (Figs. 21.7 and 21.8). All pessaries must allow the easy passage of an examining finger between the pessary and the vaginal wall in all areas. Only pessaries designed to control urinary incontinence should exert any substantial pressure beneath the urethra (Fig. 21.9).

Special Notes

Patients fitted with a pessary need careful initial monitoring. Examination 5–7 days after initial fitting is required to confirm proper placement, hygiene, and the absence of

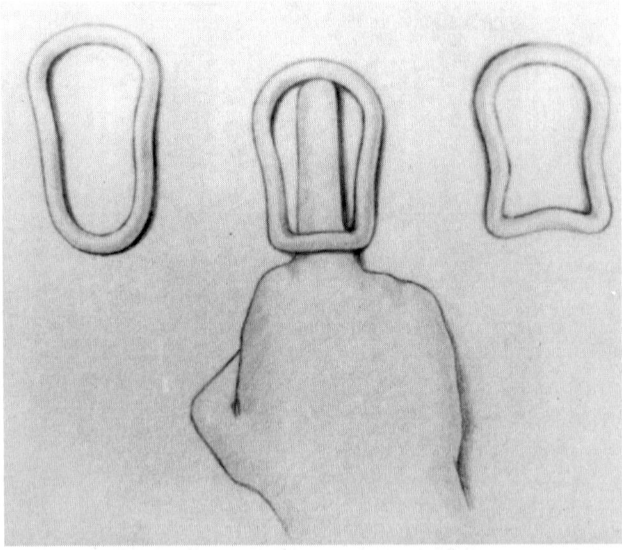

FIGURE 21.3.
The selection of pessary size and shape is primarily gauged on the basis of vaginal length. (Courtesy of Milex Products, 5915 Northwest Highway, Chicago, IL 60631.)

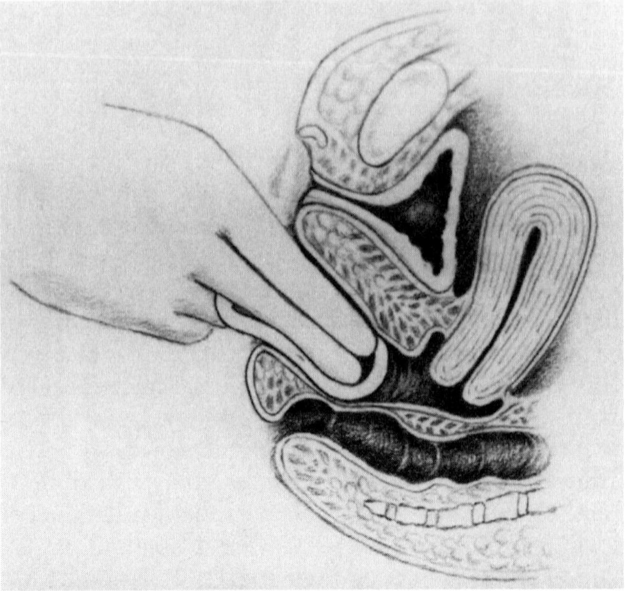

FIGURE 21.4 (*continued*).
The lubricated pessary is inserted into the vagina (continued)

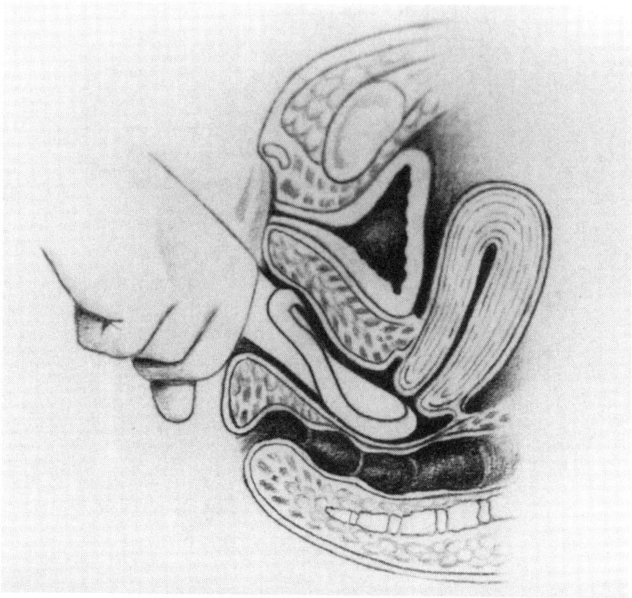

FIGURE 21.4 (*continued*). *and its placement adjusted so that the pessary is properly positioned. (continued)*

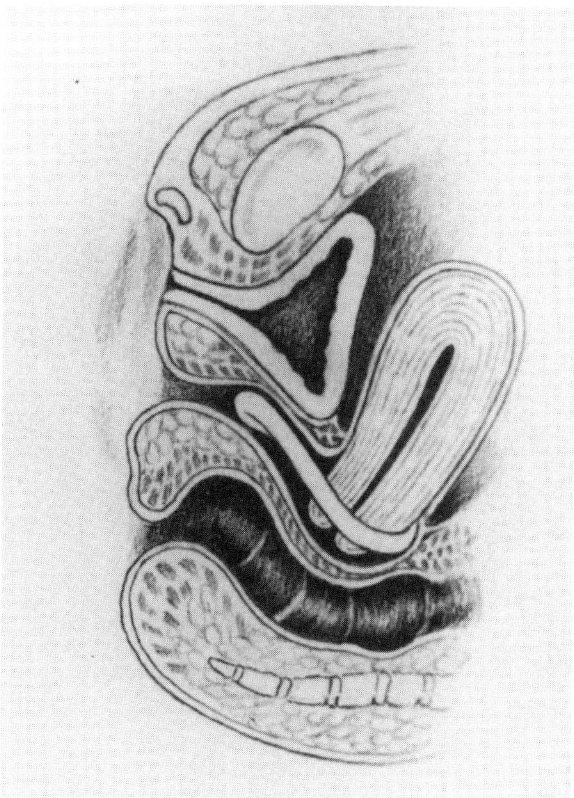

FIGURE 21.4 (*continued*). *Ring and lever pessaries should fit behind the cervix and rest in the retropubic notch. (Courtesy of Milex Products, 5915 Northwest Highway, Chicago, IL 60631.)*

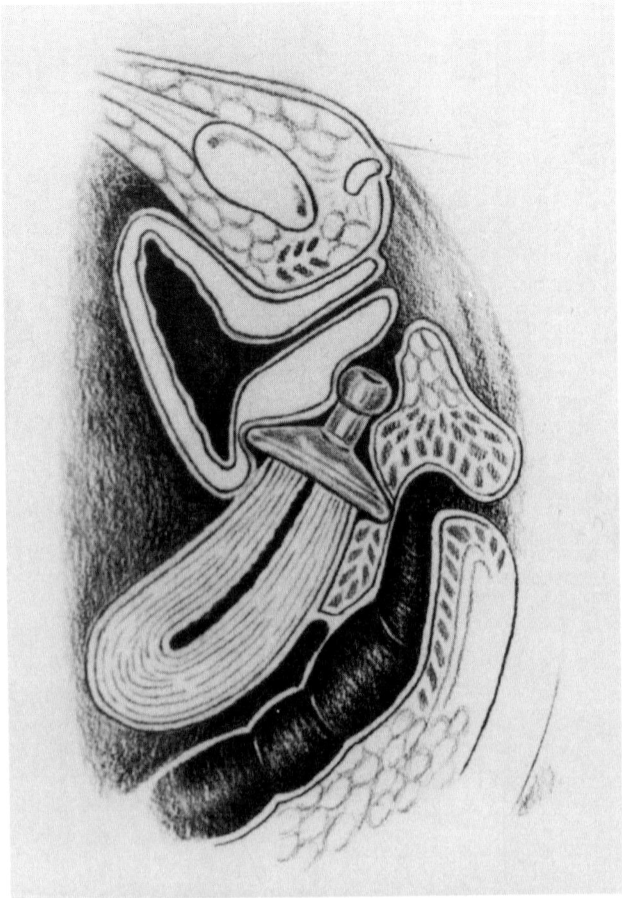

FIGURE 21.5.
The Gellhorn pessary is excellent for treating uterine prolapse. When properly fitted, the Gellhorn pessary should rest with the plate above the levator plane as shown. The stem of the pessary should be contained entirely within the vagina. (Courtesy of Milex Products, 5915 Northwest Highway, Chicago, IL 60631.)

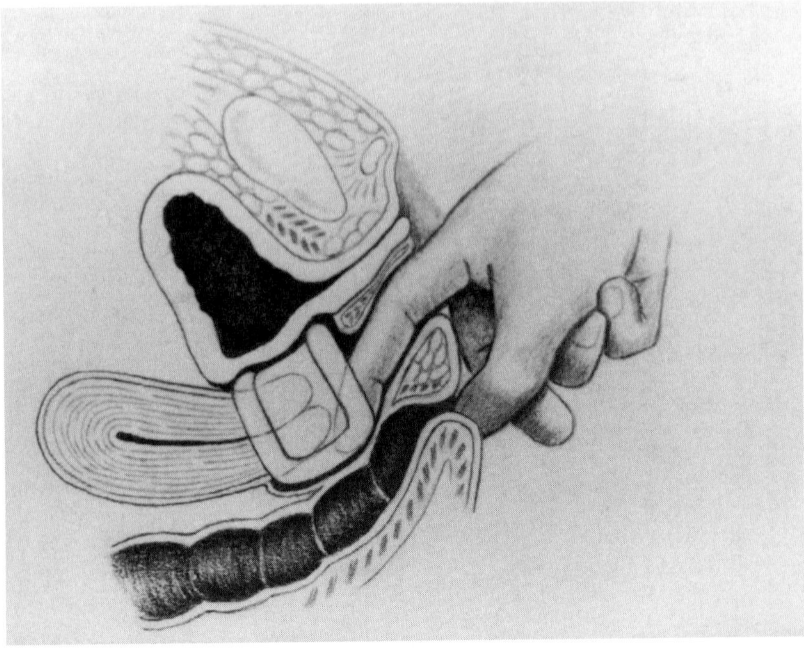

FIGURE 21.6.
The limbs of the Gehrung should sit on the levator plate lateral to the cervix at the apex of the vagina. (Courtesy of Milex Products, 5915 Northwest Highway, Chicago, IL 60631.)

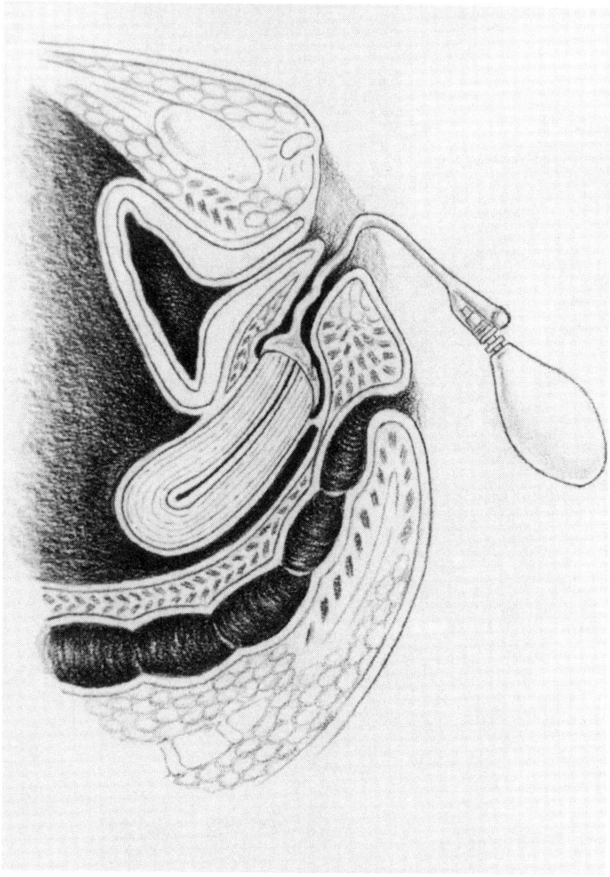

FIGURE 21.7 (*continued*).
The inflatable ball pessary should be placed into the upper vagina while deflated. (continued)

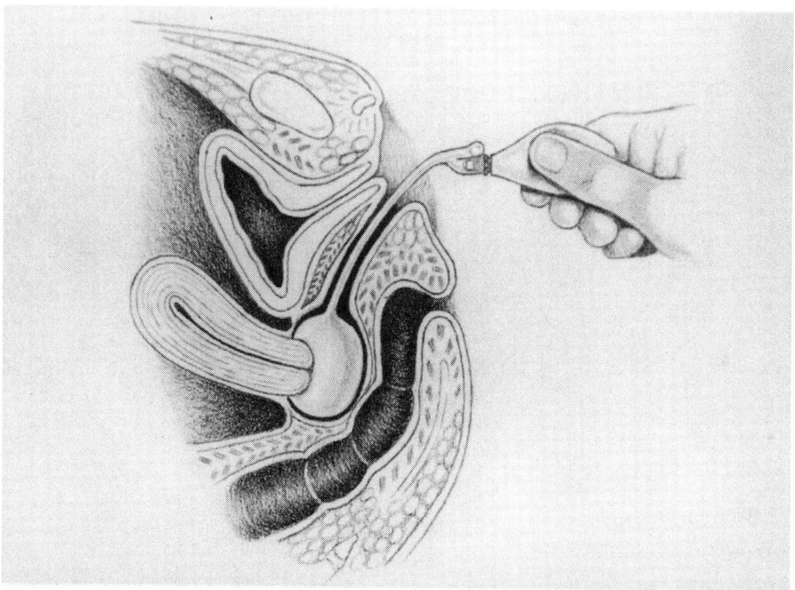

FIGURE 21.7 (*continued*).
Once in position, the ball is inflated to gently occlude the upper vagina, thereby lifting the vaginal apex and uterus. (Courtesy of Milex Products, 5915 Northwest Highway, Chicago, IL 60631.)

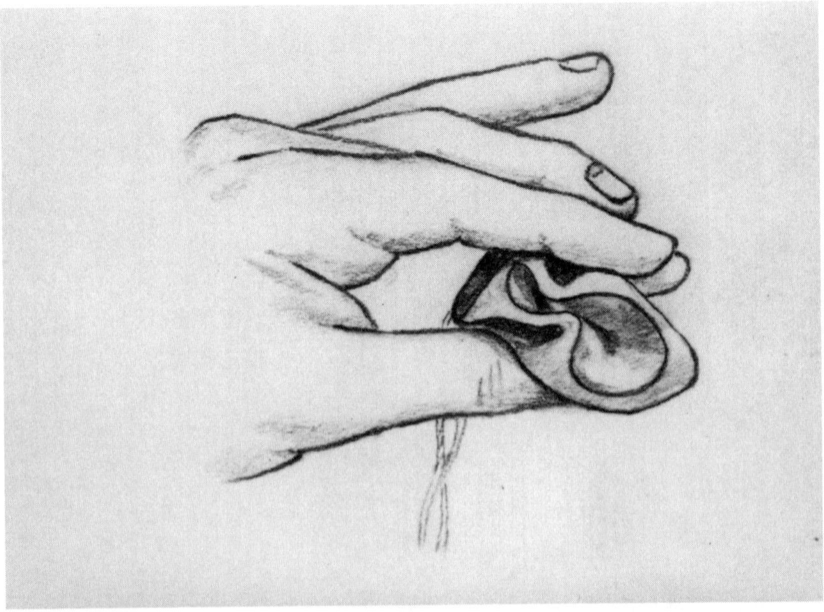

FIGURE 21.8 (*continued*).
The cube pessary must be compressed before it is inserted into the vagina. (continued)

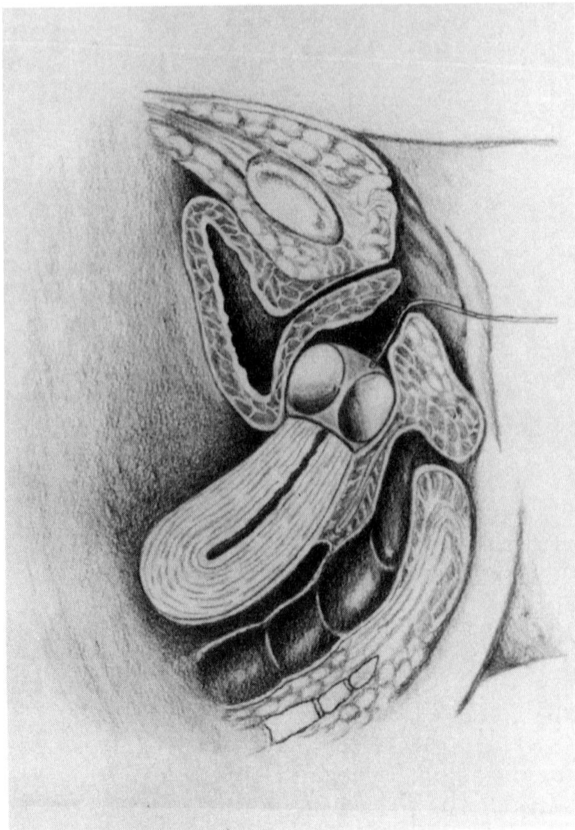

FIGURE 21.8 (*continued*).
When correctly positioned, the cube pessary should occupy the upper vagina and rest against the cervix (when present). (Courtesy of Milex Products, 5915 Northwest Highway, Chicago, IL 60631.)

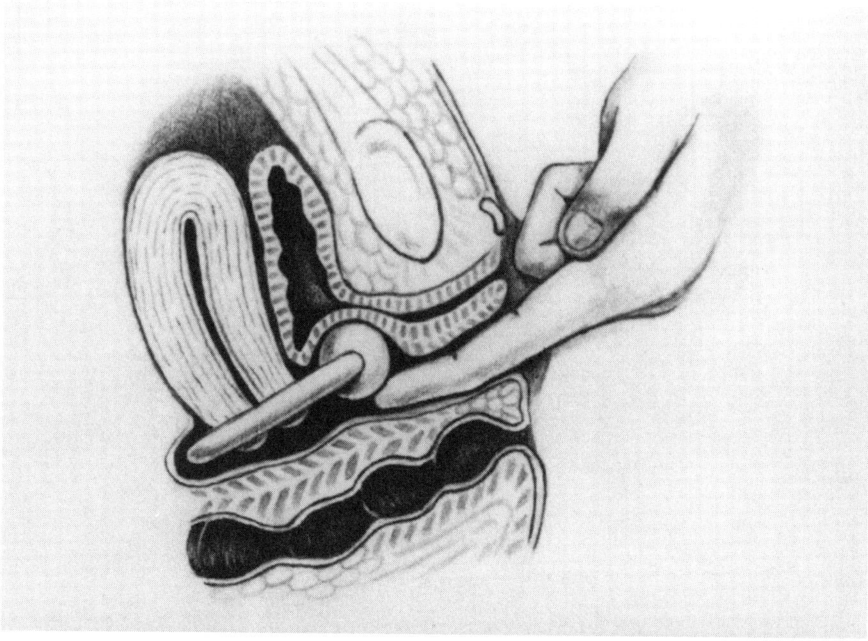

FIGURE 21.9 (*continued*).
Pessaries specifically designed to help control urinary incontinence should provide more support to the urethra and periurethral tissues. Types of pessary designed for this purpose include the ring incontinence. (continued)

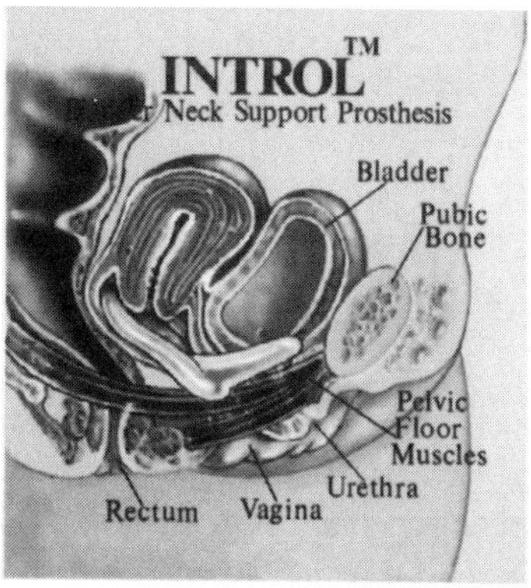

FIGURE 21.9 (*continued*).
and Introl devices. (The ring incontinence device is provided by courtesy of Milex Products, 5915 Northwest Highway, Chicago, IL 60631; the Introl device is provided by courtesy of Introl, Johnson & Johnson Medical, Arlington, TX 76004.)

pressure-related problems (vaginal trauma or necrosis). Earlier evaluation (in 24–48 hours) may be advisable for patients who are debilitated or require additional assistance.

Pessaries are not well tolerated and will not provide optimal support in patients with estrogen deficiency. For this reason, many physicians suggest that estrogen therapy be given for at least 30 days (for menopausal patients not already receiving estrogen replacement therapy) before a pessary is used.

Patients who are to use a pessary should be instructed on the proper insertion and removal techniques. Ring pessaries should be removed by hooking a finger into the pessary's opening, gently compressing the device, and then withdrawing the pessary with gentle traction (Fig. 21.10). Cube pessaries must also be compressed, but the suction created between the faces of the cube and the vaginal wall must be broken by gently separating the device from the vaginal side wall. The locator string often attached

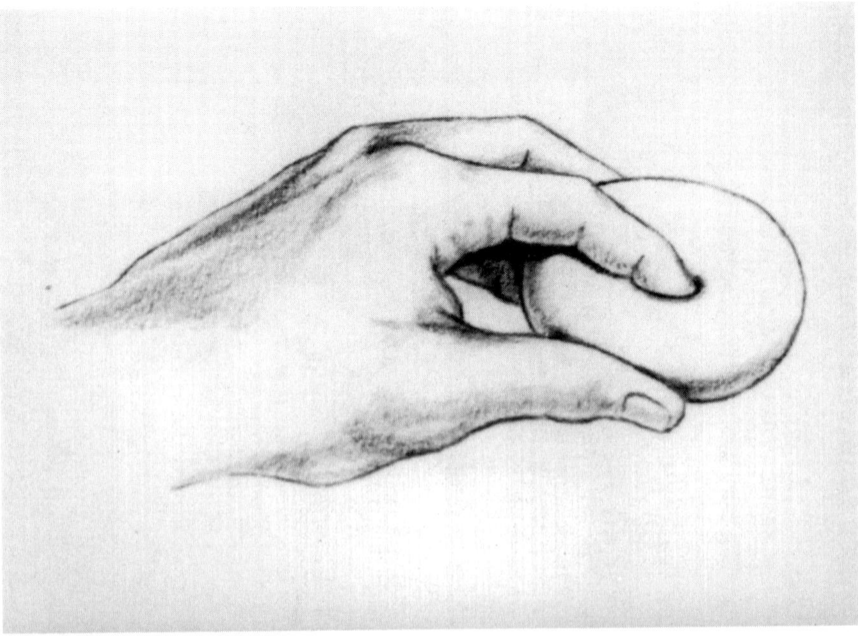

FIGURE 21.10.
To remove a ring pessary, the index finger hooks the opening and the thumb and fingers compress the sides. Gentle traction then results in easy removal. (Courtesy of Milex Products, 5915 Northwest Highway, Chicago, IL 60631.)

to these pessaries should not be used for traction. Inflatable pessaries should be deflated before removal. Gellhorn and Gehrung pessaries are removed by a reversal of their insertion procedures.

Suggested Readings

Bergman A, Bhatia NN. Pessary test: simple prognostic test in women with stress urinary incontinence. *Urology* 1984;24:109.

Bhatia NN, Bergman A. Pessary test in women with urinary incontinence. *Obstet Gynecol* 1985;65:220.

Deger RB, Menzin AW, Mikuta JJ. The vaginal pessary: past and present. *Postgrad Obstet Gynecol* 1993;13:1.

Greenhill JP. The nonsurgical management of vaginal relaxation. *Clin Obstet Gynecol* 1972;15:1083.

Miller DS. Contemporary use of the pessary. In: Sciarra JJ, ed. *Obstetrics and Gynecology*. Philadelphia: JB Lippincott, 1992:1.

Sulak PJ, Kuehl TJ, Shull BL. Vaginal pessaries and their use in pelvic relaxation. *J Reprod Med* 1993;38:919.

Williams GA. Gellhorn pessary modified to facilitate removal. *Obstet Gynecol* 1969;33:860.

Zeitlin MP, Lebherz TB. Pessaries in the geriatric patient. *J Am Geriatr Soc* 1992;40:635.

Chapter 22

SONOHYSTEROGRAPHY

Ultrasonography has fundamentally changed the practice of office obstetrics and gynecology. One limitation of traditional ultrasonographic techniques has been the detailed assessment of the endometrial cavity. The development of ultrasound studies augmented by the use of sonographic contrast holds the promise of overcoming this restriction. The application of these advanced ultrasonographic techniques is well suited to the office setting.

Equipment

- Ultrasonography unit with transvaginal probe (5–7.5 MHz), with real-time display
- Probe covers or unlubricated condoms
- Water-soluble lubricant
- Sterile infant feeding tube or other small catheter
- 35- to 50-mL sterile syringe (with adapter, if necessary, to fit feeding tube or catheter)
- Sterile saline solution (50–100 mL is usually sufficient)
- Sterile operating vaginal speculum (open-sided)
- Skin preparation materials (generally an iodine-based antibacterial solution such as Betadine)
- Sterile gloves
- Light source (for catheter placement)
- Sterile single-tooth tenaculum (optional)
- Sterile uterine sound or blunt probe (optional)

Training/Credentialing

No special credentialing needed; office procedure only. Because of the skill required to obtain good studies and interpret the results, some form of preceptorship or advanced training is desirable.

Coding

76856 Echography, pelvic (nonobstetric), B-scan and/or real time with image documentation; complete

76857 limited or follow-up (e.g., for follicles)

Technique

The main difference between sonohysterography and other forms of ultrasonography is the use of sonographic contrast material. Because of the way ultrasound waves are used to form images of body structures, any material that transmits sound at a different velocity and can intercede between the structures of interest may be used as a contrast media. When the uterine cavity is to be imaged, the simplest contrast material is sterile saline.

To perform sonohysterography, the patient should be prepared and positioned as for transvaginal imaging (see Chapter 23, Transvaginal Ultrasonography). A sterile operating (open-sided) speculum should be inserted into the vagina and the cervix brought into clear view. The cervical os should be cleansed with an appropriate solution (e.g., povidone iodine) as for endometrial biopsy (see Chapter 16, Endometrial Biopsy). If necessary, the cervix may be grasped with a tenaculum and the os probed. Because both of these steps may produce substantial discomfort, they should be used with caution.

A pediatric feeding tube, umbilical catheter, or other similar small sterile tube is then introduced into the endocervical canal. The catheter or tube should be advanced no further than the inner cervical os. The proximal end of the tube should be brought out the side of the vaginal speculum and secured with tape. The speculum (and tenaculum if used) should be removed; care should be taken not to displace the cervical catheter. Sterile saline is drawn up in a suitable syringe and attached to the catheter.

The transvaginal ultrasonography transducer should be placed in a sterile probe cover, condom, or latex glove finger. A water-soluble lubricant or ultrasound coupling gel should be liberally applied to the top of the covered probe and the probe gently inserted into the vagina. The ultrasound probe is advanced along side of the cervical catheter and advanced until it is against the apex of the vagina. The probe may be adjusted as needed to obtain an optimal view of the body of the uterus.

While the ultrasound display screen is being observed, a small amount of sterile saline is gently introduced into the uterine cavity. The amount used should be just sufficient to separate the walls of the cavity and provide contrast for the ultrasound image. Too much volume or too high a pressure during infusion results in uterine cramping and discomfort. In general, only small amounts of fluid are required.

The endometrial cavity, endometrial lining, and the myometrium should be inspected. The transducer may be angled, rotated, or both as needed to obtain the images required. The extent and vigor of these maneuvers must be tempered by the physical constraints of the vaginal tissues and patient comfort.

At the close of the procedure, appropriate documentation of the study, including photographs, video tapes, computer-based images, or notes, should be entered into the patient's chart.

Normal Findings

The normal endometrial cavity should be uniform and symmetric when viewed by ultrasonography. There should be a smooth interface between the endometrial lining and the contrast media (saline) and between the endometrium and the myometrium beneath.

A full discussion of normal and abnormal findings is beyond the scope of this book. The reader is directed to one of several very good reference and atlas works, some of which are referenced in the list of suggested readings at the end of this chapter.

Selected Abnormal Findings

Irregularities in the surface of the endometrium suggest hyperplasia or neoplasia that require further investigation. When these irregularities overlie a similar distortion in the endometrial–myometrial interface, a submucous fibroid is likely. Endometrial polyps will generally be sharply visible on sonohysterography.

Special Notes

Sonohysterography is especially well suited for distinguishing between endometrial thickenings that are global and those that are focal in origin.

If the presence of increased peritoneal fluid or blood in the cul-de-sac is of potential significance to the case being studied, the posterior cul-de-sac should be inspected for these elements at the beginning of the study before any saline has been infused. This inspection should be done because there will be retrograde passage of saline into the abdominal cavity by way of the Fallopian tubes. This saline may be detected at the end of the procedure as an increase in fluid in the dependent portions of the abdomen.

Suggested Readings

American College of Obstetricians and Gynecologists. *Gynecologic Ultrasonography. ACOG Technical Bulletin 215.* Washington, DC: American College of Obstetricians and Gynecologists, 1995.

Balen FG, Allen CM, Lees WR. Ultrasound contrast agents. *Clin Radiol* 1994;49:77.

Balen FG, Allen CM, Siddle NC, et al. Ultrasound contrast hysterosalpingography—evaluation as an outpatient procedure. *Br J Radiol* 1993;667:592.

Cullinan JA, Fleischer AC, Kepple DM, et al. Sonohysterography: a technique for endometrial evaluation. *Radiographics* 1995;15:501.

Deichert U, Schlief R, van de Sandt M, et al. Transvaginal hysterosalpingo-contrast sonography for the assessment of tubal patency with gray scale imaging and additional use of pulsed wave Doppler. *Fert Steril* 1992;57:62.

Gaucherand P, Piacenza JM, Salle B, et al. Sonohysterography of the uterine cavity: preliminary investigations. *J Clin Ultrasound* 1995;23:339.

Timor-Tritsch IE, Monteagudo A. Scanning techniques in obstetrics and gynecology. *Clin Obstet Gynecol* 1996;39:167.

Timor-Tritsch IE, Rottem S, Thaler I. Review of transvaginal ultrasonography: a description with clinical application. *Ultrasound Q* 1988;6:1.

Chapter 23

TRANSVAGINAL ULTRASONOGRAPHY

The resolution obtained by ultrasonography is directly related to the frequency of sound wave used to form the image. Unfortunately, as the frequency of sound increases, the ability of the sound to penetrate tissue and return decreases. This limits the resolution that may be obtained by transabdominal ultrasonography, which must image objects that lie 5–20 cm beyond the skin surface. By moving the transducer closer to the objects of interest, higher frequencies may be used, which enhance the detail of the image obtained. This occurs when a transvaginal technique is used to image the uterus and adnexal structures. When used to augment the information obtained from a careful history and pelvic examination, transvaginal ultrasonography becomes an important office diagnostic procedure.

Equipment

- Ultrasonography unit with transvaginal probe (5–7.5 MHz), with real-time display
- Probe covers or unlubricated condoms
- Water-soluble lubricant

Training/Credentialing

No special credentialing needed; office procedure only. Because of the skill required to obtain good studies and interpret the results, some form of preceptorship or advanced training is desirable.

Coding

76830	Echography, transvaginal
76856	Echography, pelvic (nonobstetric), B-scan and/or real time with image documentation; complete
76857	limited or follow-up (e.g., for follicles)

Technique

EQUIPMENT CONSIDERATIONS

Two main types of transvaginal probes available: mechanical sector scanner or phased array scanners. The former uses a mechanical device to rock the sound transducer back and forth to sweep the pelvis and form an image. The phased array transducer uses a group of transducers that are energized in a sequence that causes the sound waves generated to be moved in a direction without a mechanical change in the transducer.

Both types of transducer provide an adequate view of near-pelvic structures. The mechanical type provides views that are symmetric about the axis of the transducer. Phased-array transducers often provide a field of view that is slightly off axis. This may be of help when structures of interest lie at the extremes of the field of view. In these cases, the transducer may be rotated to take advantage of its asymmetry, allowing these areas to be seen without undue angling of the transducer in the vagina. In either case, the field of view provided is cone shaped and oriented horizontally rather than vertically (Fig. 23.1).

SCANNING PROCEDURES

Unlike transabdominal ultrasonography, imaging of pelvic structures using transvaginal scanning does not require a full bladder. As a result, most patients are more comfortable with the bladder empty. Because of the more intimate nature of transvaginal scanning, extra sensitivity to patient comfort and modesty should be exercised. A chaperone is advisable during this examination.

The patient should be positioned as for a routine pelvic examination: supine with feet comfortably supported in the lithotomy position. If no examination table is available, the patient may be examined in the frog-leg position with a cushion, bed pan, or other support used to elevate the hips 8–10 inches to allow for transducer manipulation.

Before use, the transducer should be placed in a sterile probe cover, condom, or latex glove finger (Fig. 23.2). A water-soluble lubricant or ultrasound coupling gel should be liberally applied to the top of the covered probe. The probe is gently inserted into the vagina and advanced until it is against the apex. The probe may be adjusted so that

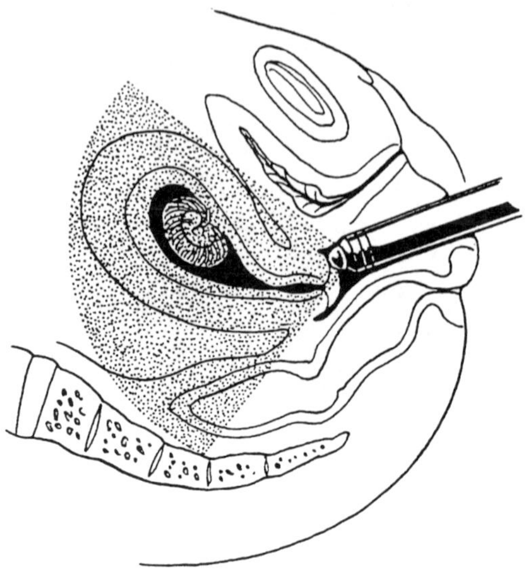

FIGURE 23.1.
Transvaginal ultrasonography provides a high-resolution, cone-shaped view of the structures near the apex of the vagina. (Reproduced with permission from Beckman RB, Ling FW, Barzansky BM, et al. Obstetrics and Gynecology. *2nd ed. Baltimore: Williams & Wilkins, 1995:23.)*

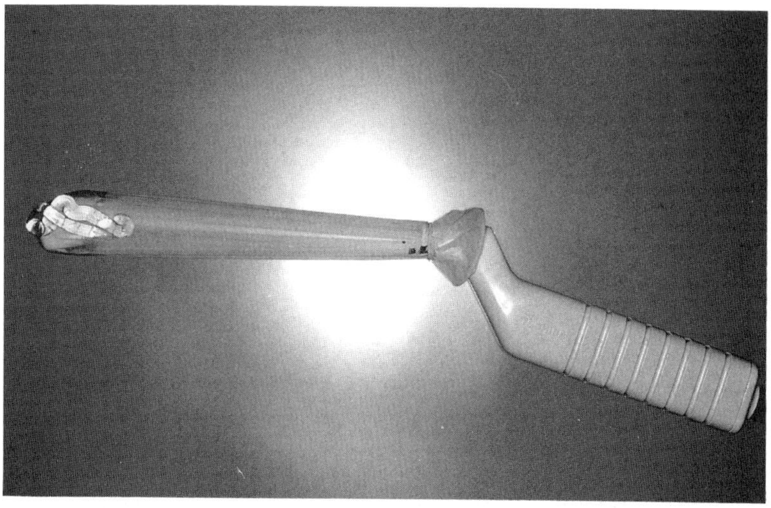

FIGURE 23.2.
Prepared probe with condom covering secured to shaft with rubber bands and gel placed on the outer surface of the condom. (Reproduced with permission from Winfield AC, Wentz AC. Diagnostic Imaging in Infertility. *2nd ed. Baltimore: Williams & Wilkins, 1992:244.)*

it lies in either the anterior or posterior fourchette as needed to obtain a better view of structures in front or in back of the uterus, respectively.

SCANNING TECHNIQUES

The initial step for most transvaginal ultrasound studies is to identify the bladder anteriorly. The bladder is easily identified because of its echo-free appearance, and it provides a consistent landmark for the identification of other structures. The uterus should be seen extending from the transducer. When normal, it has a uniform appearance, although a central endometrial stripe may be seen when the endometrium is thickened (as before menstruation). Palpation by a hand placed on the abdomen may be used to assess mobility of structures. Palpation may also be used to evaluate the relationship between the structures seen and the uterus, based on their relative motion.

The myometrium may be evaluated by transvaginal ultrasonography. The presence of leiomyomata should be noted. The location and size of these common tumors may be recorded and followed sequentially. Of special concern are tumors located just below the endometrial lining. Transvaginal studies may be able to demonstrate distortion of the endometrium overlying these fibroids, helping to support their role in bleeding symptoms. These findings may be further evaluated by the instillation of a small amount of sterile saline into the uterine cavity (see Chapter 22, Sonohysterography).

The endometrium is seen as two stripes of variable thickness, separated by a thin echogenic line (Fig. 23.3). Although the thickness of the endometrium changes over the menstrual cycle, the resolution provided by transvaginal ultrasonography allows the endometrium to be evaluated throughout the month. The thickness of the endometrium should be measured using measures from both the long axis of the uterus and the anterior-posterior dimension. Any fluid in the endometrial cavity should be noted and measured. Irregularities in the surface of the endometrial stripe or in the interface between the endometrium and the myometrium should raise suspicion of possible pathologic abnormality that may warrant further evaluation. Endometrial polyps may be seen as an irregularity or separate bulge in the endometrial cavity. The

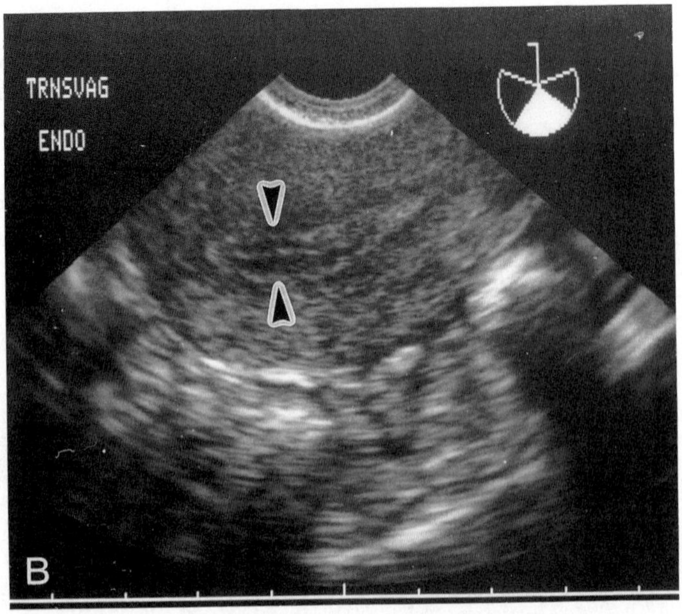

FIGURE 23.3.
The endometrium in the preovulatory period is seen as having a multilayered appearance (between arrows). (Reproduced with permission from Winfield AC, Wentz AC. Diagnostic Imaging in Infertility. *2nd ed. Baltimore: Williams & Wilkins, 1992:246.)*

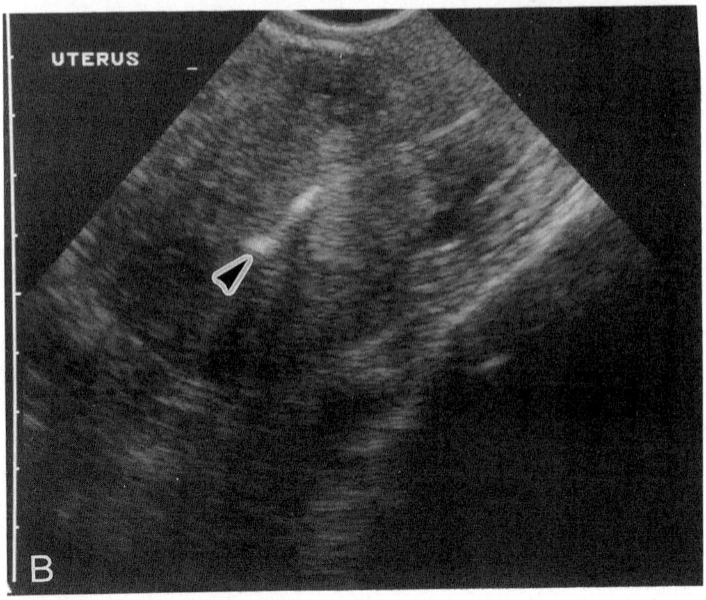

FIGURE 23.4.
A Cu-7 intrauterine contraceptive device is seen in its correct location within the endometrial cavity. (Reproduced with permission from Winfield AC, Wentz AC. Diagnostic Imaging in Infertility. *2nd ed. Baltimore: Williams & Wilkins, 1992:266.)*

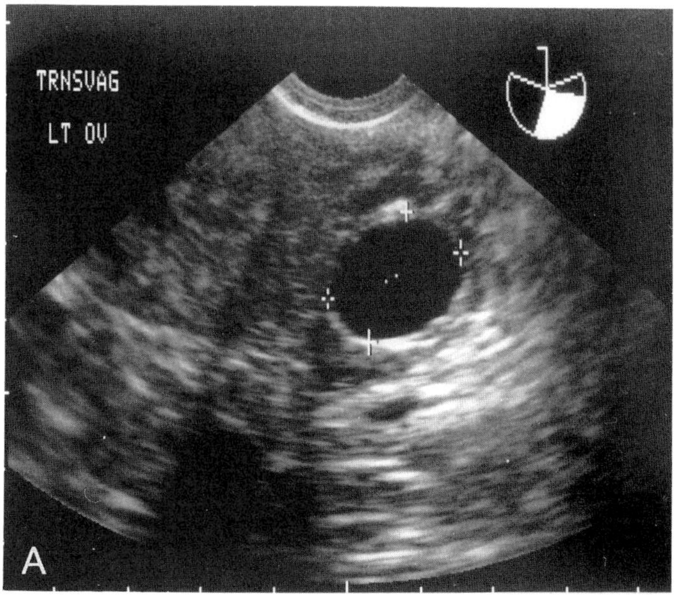

FIGURE 23.5.
The ovary is often difficult to visualize separately from the surrounding tissue. When a follicle is present, as in this view of the left ovary just before ovulation, the cystic nature of the follicle can help identify the ovary. (Reproduced with permission from Winfield AC, Wentz AC. Diagnostic Imaging in Infertility. *2nd ed. Baltimore: Williams & Wilkins, 1992:246.)*

presence and location of an intrauterine contraceptive device may also be ascertained (Fig. 23.4).

The character of the cervix should next be assessed. The high resolution provided by transvaginal assessment of the cervix has changed the role of ultrasonography in the evaluation of cervical abnormalities. Nabothian cysts, cervical fibroids, the rare occurrence of cervical pregnancy, or a distorting cervical cancer may all be detected by ultrasonographic changes.

Once the uterus has been completely evaluated, the transducer may be angled upward and to the side to allow the adnexa to come into the sound field. Because of the location of the adnexal structures and the surrounding tissues, the ovary, fallopian tube, and parametrial area are often difficult to image (Fig. 23.5). The examiner should be familiar with the sonographic appearance of the adjacent structures, including the bowel, vessels (external and internal iliac artery and vein), the ureter, and the muscles of the pelvic back and side walls. The ovaries should be found along the lateral pelvic wall, just below the pulsatile external iliac artery.

The ovary may contain several small cystic (echo-free) areas. This is normal, will be more pronounced in women of reproductive age, and will be maximal around the time of ovulation. The size of the ovary should be measured in three planes. Ovarian volume may be calculated by multiplying these three measures together and dividing by two [(length × width × height)/2]. The normal ovarian volume for reproductive age women is less than 14 cm^3. This value decreases to less than 2.5 cm^3 for postmenopausal women.

Before the examination is terminated, the posterior cul-de-sac should be inspected for the presence of masses or fluid. Appropriate documentation of the ultrasound study, by way of photographs, video tapes, computer-based images, or notes, should be made and entered into the patient's chart.

Normal Findings

Symmetry and consistency are the hallmarks of most pelvic structures when viewed by ultrasonography. A full discussion of normal and abnormal findings is beyond the scope of this book. The reader is directed to one of several very good reference and atlas works, some of which are referenced in the list of suggested readings at the end of this chapter.

Selected Abnormal Findings

Leiomyomata tend to be multiple and spherical and cause a "shadow" effect behind them. This apparent shadowing is caused by scattering of sound by the whorled structure of fibroids. As a result, little or no sound passes through the fibroid to the structures beyond, and even less sound can return as an echo that the ultrasound transducer can detect. Therefore, the area beyond these tumors appears echo-free on the display screen, mimicking a shadow.

Adenomyosis may be suspected on the basis of the presence of an echo-free (sonolucent) area within the myometrium. The final diagnosis, however, remains histologic.

Although the exact role of endometrial thickness measurements in clinical management remains the subject of debate, studies support a lack of significant tissue on biopsy when the endometrial thickness is less than 4–5 mm (maximal anterior–posterior thickness).

Calcification in tissues creates intense echo patterns. This may be seen in degenerating fibroids or in cases of Asherman's syndrome, in which calcification in uterine scarring may occur.

A gestational sac may generally be identified by the fourth–fifth week of pregnancy (Fig. 23.6). When a sac is not seen by 35 days after the last menstrual period, or when

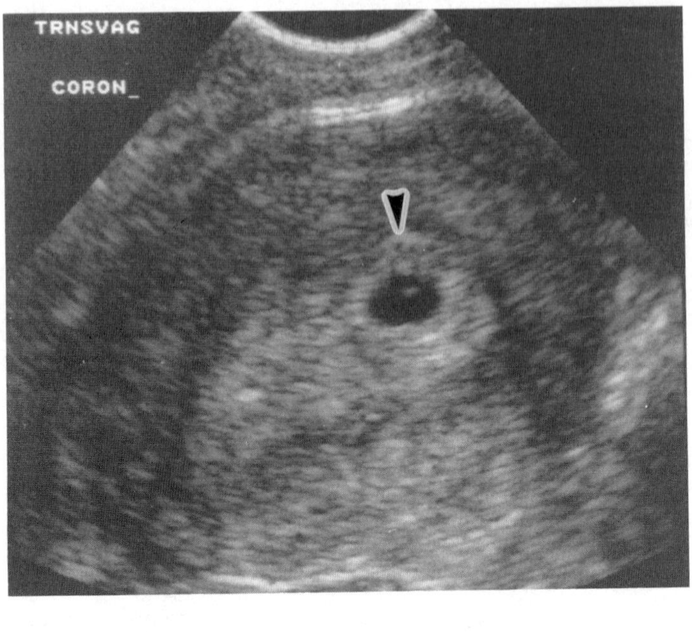

FIGURE 23.6.
Coronal transvaginal scan showing a chorionic mass (arrowhead) within the thickened chorio-decidua in a 5-week intrauterine pregnancy. (Reproduced with permission from Winfield AC, Wentz AC. Diagnostic Imaging in Infertility. *2nd ed. Baltimore: Williams & Wilkins, 1992:271.)*

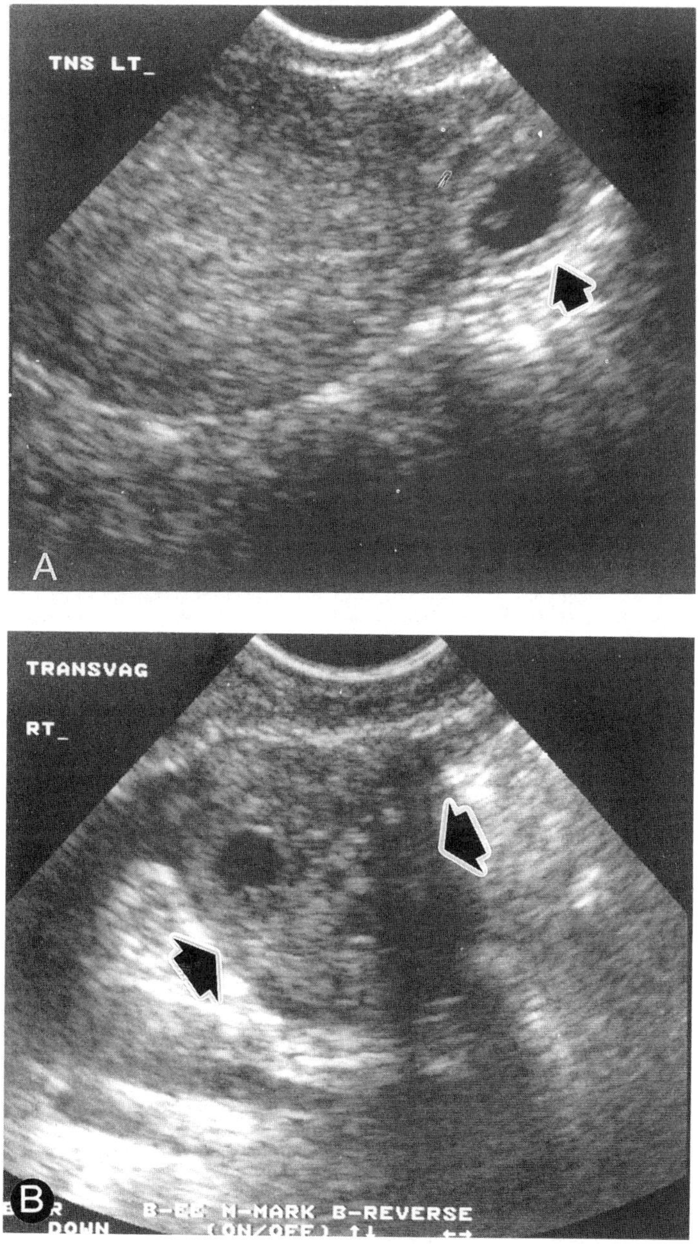

FIGURE 23.7.
Transvaginal ultrasonography of ectopic pregnancy—adnexal and cul-de-sac findings. ***A.*** *"Tubal ring" (arrow) representing an unruptured ectopic pregnancy.* ***B.*** *Ruptured ectopic pregnancy associated with hematosalpinx and hemoperitoneum. (continued)*

human chorionic gonadotropin β levels are greater than 2500 mIU/mL, the sac is considered abnormal.

Ectopic pregnancies are typified by an empty uterus and a cystic enlargement in one adnexa (Fig. 23.7). The decidual changes of early pregnancy may result in some endometrial thickening, but this is generally easy to distinguish from the ring-like gestational sac of early pregnancy (Fig. 23.6). The presence of a fetal heart beat in the adnexa is diagnostic.

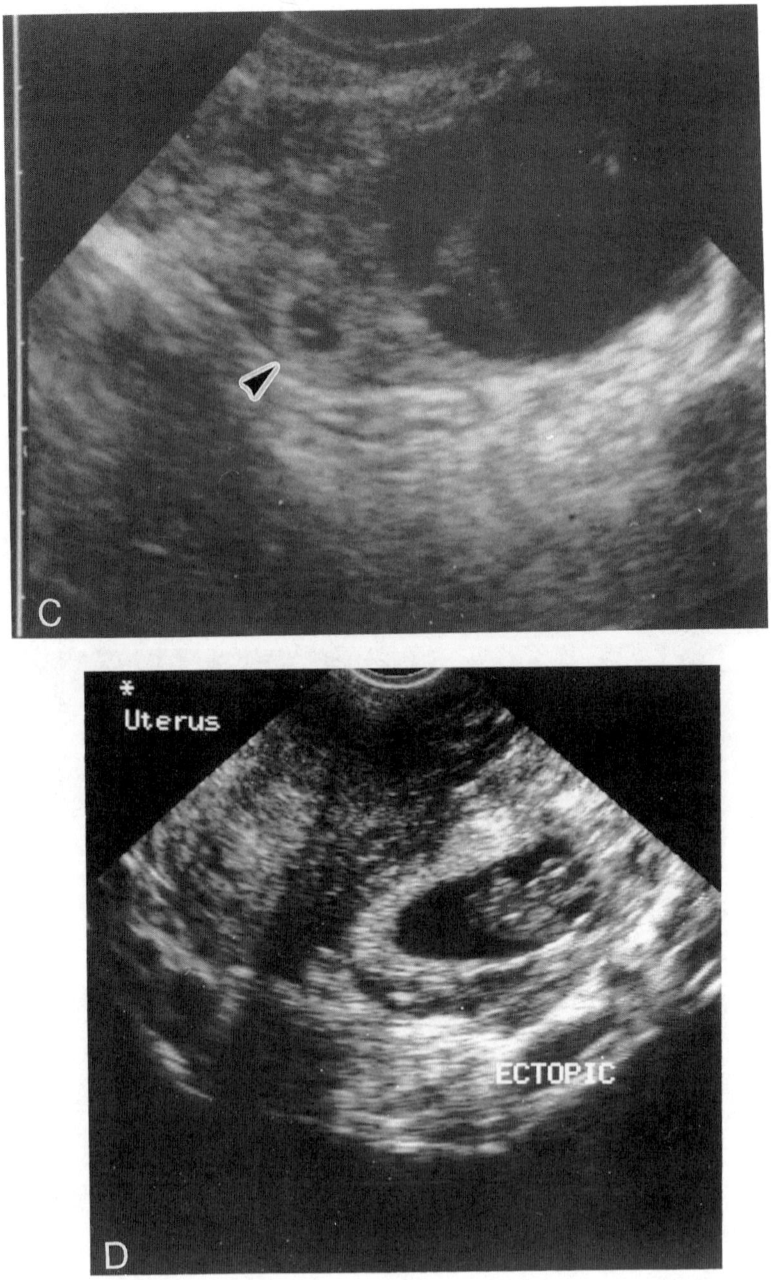

FIGURE 23.7 (*continued*).
C. *Corpus luteum containing a thin septation adjacent to an unruptured ectopic pregnancy (arrowhead).* **D.** *Living 7-week embryo within the tubal sac. (Reproduced with permission from Winfield AC, Wentz AC.* Diagnostic Imaging in Infertility. *2nd ed. Baltimore: Williams & Wilkins, 1992:284–285.)*

Special Notes

Neither transabdominal ultrasonography, transvaginal ultrasonography, nor sonohysterography can establish the diagnosis of genital tract cancer. No diagnosis should be rendered solely on the basis of sonographic findings.

Transvaginal ultrasonography is somewhat limited by the amount of transducer movement allowed by the vaginal barrel and introitus. Care must be used that attempts to visualize the pelvic structures do not induce trauma or discomfort in the pelvic structures.

Structures that lie more than 6–8 cm above the vaginal apex are poorly imaged if they are seen at all. This poor imaging is the result of the limited penetration afforded by the higher frequencies of sound used by this method.

Despite the use of transducer covers, the vaginal transducer should be disinfected after each use. The manufacturer's instructions on disinfection techniques and solutions should be followed to avoid damage.

Many ultrasound coupling gels and vaginal lubricants can interfere with sperm motility and should be avoided for couples attempting pregnancy. This is most acute for studies performed around the time of ovulation.

Suggested Readings

American College of Obstetricians and Gynecologists. Gynecologic Ultrasonography. ACOG Technical Bulletin 215. Washington, DC: American College of Obstetricians and Gynecologists, 1995.

American College of Obstetricians and Gynecologists. Ultrasonography in pregnancy. ACOG Technical Bulletin 187. Washington, DC: American College of Obstetricians and Gynecologists, 1993.

Anonymous. Recommendations on the use of ultrasound and Doppler technology in clinical obstetrics and gynecology. FIGO Study Group on the Assessment of New Technology. *Int J Gynaecol Obstet* 1992;37:221.

Bateman BG, Nunley WC Jr, Kolp LA, et al. Vaginal sonography findings and hCG dynamics of early intrauterine and tubal pregnancies. *Obstet Gynecol* 1990;75:421.

Bernaschek G, Rudelstorfer R, Csaicsich P. Vagninal sonography versus serum human chorionic gonadotropin in early detection of pregnancy. *Am J Obstet Gynecol* 1988;158:608.

Bree RL, Edwards M, Böhm-Vélez M, et al. Transvaginal sonography in the evaluation of normal early pregnancy: correlation with hCG level. *AJR Am J Roentgenol* 1989;153:75.

Cacciatore V, Titinen A, Stenman U-H, et al. Normal early pregnancy: serum hCG levels and vaginal ultrasonography findings. *Br J Obstet Gynaecol* 1990;97:889.

Daya S, Woods S, Ward S, et al. Early pregnancy assessment with transvaginal ultrasound scanning. *Can Med Assoc J* 1991;144:441.

Fossum GT, Davajan V, Kletzky OA. Early detection of pregnancy with transvaginal ultrasound. *Fertil Steril* 1988;49:788.

Gambone JC, Munro MG. Office sonography and office hysteroscopy. *Curr Opin Obstet Gynecol* 1993;5:733.

Gjelland K, Hordnes K, Tjugum J, et al. Treatment of ectopic pregnancy by local injection of hypertonic glucose: a randomized trial comparing administration guided by transvaginal ultrasound or laparoscopy. *Acta Obstet Gynecol Scand* 1995;74:629.

Goldstein SR, ed. *Endovaginal Ultrasound*. 2nd ed. New York: Wiley-Liss, 1991.

Goldstein SR, Synder JR, Watson C, et al. Very early pregnancy detection with endovaginal ultrasound. *Obstet Gynecol* 1988;72:200.

Goldstein SR. Increasing use of gynecologic ultrasonography. *Am J Obstet Gynecol* 1992;166:1310.

Levi CS, Lyons EA, Lindsay DJ. Early diagnosis of nonviable pregnancy with endovaginal US. *Radiology* 1988;167:383.

Munn CS, Kiser LC, Wetzner SM, et al. Ovary volume in young and premenopausal adults: US determination. *Radiology* 1986;159:731.

Peisner DB. Vaginal ultrasound for the practicing clinician. Equipment selection. *Clin Obstet Gynecol* 1996;39:158.

Rodriguez MH, Platt LD, Medearis AL, et al. The use of transvaginal sonography for evaluation of postmenopausal ovarian size and morphology. *Am J Obstet Gynecol* 1988;159:810.

Shapiro BS, Escobar M, Makuch R, et al. A model-based prediction for transvaginal ultrasonographic identification of early intrauterine pregnancy. *Am J Obstet Gynecol* 1992;166:1495.

Steiner H, Staudach A, Spitzer D, et al. Three-dimensional ultrasound in obstetrics and gynaecology: technique, possibilities and limitations. *Human Reprod* 1994;9:1773.

Stiller RJ, De Regt RH, Blair E. Transvaginal ultrasonography in patient at risk for ectopic pregnancy. *Am J Obstet Gynecol* 1989;161:930.

Thornton KL. Principles of ultrasound. *J Reprod Med* 1992;37:27.

Timor-Tritsch IE, Monteagudo A. Scanning techniques in obstetrics and gynecology. *Clin Obstet Gynecol* 1996;39:167.

Timor-Tritsch IE, Rottem S, Thaler I. Review of transvaginal ultrasonography: a description with clinical application. *Ultrasound Q* 1988;6:1.

Section III

COLON AND RECTAL PROCEDURES

Chapter 24

ANAL FISSURECTOMY AND LATERAL SPHINCTEROTOMY

Anal fissures are acute longitudinal tears or chronic oval ulcers of the stratified squamous epithelium of the anal canal (Fig. 24.1). The cause of these fissures is unknown, but they are thought to originate with traumatic lacerations (e.g., hard stools) that become secondarily infected. These fissures generally overlie the internal sphincter and cause it to spasm, potentially perpetuating the fissure (Fig. 24.2). The most common symptoms are pain and bleeding during and after bowel movements. The first line of therapy for anal fissures consists of stool softeners, sitz baths, bland (glycerin) suppositories, and topical soothing agents. When simple therapy fails, surgery is required.

Equipment

- #15 or #11 knife blade, thumb forceps, fine tissue scissors, operating anoscope, or anal retractor
- Fine (3-0 or 4-0) absorbable suture (optional)
- Electrosurgical generator, tip, hand piece or foot pedal control, return electrode ("ground pad") (optional)
- Sterile gloves, antiseptic solution and sterile cotton balls, or skin preparation swabs
- Sterile draping material (optional)
- Monsel's solution (optional)
- Assistant (generally required)
- Local anesthetic of choice, 25-gauge needle (may be used, but the procedure is usually performed under a regional or short general anesthetic)

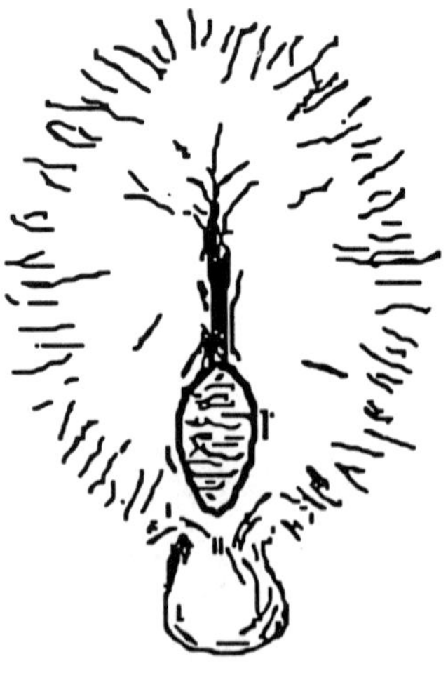

FIGURE 24.1.
When viewed in the lithotomy position with the buttocks gently parted, anal fissures are generally found in the midline posteriorly and are often accompanied by a skin tag at the distal end (sentinel pile).

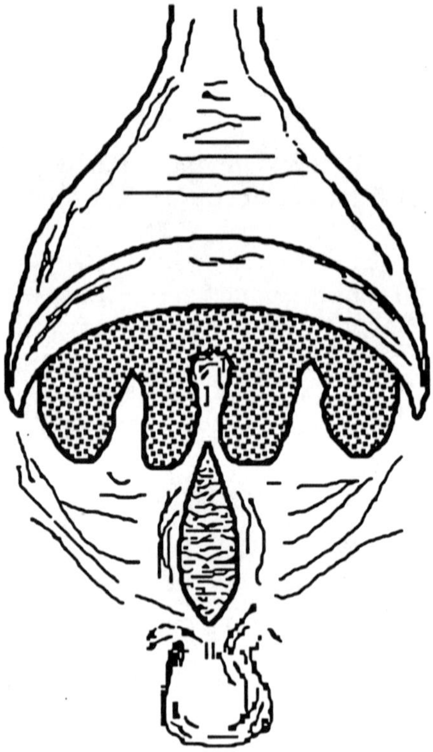

FIGURE 24.2.
When a retractor is placed in the anal opening anteriorly, the inner extent of the anal fissure can be seen. Most commonly these are found to overlie the internal sphincter and extend to the dentate line, where a hypertrophied papilla, analogous to the sentinel pile, may be found.

Training/Credentialing

Some experience is required; best to have received advanced instruction or experience before attempting alone. Improper technique may result in a loss of continence. Many hospitals or ambulatory surgery centers have special credentialing requirements.

Coding

46080 Sphincterotomy, anal, division of sphincter (separate procedure, procedure only)

46200	Fissurectomy, with or without sphincterotomy
46210	Cryptectomy; single
46211	Multiple (separate procedure)
46220	Papillectomy or excision of single tag, anus (separate procedure)
46230	Excision of external hemorrhoidal tages and/or multiple papillae
46257	Hemorrhoidectomy, internal and external, simple; with fissurectomy
46261	Hemmorrhoidectomy, internal and external, complex or extensive; with fissurectomy

Technique

PATIENT PREPARATION

Because lateral internal sphincterotomy is a surgical procedure, appropriate preparation and informed consent must be ensured. Physical preparation of the patient should include cleansing of the lower colon and, for selected patients, antibiotic prophylaxis. The bowel may be mechanically cleansed immediately before the procedure by simple enema (water or such commercial products as Fleet). These should be administered until clear fluid is returned. Generally, two enemas must be done to yield clear fluid, and 30 to 60 minutes should be allowed for adequate preparation. On the basis of the anesthetic technique chosen, there may be a need to restrict oral intake or the use of regularly prescribed medications immediately before the procedure. For patients with constipation, a laxative may be given one day before the procedure or stool softeners may be begun during the previous week. Elderly patients or those who are laxative dependent may require dietary restriction or the use of bisacodyl (Dulcolax) before the procedure.

The final steps in patient preparation include assessing the patient's status and positioning the patient. This procedure is most often performed in an ambulatory or outpatient surgical setting under local, caudal, or spinal anesthesia. The patient's status should be reassessed depending on the anesthetic method in mind. If no contraindications to the procedure are found, the patient is placed in the jackknife or prone position and appropriately prepared and draped for surgical access.

PROCEDURE

After satisfactory anesthesia is obtained, an operating anoscope or anal retractor is placed to retract the anal wall anteriorly, thereby allowing the intersphincteric groove to be clearly seen. It is vital that this landmark be identified so that only the internal sphincter is divided. Failure to limit the sphincterotomy to the internal sphincter may result in incontinence of feces or flatus. A 1-cm radial incision is made over the intersphincteric groove at about the 9 o'clock position. The edge of the incision is grasped and the sphincter is separated from the overlying anoderm through sharp and blunt dissection (Fig. 24.3). The internal sphincter is divided from the intersphincteric groove to the level of the pectinate (dentate) line (Fig. 24.4). Significantly enlarged associated anal papilla or a large skin tag at either end of the fissure may be excised at this time. The site of the fissure itself requires no specific treatment. Most authors suggest that the incision be left open to heal by secondary intention.

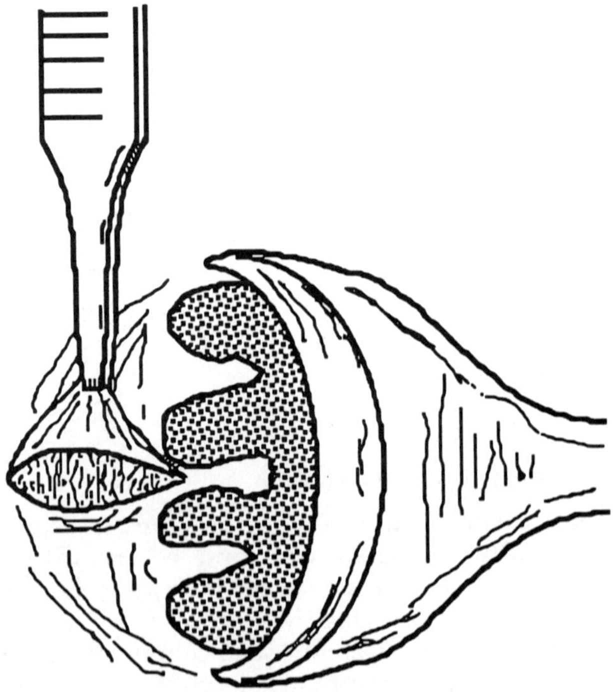

FIGURE 24.3.
Although lateral internal sphincterotomy may be carried out in the lithotomy position, it is usually performed in the jackknife or prone position, as shown here. The procedure begins with a radial incision in the anoderm, usually at the 9 o'clock (left lateral) aspect of the anus.

POSTOPERATIVE CARE

Postoperative care should include a nonconstipating pain medication (such as a nonsteroidal anti-inflammatory agent), a high-fiber diet or a fiber supplement, and topical care in the form of sitz baths and soothing wipes. Mild discomfort, slight bleeding, and minimal discharge should be expected. The discomfort experienced after this procedure is often less than that caused by the fissure itself. Bleeding or spotting with bowel movements may occur for as long as 6 weeks after the procedure.

Fissures fail to heal in approximately 5% of patients; such fissures may require repeat sphincterotomy. Infection may occur in 3–5% of cases, and the patient must be instructed to report significant pain or fever to allow this possibility to be addressed.

Normal Findings

A "sentinel pile" (skin tag) is often found at the external end of these fissures, which makes them easier to identify.

Special Notes

Chronic fissure must be differentiated from carcinoma, primary syphilis, tuberculosis, and the ulcerative lesions of Crohn's disease. Approximately 90% of fissures occur in the posterior midline; the remainder are located in the midline anteriorly. Any fissures outside of these locations should raise the suspicion of other causes.

A 5% lidocaine ointment may be used to reduce discomfort before or after surgery. This ointment also supplies additional lubrication for bowel movements. Steroid preparations may be of some help but should not be used for long periods. Suppositories and medications delivered by rectal-tipped applicators should be avoided because they worsen the patient's symptoms.

The internal sphincter is located directly beneath the internal hemorrhoidal vessels.

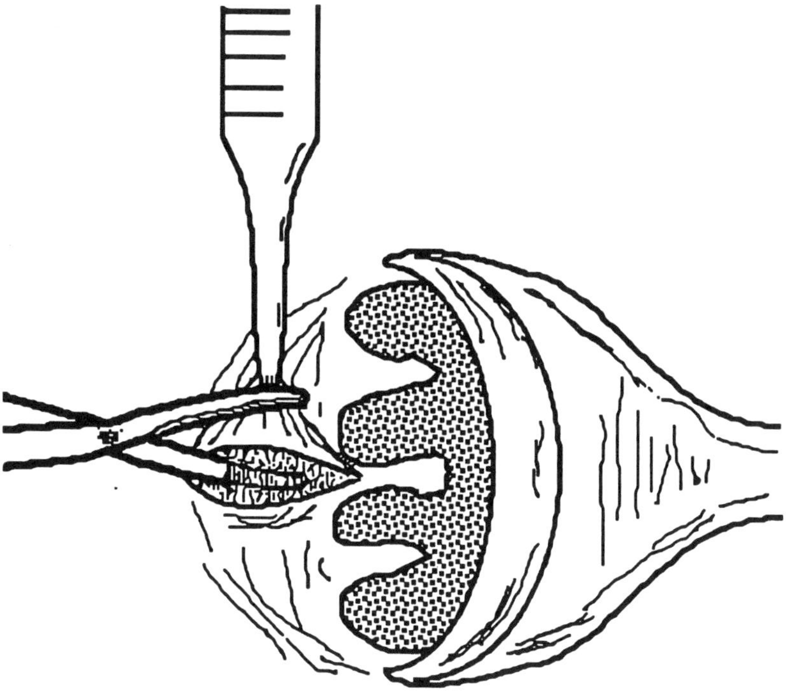

FIGURE 24.4.
Once the internal sphincter is separated from the overlying anoderm (using blunt dissection), the internal sphincter is divided. The wound may be closed with loose interrupted absorbable sutures or may be left open.

Care must be taken to minimize damage to these vessels. Should damage occur, bleeding from these vessels can be significant and may require cautery, sutures, or both to regain hemostasis.

Suggested Readings

Bassford T. Treatment of common anorectal disorders. *Am Fam Phys* 1992;45:1787.

Burke MR, Murtagh J. Anal fissure. *Aust Fam Phys* 1994;23:716.

Frezza EE, Sandei F, Leoni G, Biral M. Conservative and surgical treatment in acute and chronic anal fissure. A study on 308 patients. *Int J Colorectal Dis* 1992;7:188.

Hancock BD. ABC of colorectal diseases. Anal fissures and fistulas. *BMJ* 1992;304:904.

Isbister WH, Prasad J. Fissure in ano. *Aust NZ J Surg* 1995;65:107.

Kortbeek JB, Langevin JM, Khoo RE, et al. Chronic fissure-in-ano: a randomized study comparing open and subcutaneous lateral internal sphincterotomy. *Dis Colon Rectum* 1992;35:835.

Leong AF, Husain MJ, Seow-Choen F, et al. Performing internal sphincterotomy with other anorectal procedures. *Dis Colon Rectum* 1994;37:1130.

Mazier WP. Hemorrhoids, fissures, and pruritus ani. *Surg Clin North Am* 1994;74:1277.

Medich DS, Fazio VW. Hemorrhoids, anal fissure, and carcinoma of the colon, rectum, and anus during pregnancy. *Surg Clin North Am* 1995;75:77.

Neufeld DM, Paran H, Bendahan J, et al. Outpatient surgical treatment of anal fissure. *Eur J Surg* 1995;161:435.

Oh C, Divino CM, Steinhagen RM. Anal fissure. 20-year experience. *Dis Colon Rectum* 1995;38:378.

Pernikoff BJ, Eisenstat TE, Rubin RJ, et al. Reappraisal of partial lateral internal sphincterotomy. *Dis Colon Rectum* 1994;37:1291.

Sultan AH, Kamm MA, Nicholls RJ, et al. Prospective study of the extent of internal anal sphincter division during lateral sphincterotomy. *Dis Colon Rectum* 1994;37:1031.

Usatoff V, Polglase AL. The longer term results of internal anal sphincterotomy for anal fissure. *Aust NZ J Surg* 1995;65:576.

Wolkomir AF, Luchtefeld MA. Surgery for symptomatic hemorrhoids and anal fissures in Crohn's disease. *Dis Colon Rectum* 1993;36:545.

Chapter 25

ANAL FISTULECTOMY

Anorectal fistulae may develop spontaneously or result from the drainage of a perirectal abscess. Crohn's disease and tuberculosis are recognized risk factors, but in most patients, no predisposing cause is found. The only effective treatment is surgery.

Equipment

- Local anesthetic of choice, 25-gauge needle
- #15 or #11 knife blade, blunt probe, thumb forceps, fine tissue scissors (optional)
- Fine (3-0 or 4-0) absorbable suture
- Iodoform gauze packing (optional)
- Sterile gloves, antiseptic solution and sterile cotton balls, or skin preparation swabs
- Sterile draping material (optional)
- Large-tipped cotton swabs (such as those used for colposcopy)
- Monsel's solution (optional)
- Assistant (desirable but optional)

Training/Credentialing

Some experience is required; best to have received advanced instruction or experience before attempting alone. No special credentialing is needed for office procedure, but many hospitals or ambulatory surgery centers have special credentialing requirements.

Coding

46270	Surgical treatment of anal fistula (fistulectomy/fistulotomy); subcutaneous
46275	submuscular

46280	complex or multiple, with or without placement of seton
46285	second stage
46257	Hemorrhoidectomy, internal and external, simple; with fissurectomy
46258	Hemorrhoidectomy, internal and external, simple; with fistulectomy, with or without fissurectomy
46030	Removal of anal seton, other marker (procedure only)

Technique

PATIENT PREPARATION

Special preparation of the patient is generally not required, but mechanical cleansing of the bowel is desirable. This cleansing may be accomplished immediately before the procedure by simple enema (water or such commercial products as Fleet). Enemas should be administered until clear fluid is returned.

On the basis of the needs and desires of the patient, premedication with 800 mg of ibuprofen or an equally effective dose of any other nonsteroidal anti-inflammatory agent can provide good analgesia for the procedure. Oral diazepam or intramuscular sedatives may be given but are usually not required.

PROCEDURE

Careful digital examination and anoscopy must be performed before any treatment decision is made (see Chapter 26, Anoscopy). These examinations establish the diagnosis, allow assessment of the extent of the fistula, and help determine the origin of the fistula. Gentle digital dilation of the anus facilitates identification of the anal end of the fistula and may help reduce future recurrences.

The patient should be placed in the left lateral (Sims) position or the modified knee-chest position. (A prone position may be used if assistance with retraction of the buttocks is available.) The skin of the perineum and perianal area should be cleansed using a suitable surgical preparation method (e.g., Betadine scrub and solution, Hibiclens). Sterile draping may be placed at the discretion of the operator. A field block using local anesthetic is established by infiltrating around the fistulous tract, up to the anus.

After adequate anesthesia has been established, the fistulous tract should be explored with a blunt probe (Fig. 25.1). Shallow tracts and chronic fistulae lined by squamous epithelium may be incised and left to heal by secondary intention (Fig. 25.2). Fistulous tracts may also be excised in toto, although this technique risks unnecessary discomfort and damage to the sphincters. Deeper fistulae may require division of the subcutaneous and superficial sphincters. Division of these may be done with impunity, but the internal sphincter must be assiduously protected.

Deep fistulae may be treated by placing a suture through the tract (from one opening to the other) (Fig. 25.3). The suture is then tied and allowed to erode through the tissues over time, opening the roof of the tract in a controlled manner (seton procedure). The suture may later be removed as necessary. Most surgeons have abandoned this technique in favor of direct fistulotomy.

Normal Findings

Most fistulae involve the posterior midline and arise in the anorectal crypts.

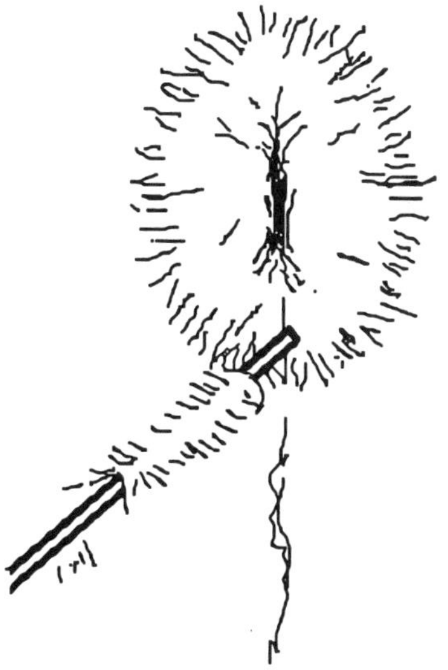

FIGURE 25.1.
The fistulous tract is identified with the help of a blunt probe (as seen in the lithotomy position).

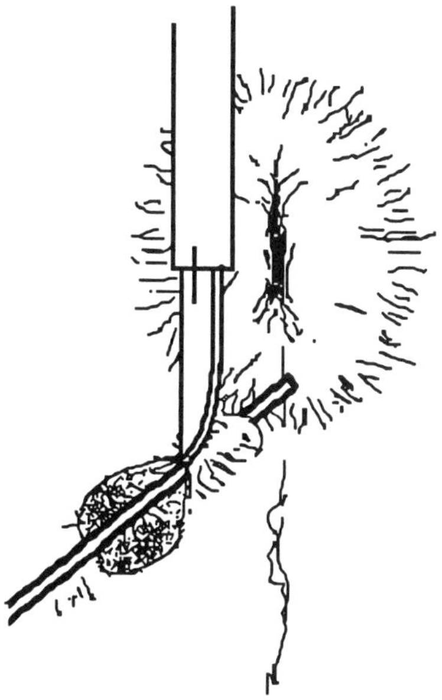

FIGURE 25.2.
Superficial fistulous tracts may be opened by incising directly over the probe. These tracts may be left to heal by secondary intention. Deeper tracts may require division of the subcutaneous or superficial anal sphincter. The internal sphincter should not be damaged.

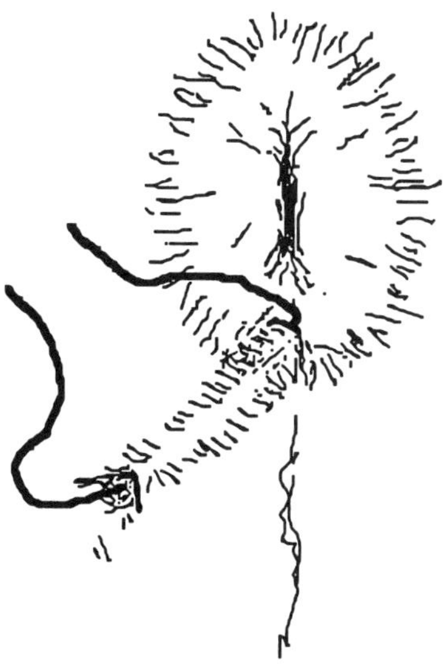

FIGURE 25.3.
Deep fistulae may be managed by passing a medium to heavy suture along the tract. The suture is tied and allowed to erode through the tissues with time. This technique has generally been superseded by direct fistulotomy.

Special Notes

Anal fistulectomy is often performed under general or spinal anesthesia in an ambulatory surgery unit. The presence of a sentinel pile should suggest the presence of an anal fissure rather than a fistula. Patients with anal fistulae should be evaluated for the possibility of inflammatory bowel disease. Fistulectomy or fistulotomy should not be performed in patients who have diarrhea or active inflammatory bowel disease.

Suggested Readings

Bassford T. Treatment of common anorectal disorders. *Am Fam Phys* 1992;45:1787.
Hancock BD. ABC of colorectal diseases. Anal fissures and fistulas. *BMJ* 1992;304:904.

Chapter 26

ANOSCOPY

Anoscopy is a useful procedure for diagnosis in both the office and emergency department. It is generally included as a part of colonoscopy or sigmoidoscopy and is useful for evaluating rectal pain, bleeding, or itching and assessing fissures, fistulae, or hemorrhoids.

Equipment

- Anoscope and light source (these vary from 7 to 10 cm in length and may have a light source that is attached or separate; some units are solid cylinders, whereas others have one or more open sides to allow direct inspection of the rectal epithelium without compression; disposable and reusable units are available)
- Examination gloves
- Water-based lubricant
- Large-tipped cotton swabs (such as those used for colposcopy)
- Biopsy forceps and Monsel's solution (optional)
- Assistant (desirable)

Training/Credentialing

Some experience is required; best to have received advanced instruction or experience before attempting alone. No special credentialing is needed for office procedure, but many hospitals or ambulatory surgery centers have special requirements for training or proficiency.

Coding

46600	Anoscopy
46606	Anoscopy with biopsy, single or multiple
46615	Anoscopy with ablation of tumor(s), polyp(s), or other lesion(s)

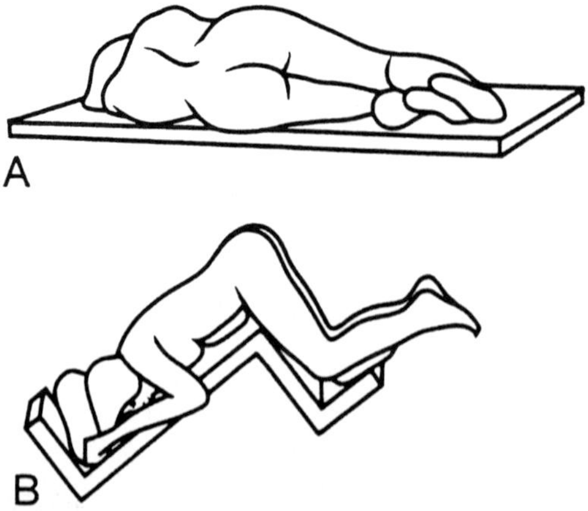

A

B

FIGURE 26.1.
A, *The left lateral (Sims) position may be used for anoscopy, flexible sigmoidoscopy, and hemorrhoidal or other anal surgery.* ***B,*** *When an adjustable table is available, the modified knee-chest position may be preferable. (Reproduced with permission from Simon RR, Brenner BE.* Emergency Procedures and Techniques. *3rd ed. Baltimore: Williams & Wilkins, 1994:19.)*

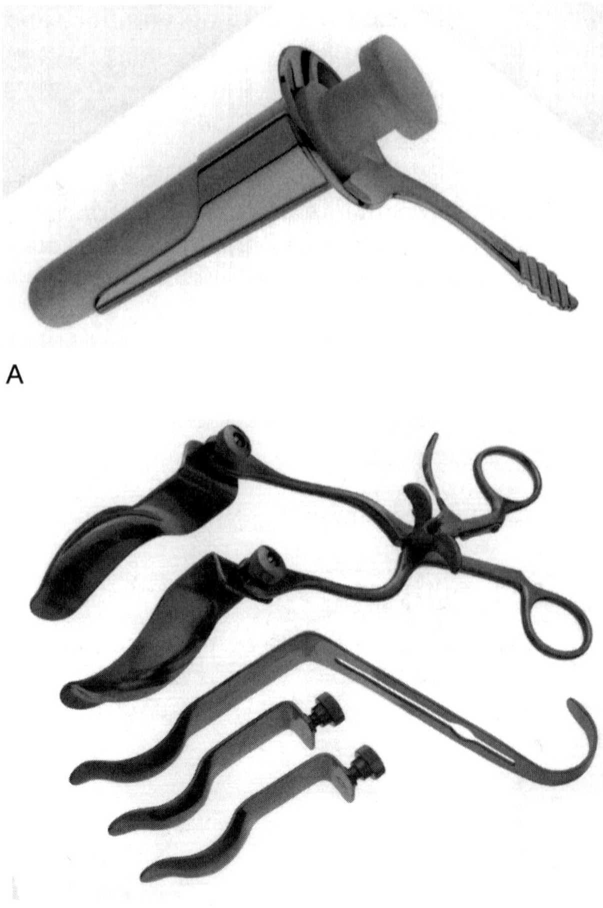

A

B

FIGURE 26.2.
*If a solid anoscope is used (**A**), it should always be inserted with the obturator in place. Open anoscopes (**B**) should be inserted in the closed position, with care being taken to avoid pinching the tissues in the blades during insertion or withdrawal. (part A, Ives Anoscope; part B, Parks Anal Retractor). (Courtesy of Baxter HealthCare, V. Mueller Division, 1435 Lake Cook Road, Deerfield, IL 60015.)*

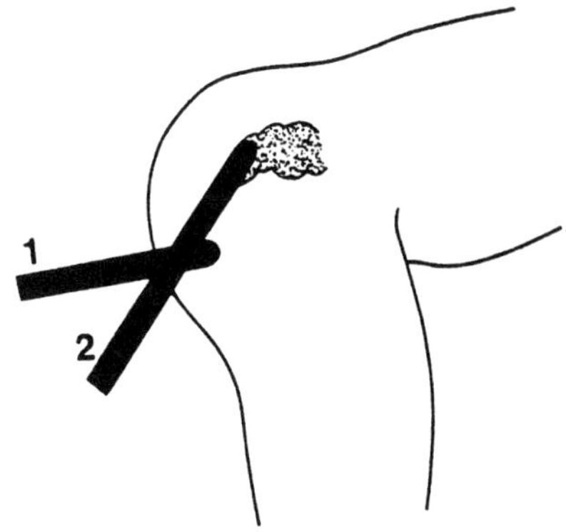

FIGURE 26.3.
The anoscope is first advanced in the direction of the umbilicus. Once the anal canal is traversed (as in proctoscopy or flexible sigmoidoscopy), the instrument should be directed posteriorly, toward the sacrum. (Reproduced with permission from Simon RR, Brenner BE. Emergency Procedures and Techniques. *3rd ed. Baltimore: Williams & Wilkins, 1994:19.)*

Technique

The patient should be placed in the left lateral (Sims') position and draped appropriately (Fig. 26.1*A*). If an adjustable table (such as that used for sigmoidoscopy) is available, the modified knee-chest position may be preferable (Fig. 26.1*B*). The glutei are separated laterally by the assistant or through the use of wide adhesive tape (the latter is less desirable). The examination begins with external inspection with the patient relaxed and with use of the Valsalva maneuver. Digital examination in which the finger is lubricated with water-based lubricant or topical anesthetic jelly (such as 2% lidocaine) should be done.

The anoscope (Fig. 26.2), with obturator in place, is lubricated and placed against the anal opening. Gentle pressure is applied until the resistance of the sphincters is overcome. The anoscope is gently advanced in the direction of the umbilicus until the full length has been inserted, or as tolerated by the patient (Fig. 26.3). The insertion process may be facilitated if the patient takes slow, deep breaths. Once the anoscope is in place, the obturator is removed and the anal canal inspected. Fecal matter may be removed with large cotton-tipped swabs. The tissues are inspected as the anoscope is gradually removed. With open-sided anoscopes, a side-to-side rotation of the instrument as it is withdrawn facilitates inspection of the anal sidewalls; however, repeated insertion and withdrawal may be needed to inspect all four quadrants.

Superficial biopsy specimens may be obtained using the same biopsy forceps used for cervical samples. Bleeding may be controlled with Monsel's solution if necessary.

Normal Findings

Inspection should include the condition of the mucosa, the pectinated line, internal hemorrhoids, and any vascular changes.

Selected Abnormal Findings

Blood, mucous, or pus is abnormal and should prompt further investigation or referral.

Special Notes

Because patients dread anoscopy, care in the preparation of patients is paramount. The patient should be reassured that although the procedure may be embarrassing, unpleasant, or even uncomfortable, it should not be painful and that few if any complications ever arise. Having the patient use an enema before the examination is not required but is helpful.

Suggested Readings

Cosman BC, Lennon SE, Perkash I. Hinged anoscope. *Dis Colon Rectum* 1993;36:1069.

Farmer KC, Church JM. Open sesame: tips for traversing the anal canal. *Dis Colon Rectum* 1992;35:1092.

Lazas DJ, Moses FM, Wong RK. Videoendoscopic anoscopy: a new technique for examining the anal canal. *Gastrointest Endos* 1995;42:351.

Rosen L. Physical examination of the anorectum: a systematic approach. *Dis Colon Rectum* 1990;33:439.

Said S, Huber P, Pichlmaier H. Technique and clinical results of endorectal surgery. *Surgery* 1993;113:65.

Chapter 27

DRAINAGE OF THROMBOSED HEMORRHOIDS

Thrombosed hemorrhoids produce substantial pain but pose little risk. Evacuation of the thrombosis rapidly relieves pain.

Equipment

- Local anesthetic of choice, 25-gauge needle
- #15 knife blade
- Fine (3-0 or 4-0) absorbable suture
- Sterile gloves, antiseptic solution, and sterile cotton balls or skin preparation swabs
- Assistant (desirable)

Training/Credentialing

Minimal experience: it is best to have observed or assisted on a few before attempting alone. No special credentialing is needed; office procedure only.

Coding

46083	Incision of thrombosed hemorrhoid, external

Technique

The patient should be placed in the knee-chest position as for anoscopy (Figure 17.1*B*) and draped as appropriately for access and modesty. The left lateral Sims' position may be used but is generally less satisfactory. To aid in gaining access to the anus and the involved hemorrhoid, an assistant can retract the buttocks; the buttocks can also be retracted through the use of tape (Fig. 27.1).

The base of the thrombosed hemorrhoid should be infiltrated with local anesthetic

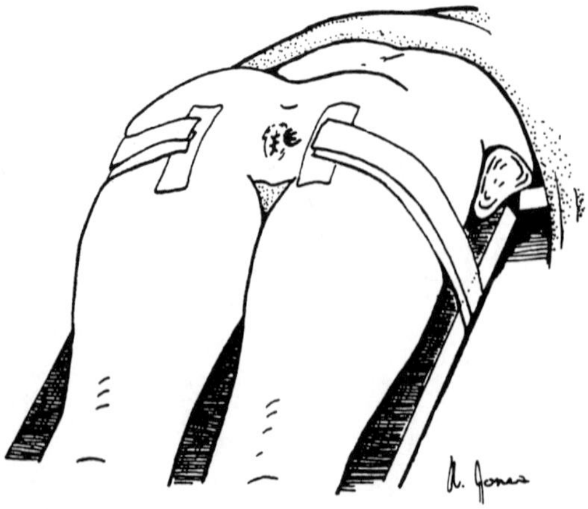

FIGURE 27.1.
When a thrombosed external hemorrhoid is being excised, separating the buttocks using 3-inch adhesive tape provides optimal exposure. (Reproduced with permission from Simon RR, Brenner BE. Emergency Procedures and Techniques. *3rd ed. Baltimore: Williams & Wilkins, 1994:26.)*

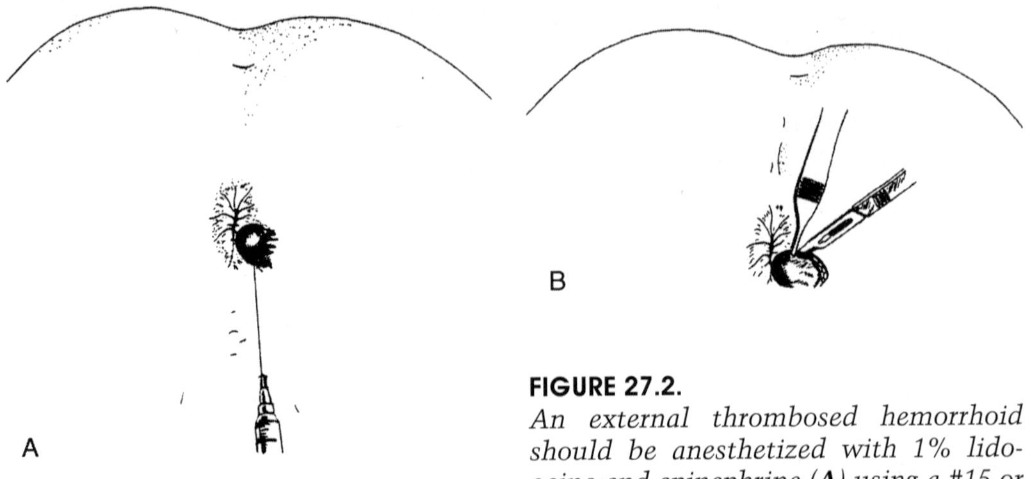

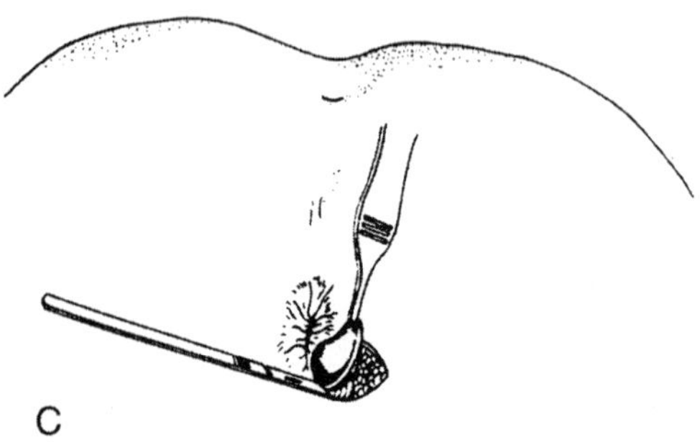

FIGURE 27.2.
*An external thrombosed hemorrhoid should be anesthetized with 1% lidocaine and epinephrine (**A**) using a #15 or #11 blade. The hemorrhoid is excised in an elliptical fashion at its base (**B**). A wedge of skin and the subcutaneous tissue that contain additional clots should also be excised (**C**). (Reproduced with permission from Simon RR, Brenner BE.* Emergency Procedures and Techniques. *3rd ed. Baltimore: Williams & Wilkins, 1994:23.)*

(Fig. 27.2*A*). The apex of the hemorrhoid is incised longitudinally, and pressure is applied to the base of the hemorrhoid to expel the clot. An instrument, such as a curved hemostat or small curette, may also be used to evacuate the clot. If needed, the incision may be closed with a running suture. The thrombosed hemorrhoid may also be excised in its entirety by using an elliptical incision (Figs. 27.2*B–C*).

Normal Findings

One or more hemorrhoids may be thrombosed. The removed clot is generally linear and well organized.

Selected Abnormal Findings

Histologic evaluation must be done if the tissue overlying the hemorrhoid is abnormal or if tissue other than clot is present in the material removed.

Suggested Readings

Bleday R, Pena JP, Rothenberger DA, et al. Symptomatic hemorrhoids: current incidence and complications of operative therapy. *Dis Colon Rectum* 1992;35:477.

MacRae HM, McLeod RS. Comparison of hemorrhoidal treatment modalities. A meta-analysis. *Dis Colon Rectum* 1995;38:687.

Medich DS, Fazio VW. Hemorrhoids, anal fissure, and carcinoma of the colon, rectum, and anus during pregnancy. *Surg Clin North Am* 1995;75:77.

Chapter 28

ENDOSCOPIC COLON BIOPSY

Many practitioners choose not to consider a biopsy at the time of flexible sigmoidoscopy or colonoscopy; however, when limited to superficial pinch biopsy, the technique is safe and effective.

Equipment

- Basic equipment for proctosigmoidoscopy (see Chapter 29, Flexible Sigmoidoscopy)
- Endoscopic biopsy forceps
- Electrosurgical generator and instruments (optional and recommended only for persons with advanced training or experience)
- Buffered formalin or other material for specimen preservation and transport

Training/Credentialing

Similar to that required for flexible sigmoidoscopy.

Coding

45330	Sigmoidoscopy, flexible; diagnostic, with or without collection of specimen(s) by brushing or washing (separate procedure)
45331	with biopsy, single or multiple
45332	with removal of foreign body
45334	with control of bleeding, any method
45379	Colonoscopy, flexible, proximal to splenic flexure; with removal of foreign body
45380	with biopsy, single or multiple
45382	with control of bleeding, any method

Technique

The preparation of the patient and the basic technique of flexible sigmoidoscopy is presumed (see Chapter 29, Flexible Sigmoidoscopy).

To perform an endoscopic biopsy of a small polyp or lesion, the closed biopsy forceps are passed down the biopsy channel until they emerge from the endoscope tip and are in the field of view. The jaws of the forceps are opened and the instrument is advanced to the lesion under direct vision. Most biopsy forceps contain a central needle tip or hook to facilitate stabilization of the instrument before obtaining the specimen. The forceps should be firmly advanced to stabilize the tissue to be sampled. The jaws of the device are closed and it is sharply withdrawn, separating the sample from the underlying tissue. The forceps (with specimen) are then withdrawn from the endoscope. If several biopsy samples are to be obtained, the action is repeated. The biopsy site must be inspected for bleeding, and adequate hemostasis should be established before the procedure is completed. Any tissue obtained must be placed separately in formalin or other transport media. The exact location from which the tissue was obtained must be documented.

Normal Findings

Most benign polyps have a smooth appearance, somewhat similar to that of endocervical polyps.

TABLE 28.1. Considerations in the Decision to Offer Endoscopic Colon Biopsy

Training	Gynecologists are inadequately trained for endoscopic colon biopsy	Endoscopic colon biopsy is little different from procedures performed by other endoscopic techniques
Risk	Endoscopic biopsy increases the risk of the procedure	When biopsy is performed with biopsy forceps and involves only the superficial 2 to 3 mm of mucosa, perforation or other complication is rare
	Performing a biopsy may increase malpractice exposure	Failure to establish a diagnosis may increase malpractice exposure
Futility	Many biopsies will have to be repeated Follow-up colonoscopy by a specialist is almost always warranted despite the biopsy findings	Many findings (e.g., hyperplasia) will obviate further evaluation or biopsy; when abnormalities are demonstrated, they may direct further evaluation in a more efficient manner
	Biopsy need not be done on small polyps	Small lesions are often difficult to diagnose without biopsy

TABLE 28.2. Relative Contraindications to Endoscopic Colon Biopsy

- Blood dyscrasia
- Inability to fully visualize entire lesion
- Incompletely prepared bowel
- Lesions inside a diverticulum
- Ulcerated lesions
- Vascular lesions

Special Notes

Unresolved debate surrounds the decision to offer endoscopic colon biopsy and, specifically, the point at which biopsy should be done (Table 28.1). If the practitioner is considering offering biopsy, additional tutelage, instruction, or proctored experience is advisable. Relative contraindications to biopsy are shown in Table 28.2.

If a biopsy may be performed, preoperative bowel preparation must be done more rigorously. This is especially true if an electrosurgical generator is to be used; bowel gas is potentially explosive. Therapy with anticoagulant agents and aspirin should be discontinued, reduced, or monitored to ensure adequate hemostasis.

Suggested Readings

DeCosse JJ, Tsioulias GJ, Jacobson JS. Colorectal cancer: detection, treatment, and rehabilitation. *CA Cancer J Clin* 1994;44:27.

Forde KA, Treat MR, Tsai JL. Initial clinical experience with a bipolar snare for colon polypectomy. *Surg Endos* 1993;7:427.

Varma JR, Mills LR. Colon polyps. *J Fam Pract* 1992;35:194.

Chapter 29

FLEXIBLE SIGMOIDOSCOPY

Flexible sigmoidoscopy has almost completely replaced the use of rigid sigmoidoscopy for screening and biopsy. With proper preparation, it may be performed in the office, an endoscopy suite, or an ambulatory surgery unit.

Equipment

- Flexible sigmoidoscope (60 or 65 cm), including body with controls, shaft, tip, and apertures (Fig. 29.1)
- Light source (compatible with sigmoidoscope chosen)
- Source of suction and air supply (if not part of a self-contained light unit designed for endoscopy [Fig. 29.2])
- Water-based lubricant
- Water for cleaning the instrument and suction channel
- Anoscopy supplies (anoscope, unsterile gloves, gauze pads)
- Biopsy forceps and fixative if biopsy is to be considered
- Video camera, monitor, videotape recorder, or film recorder (all are optional but common and useful for documentation and patient counseling)
- Disposable cover or sheath for the endoscope (advisable if available for the type and brand of sigmoidoscope used)

Training/Credentialing

Some experience is required; it is best to have received advanced instruction or experience before attempting on your own. No special credentialing is needed for office procedure, but many hospitals or ambulatory surgery centers have special requirements for training or proficiency.

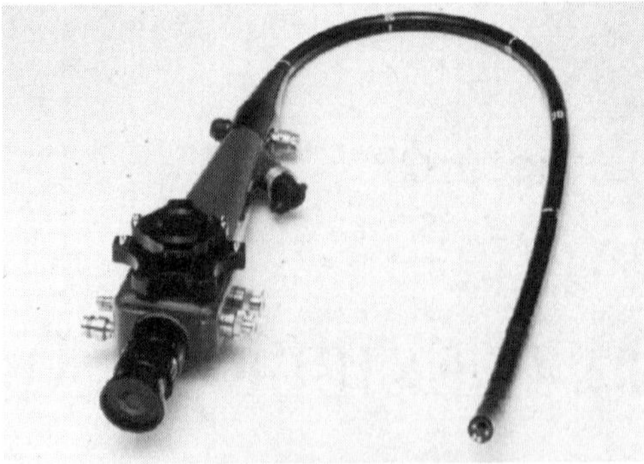

FIGURE 29.1.
Flexible sigmoidoscopes are available from several suppliers. All have some degree of similarity, but the operator should be familiar with the specifics of connections and control peculiar to the device being used. (Courtesy of Olympus America, Two Corporate Center Drive, Melville, NY 11747.)

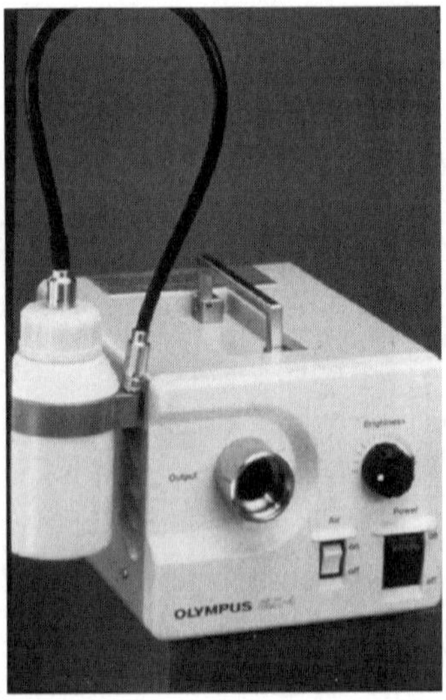

FIGURE 29.2.
Although connections vary by manufacturer, many sigmoidoscopes have systems that can supply integrated support functions such as light and suction. (Courtesy of Olympus America, Two Corporate Center Drive, Melville, NY 11747.)

Coding

45330	Sigmoidoscopy, flexible; diagnostic, with or without collection of specimen(s) by brushing or washing (separate procedure)
45331	with biopsy, single or multiple
45332	with removal of foreign body
45333	with removal of tumor(s), polyp(s), or lesion(s) by hot biopsy forceps or bipolar cautery
45334	with control of bleeding, any method
45338	with removal of tumor(s), polyp(s), or other lesion(s) by snare technique
45339	with ablation of tumor(s), polyp(s), or other lesion(s) not amenable to removal by hot biopsy forceps, bipolar cautery, or snare technique (e.g., laser)
45378	Colonoscopy, flexible, proximal to splenic flexure; diagnostic, with or without collection of specimen(s) by brushing or washing, with or without colon decompression (separate procedure)
45379	with removal of foreign body

45380	with biopsy, single or multiple
45382	with control of bleeding, any method
45383	with ablation of tumor(s), polyp(s), or other lesion(s) not amenable to removal by hot biopsy forceps, bipolar cautery, or snare technique (e.g., laser)
45384	with removal of tumor(s), polyp(s), or lesion(s) by hot biopsy forceps or bipolar cautery
45385	with removal of tumor(s), polyp(s), or other lesion(s) by snare technique

Technique

PATIENT PREPARATION

The perceived invasive nature of proctosigmoidoscopy makes education and counseling before the procedure highly desirable. This should include information on the procedure required for informed consent but also must address the issues of embarrassment and discomfort that accompany the procedure.

Physical preparation of the patient includes cleansing of the bowel and antibiotic prophylaxis for specific patients. The bowel may be mechanically cleansed immediately before the procedure by simple enema (water or such commercial products as Fleet). This should be administered until clear fluid is returned. Generally, two enemas must be done to yield clear fluid, and 30–60 minutes should be allowed for adequate preparation. There is no need to restrict oral intake or the use of regularly prescribed medications.

Premedication with 800 mg of ibuprofen or an equally effective dose of any other nonsteroidal anti-inflammatory agent can provide good analgesia for the procedure. Oral diazepam or intramuscular sedatives may be given but are often not required.

The final steps in patient preparation include assessment of the patient's status and patient positioning. Immediately before the procedure is started, vital signs (including temperature, pulse, respiration, and blood pressure) should be taken. The heart and lungs should be examined by auscultation and the abdomen examined by both auscultation and palpation. If no contraindications to the procedure are found, the patient is placed in the left lateral Sims' position and appropriately draped for modesty and access.

ENDOSCOPY PROCEDURE

Both the endoscopist and assistant should don gloves and the endoscope prepared by lubricating the distal 3–4 cm with a water-soluble surgical lubricant, taking care to avoid the distal optics of the device. If a disposable cover is available, it should be used to facilitate clean-up after the case. The endoscope should be straightened and the position of the control dials noted. Appropriate connections to sources of light, air, water, and suction should be made and tested (Fig. 29.3).

To begin the procedure, the gluteal folds are retracted and a rectal examination is performed using a lubricated finger. This allows an initial assessment, alerts the examiner to possible obstruction, stool, or lesions; relaxes the anal sphincter; and lubricates the distal rectum. Anoscopy may be performed at this point, if desired.

The body (control portion) of the endoscope is held in the left hand with the palm upward, while the right hand grasps the shaft with one or more extended fingers stabilizing the tip. Because of the design of most endoscopes, these hand positions should

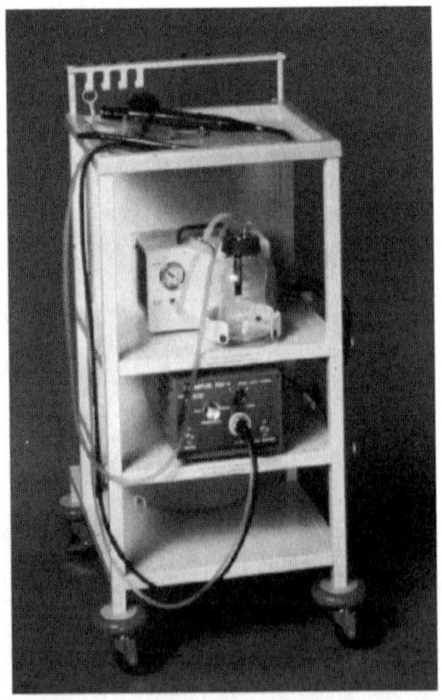

FIGURE 29.3.
Flexible sigmoidoscopy can be facilitated by combining the necessary equipment and supplies onto one rolling cart. (Courtesy of Olympus America, Two Corporate Center Drive, Melville, NY 11747.)

be used for both right- and left-handed endoscopists. The tip of the sigmoidoscope is inserted through the sphincter and advanced blindly, being directed somewhat posteriorly. Once the instrument has been advanced 8–10 cm, the light source is activated and the view checked.

Under direct vision, the endoscope is gently advanced by the right hand while the left hand operates suction, air, and water controls and directs the flexible portion of the tip through manipulation of the dials located on the side of the control head. As an alternative, the assistant may gently advance the shaft of the sigmoidoscope while the endoscopist's right hand is used to manipulated the dials. With this technique, any advancement of the shaft by the assistant must be under the direction of the endoscopist and must never be pursued in the face of resistance.

To obtain the best view and to allow advancement of the endoscope, the lumen of the bowel must be gently distended with air. This may be accomplished with a bulb insufflator or the mechanical air supply available with many endoscopy light sources. Only an amount of air sufficient to allow vision and scope advancement should be used. Over-distention produces discomfort and may result in damage to the bowel (including perforation).

With a clear view forward, the endoscope is gently advanced. This should be accomplished by the repetitive sequence of insufflation, alignment of the tip of the endoscope with the axis of the lumen, and advancement of the body of the endoscope. If the tip of the endoscope comes in contact with the wall of the bowel, the field of view becomes opaque red or white with no details visible and no lumen apparent. If this occurs, the endoscope should be slightly withdrawn, additional air introduced, and advancement again attempted. Other techniques that are useful when insertion is particularly difficult are summarized below. Advancement should continue as far as possible without any effort to carefully examine the bowel in the process; careful inspection is reserved for the withdrawal phase of the examination.

The withdrawal portion of the examination is the easiest phase mechanically but the most important for diagnosis and screening. As the sigmoidoscope is withdrawn, the tip should be flexed back and forth and the shaft of the endoscope rotated to and fro to allow the entire circumference of the lumen to be inspected. Extra care must be exerted to inspect portions of the bowel wall that fall behind fold or turns. Inspection of these areas may require additional distention or slight readvancement and withdrawal of the endoscope. This continues until the rectum is reached. Polyps or lesions that are encountered should be documented; biopsy specimens may be taken on the basis of need, the experience of the operator, and the availability of equipment (see Chapter 28, Endoscopic Colon Biopsy).

The procedure is completed by inspecting the anal canal. This may be accomplished by hooking the flexible tip of the sigmoidoscope back onto itself to allow visualization or by separately performing anoscopy. (See the section on anoscopy for a description of this procedure.) As the sigmoidoscope is removed from the anus, care must be taken to avoid dropping or otherwise damaging the delicate tip and associated optics.

Once the procedure has been completed, soapy water should be aspirated through the suction port, debris expelled from the air port, and the exterior of the endoscope wiped with soap and water to facilitate final cleanup.

THE DIFFICULT ADVANCEMENT

Insertion of a sigmoidoscope may be difficult in older patients and in those who have postoperative or other adhesions. Redundancy or fixation of sigmoid may make advancement of the endoscope by simple pressure difficult or ineffective. A view that does not change as the shaft is advanced or increased resistance to insertion suggests that a problem is present and that an alternative technique should be used.

One of the simplest alternatives consists of to-and-fro advancement coupled with twisting of the shaft. In this technique, the shaft is withdrawn by 5–10 cm while the shaft is rotated 45–60° in a clockwise direction. This twisting motion is reversed (counterclockwise) as the endoscope is readvanced. This combination of retreat, advance, and twisting tends to straighten the sigmoid and allow the endoscope to pass in an accordion-like fashion. This series of maneuvers is most successful when a redundant sigmoid is the problem (e.g., in elderly persons). This technique is generally well tolerated by the patient and, with care, is safe.

Another method that may help with a difficult insertion is to hook a mucosal fold, pull back, release, and advance. To perform this technique, the tip of the endoscope is flexed 30–90° to catch a mucosal fold and draw it downward as the endoscope is slightly withdrawn. This will straighten out a short segment of the colon, enabling the sigmoidoscope to then be advanced. This maneuver must only be done in the face of minimal or no resistance to the withdrawal phase.

Other more involved (and dangerous) techniques have been described, but these are best left for experienced endoscopists.

Normal Findings

Three "valves" of Houston will be encountered at approximately 6, 9, and 12 cm. These will appear as semilunar ridges that may hamper the advancement of the sigmoidoscope. Advancement past these valves may be facilitated by directing the flexible tip of the instrument toward the axis of the lumen and away from the valve.

Selected Abnormal Findings

A red field of view indicates contact with the wall, whereas a white field of view indicates that the endoscope tip provides pressure sufficient to cause ischemia. In both cases, the sigmoidoscope must be slightly withdrawn until the axis of the lumen can be reacquired.

If the field of view becomes dark with no indication of direction, overdistension of the bowel lumen is probable. Release of some of the distending air allows the lumen to collapse, making the axis of movement again apparent. This is most likely to occur in the area of the rectal vault.

Special Notes

Routine screening through flexible sigmoidoscopy is recommended for all patients older than 50 years of age, with follow-up examinations every 3–5 years. Screening should begin at age 35–40 years for patients with significant risk factors, including a family history of colon cancer. Common indications for flexible sigmoidoscopy are shown in Table 29.1 and contraindications are shown in Table 29.2.

Flexible fiberoptic sigmoidoscopes are available in 35-cm lengths in addition to the 60- and 65-cm types discussed above. In general, these shorter instruments have limited utility, making the investment in the longer instruments more advisable.

Some authors suggest that the use of aspirin should be discontinued 2 weeks before sigmoidoscopy.

Once the sigmoidoscope has been withdrawn from the patient, some authors suggest reinserting it 5–8 cm and using the suction to help remove any residual air. If suction is used, care must be taken that it be applied only intermittently and that the bowel wall is not inadvertently damaged by being drawn into the suction opening.

TABLE 29.1. Common Indications for Flexible Sigmoidoscopy

Abdominal pain
Change in bowel habits
Crohn's disease
New or persistent constipation
Protracted diarrhea
Follow-up of previous polypectomy
Occult blood in stool
Rectal bleeding
Ulcerative colitis
Unexplained weight anemia
Unexplained weight fever
Unexplained weight loss

TABLE 29.2. Contraindications to Flexible Sigmoidoscopy

- Absolute
  - Active diverticulitis
  - Acute abdomen
  - Blood dyscrasia or coagulopathy
  - Acute or severe cardiopulmonary disease
  - Inadequate bowel preparation
  - Subacute bacterial endocarditis or prosthetic heart valve without adequate antibiotic prophylaxis
  - Suspected bowel perforation
- Relative
  - Active infection
  - Peritonitis
  - Pregnancy
  - Recent abdominal surgery

Suggested Readings

Ballas MT, Markert RJ, Oler MJ. Screening flexible sigmoidoscopy and insurance reimbursement. *J Fam Pract* 1995;40:535.

Coller JA. Technique of flexible fiberoptic sigmoidoscopy. *Surg Clin North Am* 1980;60:456.

DeCosse JJ, Tsioulias GJ, Jacobson JS. Colorectal cancer: detection, treatment, and rehabilitation. *CA Cancer J Clin* 1994;44:27.

Lee MG. Comparison of three bowel preparations for sigmoidoscopy. *West Ind Med J* 1993;42:118.

Levine R, Tenner S, Fromm H. Prevention and early detection of colorectal cancer. *Am Fam Phys* 1992;45:663.

Moran JA. Flexible fibreoptic sigmoidoscopy. Safe and effective for family practice. *Can Fam Phys* 1993;39:1927.

Preston KL, Peluso FE, Goldner F. Optimal bowel preparation for flexible sigmoidoscopy—are two enemas better than one? *Gastrointest Endos* 1994;40:474.

Ransohoff DF, Lang CA. Sigmoidoscopic screening in the 1990s. *JAMA* 1993;269:1278.

Reed DN, Collins JD, Wyatt WJ. Can general surgeons perform colonoscopy safely? *Am J Surg* 1992;163:257.

Renneker M, Saner H. Low-cost flexible sigmoidoscopy screening: a community demonstration and education project. *J Cancer Ed* 1995;10:25.

Rex DK, Mark D, Clarke B, et al. Flexible sigmoidoscopy plus air-contrast barium enema versus colonoscopy for evaluation of symptomatic patients without evidence of bleeding. *Gastrointest Endos* 1995;42:132.

Rothstein RI, Littenberg B. Disposable, sheathed, flexible sigmoidoscopy: a prospective, multicenter, randomized trial. The Disposable Endoscope Study Group. *Gastrointest Endos* 1995;41:566.

Singh S, Bowditch M, Dennison A, et al. Sigmoidoscopy with a view. *Br J Surg* 1994;81:1795.

Twist MH, Vipond MN, Veitch PS. Flexible sigmoidoscopy in addition to contrast enema in the diagnosis of left-sided large bowel obstruction. *Br J Surg* 1994;81:1670.

Varma JR, Mills LR. Colon polyps. *J Fam Pract* 1992;35:194.

Chapter 30

HEMORRHOID BANDING

Hemorrhoids occur in an estimated 50–80% of all Americans. As a result, the ability to offer simple office-based therapy for these problems has become an important part of the primary care of women. Although the first line of therapy for symptomatic hemorrhoids remains medical (stool softeners, bowel movement regulation, and topical medications), surgical therapy is appropriate for patients with debilitating symptoms or failed medical therapy (15–20% of cases). Banding of internal hemorrhoids is better accepted by patients than is traditional surgical therapy. Hemorrhoidal banding requires a minimum of equipment and is well suited to the office or outpatient surgical setting.

Equipment

- Anoscope (operating or open-sided) and light source
- Band applier (e.g., Barron or McGivney ligator), similar to that used for endoscopic tubal occlusion (Fig. 30.1)
- Alligator clamp or other grasping instrument (if the band applier does not contain its own grasping device)
- Examination gloves
- Water-based lubricant
- Large-tipped cotton swabs (such as those used for colposcopy)
- Biopsy forceps and Monsel's solution (optional)
- Assistant (desirable)

Training/Credentialing

Some experience is required; it is best to have received advanced instruction or experience before attempting the procedure alone. No special credentialing is needed for office procedure, but many hospitals or ambulatory surgery centers have special requirements for training or proficiency.

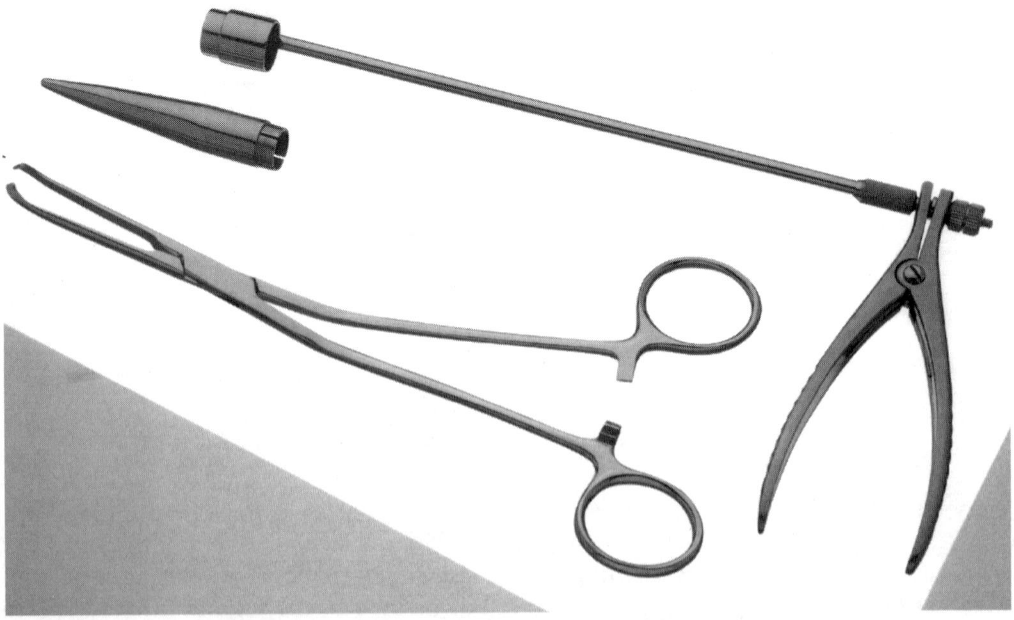

FIGURE 30.1.
The equipment used for hemorrhoid banding consists of a band applier, grasping forceps, and a cone-shaped device to facilitate loading the elastic bands. (McGivney hemorrhoidal ligator. Courtesy of Baxter HealthCare, V. Mueller Division, 1435 Lake Cook Road, Deerfield, IL 60015.)

Coding

46221	Hemorrhoidectomy, by simple ligature (e.g., rubber band)
46250	Hemorrhoidectomy, external, complete
46255	Hemorrhoidectomy, internal and external, simple
46257	with fissurectomy
46258	with fistulectomy, with or without fissurectomy
46934	Destruction of hemorrhoids, any method: internal
46935	external
46936	internal and external
46945	Ligature of internal hemorrhoids: single procedure
46946	multiple procedure

Technique

PATIENT PREPARATION

Preparation of the patient may include cleansing of the bowel and for some patients, antibiotic prophylaxis. Mechanical cleansing of the bowel is desirable but not absolutely necessary. The bowel may be cleansed immediately before the procedure by simple enema (water or such commercial products as Fleet). The enema should be administered until clear fluid is returned.

As with mechanical bowel cleansing, premedication should be at the discretion of the clinician and based on the needs and desires of the patient. Premedication with 800 mg of ibuprofen or an equally effective dose of any other nonsteroidal anti-inflammatory agent can provide good analgesia for the procedure. Oral diazepam or intramuscular sedatives may be given but are usually not required.

PROCEDURE

The patient should be placed in the left lateral (Sims') position or the modified knee-chest position. (A prone position may be used if assistance with retraction of the buttocks is available.) Anoscopy must be performed before any treatment decision (see Chapter 26, Anoscopy). Anoscopy helps establish the diagnosis to be established, assess the extent of the hemorrhoids, and determine their origin (Fig. 30.2). Banding techniques are appropriate only for the treatment of internal hemorrhoids (those arising above the pectinate line); external hemorrhoids must be treated by excision (see Chapter 31, Hemorrhoid Excision (External)). Banding is best suited for moderate to large internal hemorrhoids and those that undergo prolapse. Patient comfort and compliance are greatest if only one group of hemorrhoids is treated at any one visit. For this reason, the worst hemorrhoids are generally treated first; others are treated on return visits.

The band applier should be loaded with two elastic bands immediately before the procedure (Fig. 30.3). Most of these instruments have a cone-shaped attachment to facilitate the placement of the bands into their correct position (Fig. 30.1). (Loading is accomplished in much the same manner as that employed for the band applier used for laparoscopic sterilization procedures.)

To perform the ligation, the lubricated anoscope is inserted and the hemorrhoids to be treated are brought into clear view. The anoscope should be stabilized by the assistant, and the hemorrhoid should be grasped at its apex with grasping forceps. If the band applier used does not have such a grasping capability built in, the forceps used must be passed through the drum of the band applier before the hemorrhoid is grasped

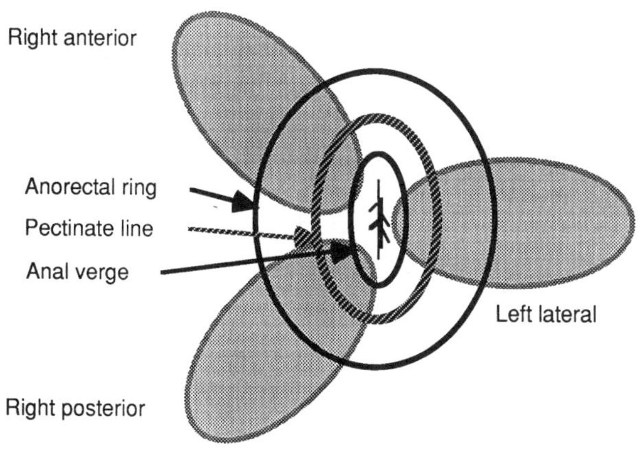

FIGURE 30.2.
ecause of vascular architecture of the anal canal, internal hemorrhoids are generally found in three positions: left lateral, right anterior, and right posterior. These positions are shown as seen during gynecologic examination in the dorsal lithotomy position. When therapy for hemorrhoids is undertaken, the patient is often placed in the left lateral decubitus (Sims') position or in a modification of the knee-chest position.

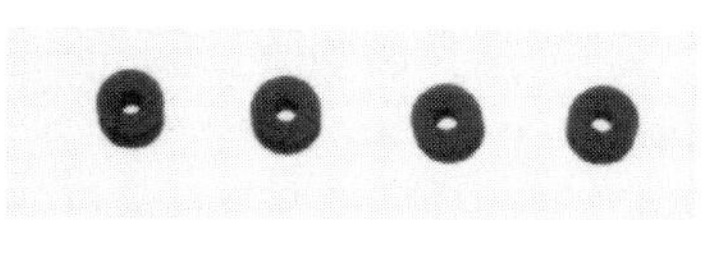

FIGURE 30.3.
Small elastic bands such as these are loaded on the tip of the applicator. Most applicators are designed to hold two bands at a time. (Latex O bands. Courtesy of Baxter HealthCare, V. Mueller Division, 1435 Lake Cook Road, Deerfield, IL 60015.)

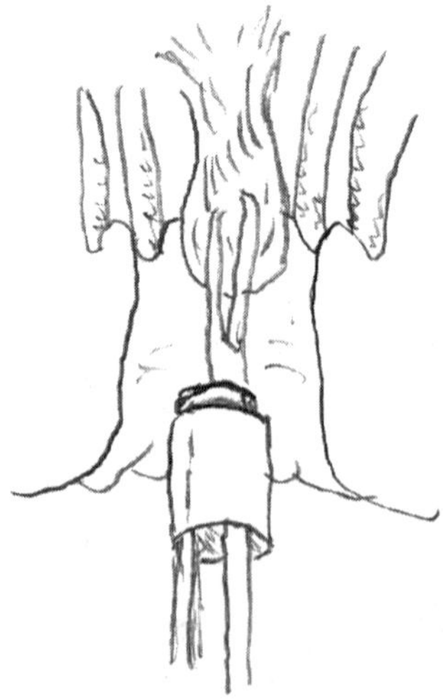

FIGURE 30.4.
The hemorrhoid to be banded should be grasped so that it may be drawn into the banding instrument.

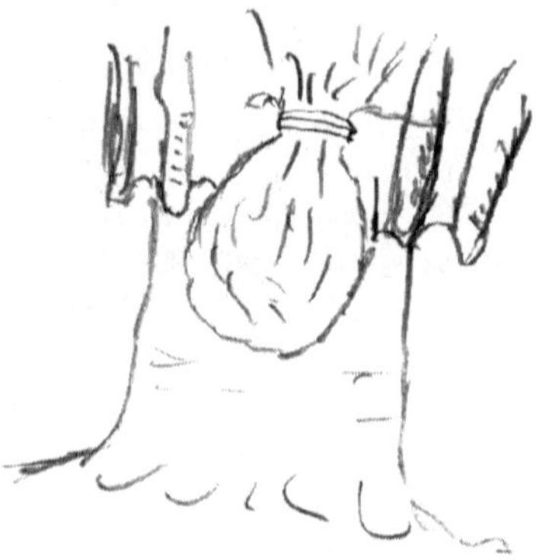

FIGURE 30.5.
When correctly placed, both elastic bands should rest near the base of the internal hemorrhoid.

(Fig. 30.4). If pain is experienced, the hemorrhoid should be released and regrasped more proximally, above the level of innervation. The hemorrhoid is then drawn into the drum of the band applier as it is advanced to rest against the base of the hemorrhoid. The handle of the ligator is squeezed, thereby releasing the bands from the tip of the instruments. Once both bands have been released, the grasping and ligating instruments may be removed. The site should be inspected to ensure adequate placement (Fig. 30.5); the anoscope should then be removed. Follow-up and further banding, if needed, should be scheduled for 3 to 4 weeks.

Normal Findings

Most patients will experience some mild aching for the first 2–3 days after surgery. Mild bleeding may be expected in 1–2 weeks as the hemorrhoidal tissue undergoes necrosis and slough. Sitz baths and topical analgesics (e.g., witch hazel, Balneol) may be used as needed. Wiping after a bowel movement using a moistened tissue or a medicated wipe, such as those used for diaper changes, may be preferable to using a dry tissue. Consumption of a high-fiber diet, use of stool softeners, and adequate fluid intake should be encouraged.

Selected Abnormal Findings

If immediate discomfort is experienced, the bands may be too close to the pectinate line (where innervation begins). The bands should be clipped with scissors and new bands applied in a more proximal location.

TABLE 30.1. Contraindications to Banding of Hemorrhoids

Acquired immunodeficiency syndrome or immunocompromise
Anorectal fissures
Bleeding diathesis or blood dyscrasia
Inflammatory bowel disease
Portal hypertension
Rectal prolapse
Undiagnosed anorectal tumor
Undiagnosed rectal bleeding

After surgery, increased pain, bleeding, or fever should be reported promptly. Urinary retention can be an early sign of perineal sepsis and should suggest immediate evaluation.

Special Notes

Hemorrhoids are classified according to their location of origin (not the most distal extension): those that arise above the dentate line are internal hemorrhoids; those that arise below the pectinate (dentate) line are external hemorrhoids. Internal hemorrhoids are void of somatic enervation and are covered only by intestinal mucosa. External hemorrhoids, by contrast, are well enervated and covered by stratified squamous epithelium, similar to the skin of other areas of the body. Unipolar or bipolar electrosurgical techniques may be used instead of banding procedures. Contraindications to hemorrhoid banding are shown in Table 30.1.

Suggested Readings

Bassford T. Treatment of common anorectal disorders. *Am Fam Phys* 1992;45:1787.

Bleday R, Pena JP, Rothenberger DA, et al. Symptomatic hemorrhoids: current incidence and complications of operative therapy. *Dis Colon Rectum* 1992;35:477.

Devine R, Ory S. Treatment of hemorrhoids in pregnancy. *J Fam Pract* 1992;17:65.

Inoue H, Takemura K, Hori H, et al. Sclerotherapy of internal hemorrhoids using newly devised transparent disposable anorectoscope. *Surg Endos* 1992;6:125.

Johanson JF, Rimm A. Optimal nonsurgical treatment of hemorrhoids: a comparative analysis of infrared coagulation, rubber band ligation, and injection sclerotherapy. *Am J Gastroenterol* 1992;87:1600.

MacRae HM, McLeod RS. Comparison of hemorrhoidal treatment modalities. A meta-analysis. *Dis Colon Rectum* 1995;38:687.

Mazier WP. Hemorrhoids, fissures, and pruritus ani. *Surg Clin North Am* 1994;74:1277.

Medich DS, Fazio VW. Hemorrhoids, anal fissure, and carcinoma of the colon, rectum, and anus during pregnancy. *Surg Clin North Am* 1995;75:77.

Morinaga K, Hasuda K, Ikeda T. A novel therapy for internal hemorrhoids: ligation of the hemorrhoidal artery with a newly devised instrument (Moricorn) in conjunction with a Doppler flowmeter. *Am J Gastroenterol* 1995;90:610.

Schussman LC, Lutz LJ. Outpatient management of hemorrhoids. *Prim Care* 1986;13:527.

Chapter 31

HEMORRHOID EXCISION (EXTERNAL)

Unlike internal hemorrhoids, which may be treated with simple surgical techniques (banding) and a minimum of discomfort, external hemorrhoids that do not respond to conservative therapy require much more extensive surgical intervention. Local anesthesia, excision of the hemorrhoid and surrounding tissue, and suture repair are all required for the successful treatment of these hemorrhoids. Despite these limitations, however, office treatment is still possible.

Equipment

- Local anesthetic of choice, 25-gauge needle
- #15 or #11 knife blade, thumb forceps, fine tissue scissors (optional)
- Fine (3-0 or 4-0) absorbable suture
- Sterile gloves, antiseptic solution and sterile cotton balls, or skin preparation swabs
- Sterile draping material (optional)
- Anoscope (operating or open-sided) and light source
- Large-tipped cotton swabs (such as those used for colposcopy)
- Monsel's solution (optional)
- Assistant (desirable)

Training/Credentialing

Some experience is required; it is best to have received advanced instruction or experience before attempting the procedure alone. No special credentialing is needed for office procedure, but many hospitals or ambulatory surgery centers have special requirements for training or proficiency.

Coding

46250	Hemorrhoidectomy, external, complete
46255	Hemorrhoidectomy, internal and external, simple
46257	with fissurectomy
46258	with fistulectomy, with or without fissurectomy
46934	Destruction of hemorrhoids, any method: internal
46935	external
46936	internal and external

Technique

PATIENT PREPARATION

Special preparation of the patient is generally not required, but mechanical cleansing of the bowel may be desirable. If desired, the bowel may be cleansed immediately before the procedure by simple enema (water or such commercial products as Fleet). If used, the enema should be administered until clear fluid is returned.

Depending on the needs and desires of the patient, premedication with 800 mg of ibuprofen or an equally effective dose of any other nonsteroidal anti-inflammatory agent can provide good analgesia for the procedure. Oral diazepam or intramuscular sedatives may be given but are usually not required.

PROCEDURE

The patient should be placed in the left lateral (Sims') position or the modified knee-chest position. (A prone position may be used if assistance with retraction of the buttocks is available.) As with hemorrhoid banding, anoscopy must be performed before any treatment decision is made (see Chapter 26, Anoscopy). Anoscopy helps establish the diagnosis, assess the extent of the hemorrhoids, and determine their origin. Banding techniques are only appropriate for treating internal hemorrhoids; external hemorrhoids must be treated by excision, whereas banding techniques are more desirable if the hemorrhoids are internal (see Chapter 30, Hemorrhoid Banding).

The skin of the perineum and perianal area should be cleansed using a suitable surgical preparation method (e.g., Betadine scrub and solution, Hibiclens). Sterile draping may be placed at the discretion of the operator. A field block using local anesthetic is established by infiltrating around the anal opening in each of the four quadrants (Fig. 31.1). After adequate anesthesia has been established, an elliptical incision is made on either side of the hemorrhoid to be removed. The long axis of this incision should be directed in a radial manner toward the anal opening (Fig. 31.2). This incision is extended downward and toward the opposite incision, and the hemorrhoid is excised. The incision should be kept as superficial as possible but still ensure complete excision of the hemorrhoid. The incision may be closed with simple fine absorbable sutures or may be left open to heal by secondary intention.

Sitz baths and topical analgesics (e.g., witch hazel, Balneol) may be used as needed. Wiping after a bowel movement using a moistened tissue or a medicated wipe, such as those use for diaper changes, may be preferable to using a dry tissue. Consumption of a high-fiber diet, use of stool softeners, and adequate fluid intake should be encouraged.

After surgery, increased pain, bleeding, or fever should be reported promptly. Uri-

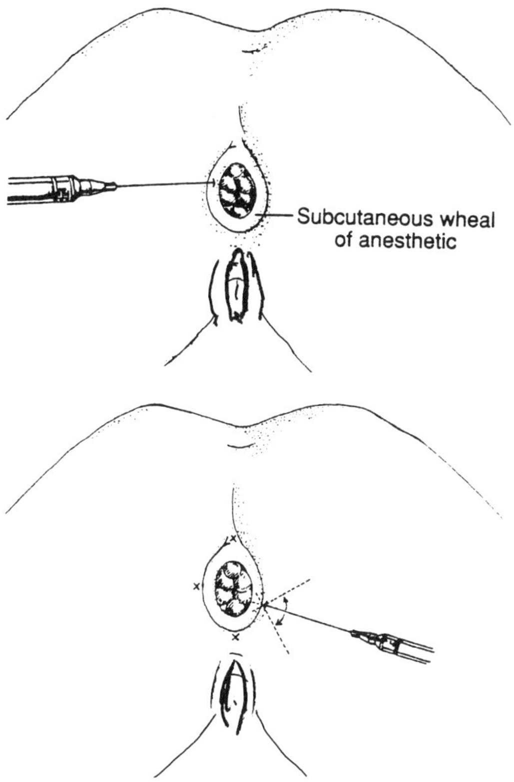

FIGURE 30.1.
An anesthetic wheal is deposited in each quadrant around the anus. This four-quadrant infiltration of anesthetic solutions is generally adequate to provide anesthesia for hemorrhoid excision. When only one relatively small hemorrhoid is to be excised, a field block involving only the area to be operated on may be used. (Modified from Simon RR, Brenner BE. Emergency Procedures and Techniques. *3rd ed. Baltimore: Williams & Wilkins, 1994:24.)*

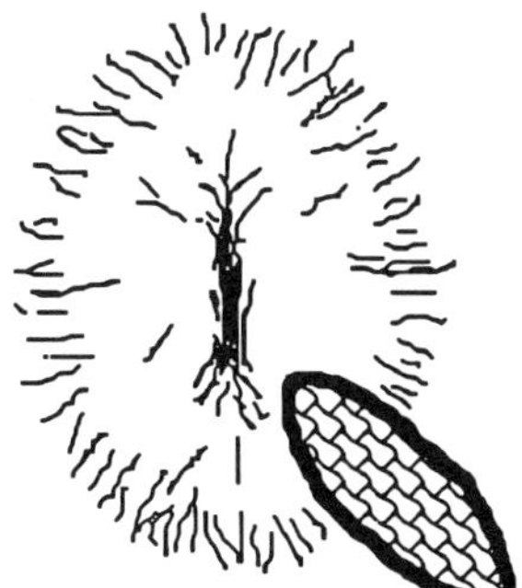

FIGURE 30.2.
When external hemorrhoids are excised, the elliptical incision should be oriented with its long axis radially aligned toward the opening of the anus.

TABLE 31.1. Contraindications to Excision of Hemorrhoids

Acquired immunodeficiency syndrome or immunocompromise
Anorectal fissures
Bleeding diathesis or blood dyscrasia
Inflammatory bowel disease
Portal hypertension
Rectal prolapse
Undiagnosed anorectal tumor
Undiagnosed rectal bleeding

nary retention can be an early sign of perineal sepsis and should suggest immediate evaluation. A follow-up appointment should be scheduled for 3 to 4 weeks.

Special Notes

External hemorrhoids are often excised under general or spinal anesthesia in an ambulatory surgery unit. Contraindications to hemorrhoid excision are shown in Table 31.1.

Suggested Readings

Bassford T. Treatment of common anorectal disorders. *Am Fam Phys* 1992;45:1787.

Bleday R, Pena JP, Rothenberger DA, et al. Symptomatic hemorrhoids: current incidence and complications of operative therapy. *Dis Colon Rectum* 1992;35:477.

Devine R, Ory S. Treatment of hemorrhoids in pregnancy. *J Fam Pract* 1992;17:65.

MacRae HM, McLeod RS. Comparison of hemorrhoidal treatment modalities. A meta-analysis. *Dis Colon Rectum* 1995;38:687.

Mazier WP. Hemorrhoids, fissures, and pruritus ani. *Surg Clin North Am* 1994;74:1277.

Medich DS, Fazio VW. Hemorrhoids, anal fissure, and carcinoma of the colon, rectum, and anus during pregnancy. *Surg Clin North Am* 1995;75:77.

Schussman LC, Lutz LJ. Outpatient management of hemorrhoids. *Prim Care* 1986;13:527.

Wolkomir AF, Luchtefeld MA. Surgery for symptomatic hemorrhoids and anal fissures in Crohn's disease. *Dis Colon Rectum* 1993;36:545.

Chapter 32

INGUINAL HERNIA REDUCTION

Indirect inguinal hernias are the most common type of groin hernia and are found most commonly in children and young adults. Indirect hernias result in a hernia sac that is lateral to the inferior epigastric vessels, whereas a direct hernia is medial to these vessels. Femoral hernias are more common in adult women and result in a hernia sac that lies beneath the inguinal ligament, just medial to the femoral vessels. The risk for incarceration is greatest in indirect hernias.

A hernia may be diagnosed by palpation in the supine and standing positions, auscultation of bowel sounds arising from the hernia sac, or transillumination. Enlarged lymph nodes or varicose veins must also be considered.

Equipment

- No special equipment required; examination gloves may be desirable

Training/Credentialing

No special credentialing needed; office procedure only.

Coding

49999 Unlisted procedure, abdomen, peritoneum and omentum

Technique

The patient should be placed in the supine Trendelenburg position to allow for gravitational assist. Analgesia and muscle relaxation, accomplished by the administration of a narcotic agent or intravenous diazepam, should be established. The patient should remain in the supine Trendelenburg position for 30–40 minutes to allow passive reduction to take place if possible. If passive reduction does not ensue, one hand should be placed over the hernia neck to help guide the contents back into the abdominal cavity while the other hand provides gentle, steady distal-to-proximal compression.

After successful reduction, the patient should undergo elective hernia repair at the earliest convenient date. External support, in the form of a truss, may reduce the risk for further episodes of incarceration but should only be used until definitive surgical repair is done.

Normal Findings

Roughly one-third to one-half of incarcerated hernias may be reduced using these methods.

Special Notes

Strangulation of hernia contents is a surgical emergency that should only be handled in the operating room. Strangulation may be suspected by the presence of fever, significant malaise, extreme tenderness of the hernia bulge, or erythema of the overlying skin. Femoral hernias are less likely to be successfully reduced and frequently must be referred for surgical reduction and repair.

Suggested Readings

Kauffman HM, O'Brien DP. Selective reduction of incarcerated inguinal hernia. *Am J Surg* 1970;119:660.

Fraser GC. Reduction of an incarcerated hernia [Letter]. *J Pediatr Surg* 1993;28:1519.

Chapter 33

PERIANAL SKIN TAG EXCISION

Perianal skin tags are not true hemorrhoids but rather a redundancy of normal perianal skin caused by stretching and enlargement. These extra flaps of tissue are minimally symptomatic; the most common symptom is fecal soiling as the result of problems with normal anal hygiene. This soiling must be differentiated from true fecal incontinence caused by other conditions. Perianal skin tags are generally not responsible for bleeding, pain, or itching. When these symptoms predominate, other causes should be sought.

Equipment

- Sterile gloves, antiseptic solution and sterile cotton balls, or skin preparation swabs
- Local anesthetic of choice (generally without epinephrine), 25-gauge needle
- Sterile forceps
- Fine scissors (or knife blade) or an electrosurgical generator and loop electrode used in large loop excision of the transformation zone
- Monsel's solution
- Fine absorbable sutures (optional)
- Assistant (desirable)

Training/Credentialing

Some experience is desirable; it is best to have received instruction or experience before the procedure is attempted alone. No special credentialing needed; office procedure only.

Coding

46230 Excision of perianal skin tag

11200 Removal of skin tags, multiple fibrocutaneous tags, any area; up to and including 15 lesions

Technique

The patient should be placed in the left lateral (Sims') position or the modified knee-chest position and draped appropriately. The glutei are separated laterally by the assistant or through the use of wide adhesive tape (Fig. 27.1). The base of the skin tag or tags to be excised should be infiltrated with 1 mL of local anesthetic (without epinephrine) using a fine needle and slow infusion technique to minimize discomfort. Once adequate anesthesia is accomplished, the skin tag is grasped with forceps and gently elevated; care should be taken not to tent the surrounding tissue, which might result in an excessively wide base of excision. If the infiltration process causes excessive edema, compression between the fingers for a few seconds restores the tissues to a more normal turgor and reduces the risk for excessive tissue removal.

The skin tag is excised by either loop electrosurgical excision or by knife incision at the base of the tag. The line of excision is made approximately 2–3 mm above the normal perianal tissues. Small bleeding sites may be cauterized using the electrosurgical unit or by applying Monsel's solution. Closure of the wound is generally not necessary and may increase the patient's discomfort. Most colon and rectal specialists recommend limiting excisions to a single skin tag at any one visit.

The patient should be advised to avoid creams and ointments applied to the anal area, to consume a high-fiber diet (to avoid constipation), and to use a mild nonsteroidal anti-inflammatory medication for postoperative discomfort. The latter should be minimal and resolve in 5–7 days. Sitz baths may be used if needed.

Special Notes

Edematous or "fleshy" appearing perianal skin tags suggest anal Crohn's disease and should prompt further investigation or referral before any excision is contemplated. Symptoms of pain, bleeding, or itching are unlikely to be resolved by removing perianal skin tags. When these symptoms are present, other causes should be sought.

Suggested Readings

Gordon P, Nivatvongs S. *Principles and practice of surgery for the colon, rectum, and anus*. St. Louis: Quality Medical Publishing, 1992.

Pirone E, Infantino A, Masin A, et al. Can proctological procedures resolve perianal pruritus and mycosis? A prospective study of 23 cases. *Int J Colorectal Dis* 1992;7:18.

Chapter 34

PILONIDAL CYST EXCISION

Pilonidal cysts generally present as one or more midline or eccentric pits or sinuses in the skin of the sacral region (Fig. 34.1). Infection may lead to abscess formation or chronically draining sinuses, which require surgical drainage or extirpation. Though these cysts are three times more common in young male patients, awareness of this problem and familiarity with its treatment are appropriate in the gynecologic setting.

Equipment

- Local anesthetic of choice, 25-gauge needle
- #15 or #11 knife blade, thumb forceps, fine tissue scissors
- Electrosurgical generator, tip, hand piece or foot pedal control, return electrode ("ground pad") (optional)
- Fine (2-0 or 3-0) absorbable suture
- Iodoform gauze packing
- Sterile gloves, antiseptic solution and sterile cotton balls, or skin preparation swabs
- Sterile draping material (optional)
- Monsel's solution (optional)
- Assistant (desirable)

Training/Credentialing

Many hospitals or ambulatory surgery centers have special credentialing requirements.

Coding

10080	Incision and drainage of pilonidal cyst; simple
10081	complicated
11770	Excision of pilonidal cyst or sinus; simple

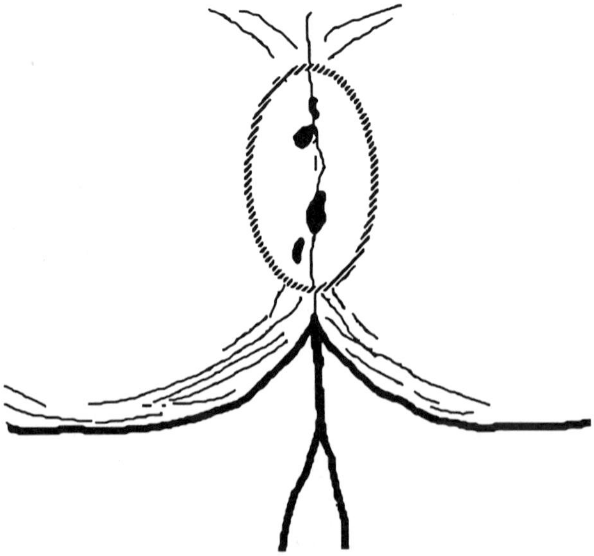

FIGURE 34.1.
Pilonidal cysts are located over the lower sacrum, 5–10 cm from the anal verge. Although their location may be identified by pits, depressions, or sinus in or adjacent to the midline, induration and infection may extend laterally (oval).

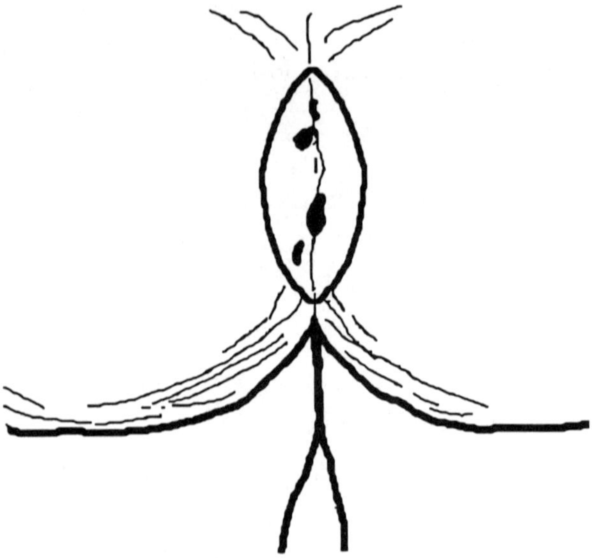

FIGURE 34.2.
An ellipse of tissue is excised; the sinus tracks and any infected tissue are incorporated.

11771	extensive
11772	complicated

Technique

The procedure of choice for pilonidal cysts is incision and drainage; the wound is left open to heal during the subsequent weeks. The operative site should be disinfected as for any surgical procedure, and sterile drapes should be applied as needed to establish a sterile field in which to work. A field block should be established using several milliliters of local anesthetic solution. When the cyst is small, the opening should be probed and the cyst unroofed by knife or electrosurgical device.

When multiple sinuses are present or significant lateral extension of the cysts or infection is present, an en block excision of the area and larger and deeper field of anesthesia are needed. The tissue involved should be excised using a ellipse whose long

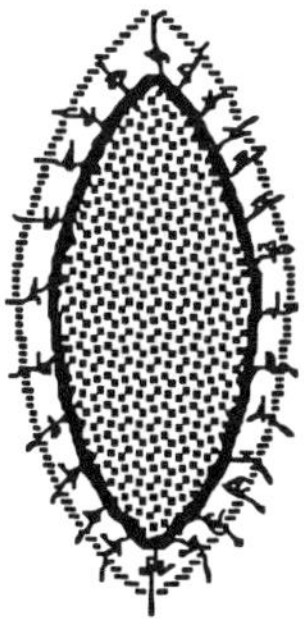

FIGURE 34.3.
The edges of the wound may be sutured with interrupted absorbable sutures to the underlying fascia. Depending on the size of the tissue defect, the wound may be packed with iodoform gauze or left open.

axis is oriented in the midline (Fig. 34.2). This incision should be carried down to the fascia and laterally to healthy, uninfected tissue. If the defect is not too deep or wide, the edges may be sewn to the underlying tissues using interrupted or continuous absorbable sutures (Fig. 34.3). The wound should be loosely packed with iodoform gauze, which should be changed periodically. The frequency of these changes should be based on the size of the wound and may be decreased as the wound heals. Daily irrigation or cleansing of the wound with water is generally sufficient.

Pilonidal cysts that extend widely may require the excision of so much tissue that a flap or graft is required to cover the defect. The surgeon must either be able to perform such a graft if it is necessary or refer the patient to a general surgeon for the excision.

Normal Findings

The almost pathognomonic symptoms of a patient with a pilonidal cyst are a history of recurrent infection and drainage at the base of the spine. Loose hairs are commonly associated with pilonidal cysts and, when present, support the diagnosis.

Selected Abnormal Findings

Pilonidal sinuses that are located near the anal canal must be differentiated from fistulae. The possibility of other causes, such as Crohn's disease, must be considered.

Special Notes

Antibiotic treatment of pilonidal cysts is only palliative and is associated with frequent recurrences; the definitive treatment is surgical. Patients with minimal drainage and no induration suggestive of infection may require no therapy at all. Because of the proximity to infected tissue, caudal and low spinal anesthesia should not be used.

Suggested Readings

Armstrong JH, Barcia PJ. Pilonidal sinus disease. The conservative approach. *Arch Surg* 1994;129:914.

Fuzun M, Bakir H, Soylu M, et al. Which technique for treatment of pilonidal sinus—open or closed? *Dis Colon Rectum* 1994;37:1148.

Isbister WH, Prasad J. Pilonidal disease. *Aust NZ J Surg* 1995;65:561.

Jones DJ. ABC of colorectal diseases. Pilonidal sinus. *BMJ* 1992;305:410

Khaira HS, Brown JH. Excision and primary suture of pilonidal sinus. *Ann Roy Coll Surg Engl* 1995;77:242.

Lundhus E, Gottrup F. Outcome at three to five years of primary closure of perianal and pilonidal abscess. A randomised, double-blind clinical trial with a complete three-year followup of one compared with four days' treatment with ampicillin and metronidazole. *Eur J Surg* 1993;159:555.

Matter I, Kunin J, Schein M, et al. Total excision versus non-resectional methods in the treatment of acute and chronic pilonidal disease. *Br J Surg* 1995;82:752.

Purkiss SF. Decision making in surgery: a pilonidal sinus. *Br J Hosp Med* 1993;50:554.

Sondenaa K, Andersen E, Soreide JA. Morbidity and short term results in a randomised trial of open compared with closed treatment of chronic pilonidal sinus. *Eur J Surg* 1992;158:351.

Sondenaa K, Nesvik I, Andersen E, et al. Bacteriology and complications of chronic pilonidal sinus treated with excision and primary suture. *Int J Colorectal Dis* 1995;10:161.

Stephens FO, Stephens RB. Pilonidal sinus: management objectives. *Aust NZ J Surg* 1995;65:558.

Surrell JA. Pilonidal disease. *Surg Clin North Am* 1994;74:1309.

Yabe T, Furukawa M. The origin of pilonidal sinus: a case report. *J Dermatol* 1995;22:696.

Chapter 35

PROCTOSCOPY

Flexible proctosigmoidoscopy has generally replaced the older technique of rigid proctoscopy. The simplicity of equipment, lack of expense, and clinical utility that proctoscopy can afford for selected patients make it a procedure that deserves mention.

Equipment

- Rigid proctoscope and light source
- Examination gloves
- Water-based lubricant
- Large-tipped cotton swabs (such as those used for colposcopy)
- Biopsy forceps and Monsel's solution (optional)
- Assistant (desirable)

Training/Credentialing

No special credentialing needed; office procedure only.

Coding

45300	Sigmoidoscopy, rigid; diagnostic, with or without collection of specimen(s) by brushing or washing (separate procedure)
45303	with dilation, any method
45305	with biopsy, single or multiple
45307	with removal of foreign body
45308	with removal of single tumor, polyp, or other lesion by hot biopsy forceps or bipolar cautery
45309	with removal of single tumor, polyp, or other lesion by snare technique
45315	with removal of multiple tumors, polyps, or other lesions by hot biopsy forceps, bipolar cautery, or snare technique

45317	with control of bleeding, any method
45320	with ablation of tumor(s), polyp(s), or other lesion(s) not amenable to removal by hot biopsy forceps, bipolar cautery or snare technique (e.g., laser)

Technique

Patient preparation should proceed as for flexible sigmoidoscopy (see Chapter 29, Flexible Sigmoidoscopy). The examination begins with external inspection, with the patient relaxed and the Valsalva maneuver used. Digital examination using a finger lubricated with water-based lubricant or topical anesthetic jelly (such as 2% lidocaine) should be done.

The proctoscope, with obturator in place, is lubricated and placed against the anal opening. Gentle pressure is applied until the resistance of the sphincters is overcome. The proctoscope is gently advanced in the direction of the umbilicus (Fig. 35.1). This insertion process may be facilitated if the patient slowly breathes in and out. Once the proctoscope has been advanced approximately 5 cm, the obturator is removed and the canal inspected. The proctoscope tip should be at the level of the anal verge. Fecal matter may be removed with large cotton-tipped swabs. The proctoscope is next angled posteriorly; gentle advancement to about 8 cm should bring the middle rectal fold into view (Fig. 35.2). This is the level of the peritoneal reflection. Extra care must be taken with further insertion because the most common site of perforation is located between this point and the superior rectal fold (10–12 cm). Beyond 12 cm, insertion becomes less difficult. Advancement from 5 cm onward should be done under direct vision. Insufflation should be sufficient to allow inspection while maintaining patient comfort.

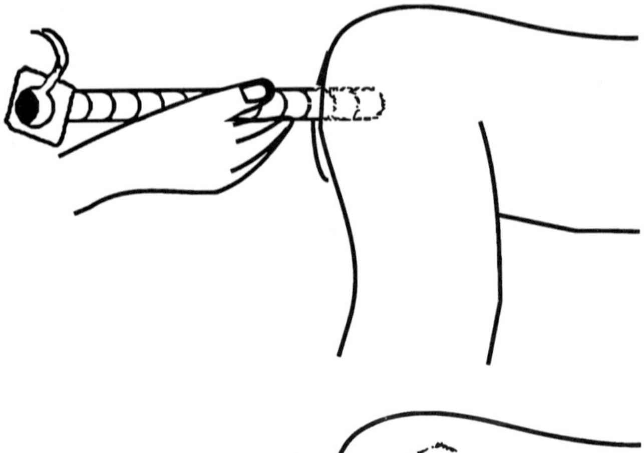

FIGURE 35.1.
When the proctoscope is first inserted, it should be directed toward the umbilicus. During this first step, the obturator is generally left in place.

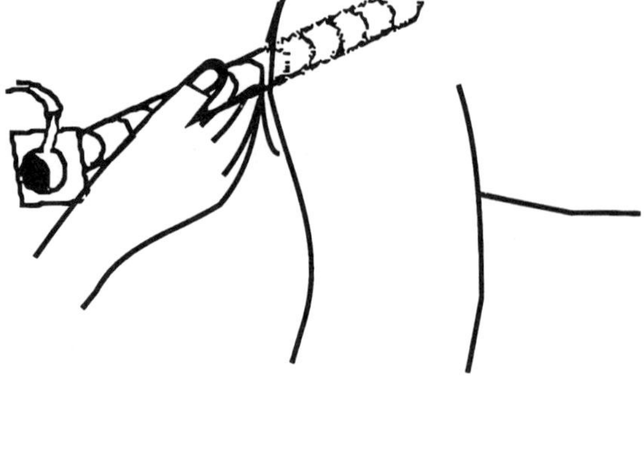

FIGURE 35.2.
Once the proctoscope has been advanced 3–4 cm into the anal canal, the obturator should be removed and the canal inspected. Further advancement must be directed posteriorly toward the hollow of the sacrum, following the course of the upper rectum and sigmoid.

Special Notes

Many providers prefer to perform anoscopy separately from proctoscopy. If this is the case, it should be performed immediately before proctoscopy (see Chapter 26, Anoscopy). Anoscopy combined with proctoscopy is generally not billed as a separate charge.

Suggested Readings

DeCosse JJ, Tsioulias GJ, Jacobson JS. Colorectal cancer: detection, treatment, and rehabilitation. *CA Cancer J Clin* 1994;44:27.

Farmer KC, Church JM. Open sesame: tips for traversing the anal canal. *Dis Colon Rect* 1992;35:1092.

Kockelbergh RC, Nash JR. The transanal resectoscope: an under-used instrument? *Aust N Z J Surg* 1992;62:809.

Lazas DJ, Moses FM, Wong RK. Videoendoscopic anoscopy: a new technique for examining the anal canal. *Gastrointest Endos* 1995;42:351.

Said S, Huber P, Pichlmaier H. Technique and clinical results of endorectal surgery. *Surgery* 1993;113:65.

Silbertrust N. Instrumentation for transanal endoscopic surgery. *Endoscop Surg Allied Tech* 1993;1:52.

Williams CB, Nicholls RJ. Management of large rectal polyps: questions of technique, terminology, and turf. *Gastrointest Endos* 1995;41:615.

Section IV

DERMATOLOGIC PROCEDURES

Chapter 36

DERMAL BIOPSY

Histologic evaluation of dermal conditions is advisable in many situations. The same principles used to obtain biopsy samples of vulvar skin may be used to obtain tissue from other areas of the body.

Equipment

- Basic suture tray (may be replaced by sterile gloves, antiseptic solution and sterile cotton balls, or skin preparation swabs)
- Local anesthetic of choice (generally without epinephrine), 25-gauge needle
- Monsel's solution (ferric subsulfate)
- Skin closure tapes (Steri-Strips) or fine absorbable sutures
- 10% buffered formalin or other fixative
- #11, #15, or #15c knife blade or fine scissors
- Disposable dermal punch (2–10 mm punches are available; 2–4 mm are most useful)

or

- Fine forceps

Training/Credentialing

Minimal experience is required. No special credentialing needed; office procedure only.

Coding

11100	Biopsy of skin, subcutaneous tissue and/or mucous membrane (including simple closure), unless otherwise listed (separate procedure); single lesion
11101	Each separate/additional lesion

Coding varies depending on the site, number of biopsy samples taken, the technique used, and whether the lesion is malignant. Care must be taken in selecting the correct code.

Technique

PINCH BIOPSY

The site of biopsy is cleansed with antiseptic solution, and an anesthetic skin weal is created with a small amount of anesthetic agent. The center of the area in which biopsy is to be done is lifted with forceps; an elliptical incision is made at the base of the elevated tissue (Fig. 36.1). This incision should result in the removal of an ellipse of tissue; the long axis of the ellipse should be aligned with the natural skin lines and the points of the ellipse should approximate a 30° angle. The biopsy specimen should generally include the full dermal thickness. The specimen should be promptly placed in formalin or other preservation media for transport to the histology laboratory. Capillary bleeding may be controlled by pressure or the application of Monsel's solution. Small biopsy sites may be closed with skin tapes, whereas larger sites may require fine sutures.

PUNCH BIOPSY

The site of biopsy is cleansed and an anesthetic skin weal is created as for a pinch biopsy. A biopsy punch large enough to encompass the lesion or to provide a representative sample should be used (Fig. 36.2). The skin of the surrounding area is stretched in a direction perpendicular to the normal skin lines, and the biopsy punch

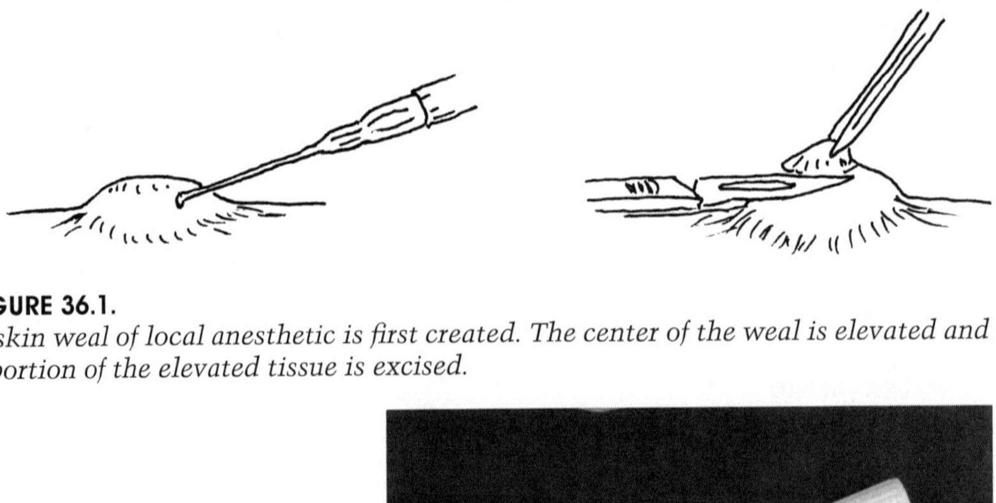

FIGURE 36.1.
A skin weal of local anesthetic is first created. The center of the weal is elevated and a portion of the elevated tissue is excised.

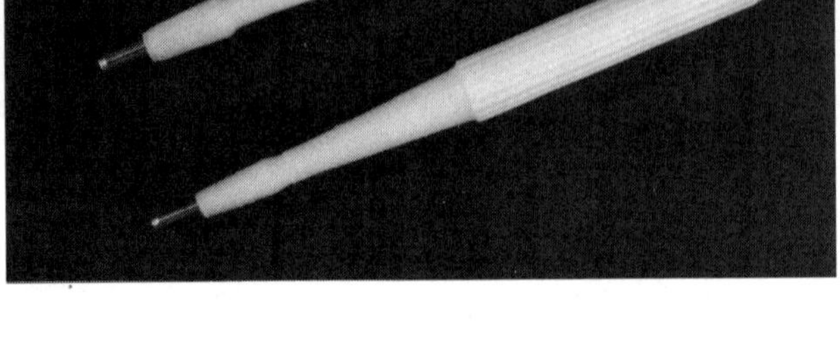

FIGURE 36.2.
Disposable dermal biopsy punches are available in many sizes.

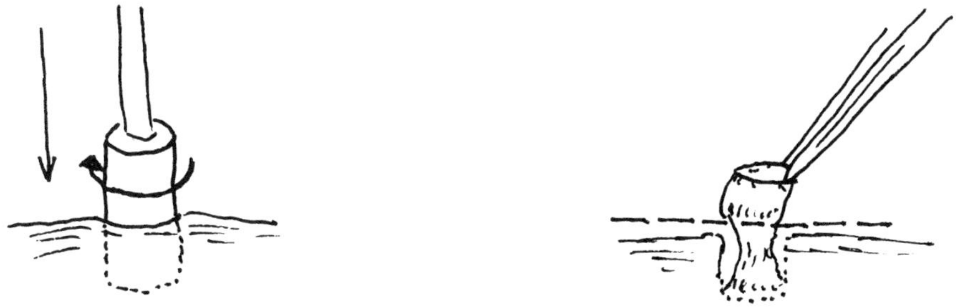

FIGURE 36.3.
Punch biopsy is accomplished by pressing the instrument downward with a slight twisting motion until a loss of resistance is felt. The core of tissue created is elevated and excised at its base.

is placed against the skin. The punch is pressed downward with a slight twisting motion until the punch has penetrated to a depth that approximates the dermal thickness (Fig. 36.3). A slight loss of resistance is often felt at this point. The punch is removed and the plug of tissue is elevated with forceps and excised at its base with a knife blade or fine scissors. The specimen should be promptly placed in formalin or other preservation media and transported to the histology laboratory. Pressure or Monsel's solution may be used to provide hemostasis. Most small biopsy sites may be closed with skin tapes.

Special Notes

If a melanoma is suspected, the depth of involvement is critical to diagnosis and treatment planning. Referral of these patients should be seriously considered to ensure that the biopsy sample is appropriate. Biopsies of the lips or eyelids should be performed by consultants. If sutures are required, synthetic delayed absorbable sutures are best, generally in sizes of 4-0 to 6-0.

Suggested Readings

Gross DA. The vertical wedge biopsy. *J Dermatol Surg Oncol* 1992;18:630.
Pariser RJ. Skin biopsy: lesion selection and optimal technique. *Modern Med* 1989; 57:82.

Chapter 37

DIGITAL BLOCK ANESTHESIA

Digital block anesthesia is useful as part of the treatment of paronychia, ingrown nails, hematoma evacuation, ring removal, or some biopsies.

Equipment

- Either antiseptic solution and sterile cotton balls or skin preparation swabs
- 5-mL syringe, 25- or 27-gauge needle
- 1% Xylocaine without epinephrine (or similar)

Training/Credentialing

No special credentialing needed; office procedure only.

Coding

01800	Anesthesia for all procedures on integumentary system of forearm, wrist, and hand
01460	Anesthesia for all procedures on integumentary system of lower limb, ankle and foot

Technique

After appropriate skin cleansing, an anesthetic weal is raised at the base of the digit near the dorsal surface. The injection is directed toward the volar or plantar surface, depositing approximately 1 mL of anesthetic in the area of the digital nerve branches on that side (Fig. 37.1). This procedure is repeated on the opposite side (medial or lateral) of the same digit. Anesthesia is generally adequate within 5–10 minutes.

As an alternative, the web between digits may be used as a site of injection (Figs. 37.2 and 37.3). When the toes are anesthetized, the needle may be inserted in the dorsal midline, over the extensor tendon, and then directed laterally to either side of the toe to deposit the anesthetic agent (Fig. 37.4).

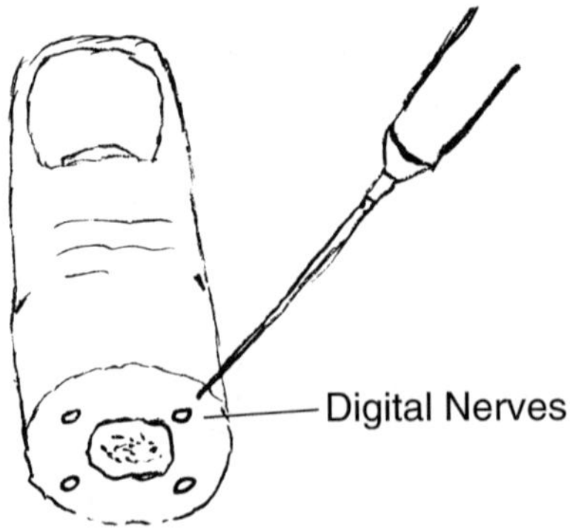

FIGURE 37.1.
A digital nerve block in the distal finger involves infiltrating anesthetic agent into both the volar and palmar branches of the nerve on both sides of the digit.

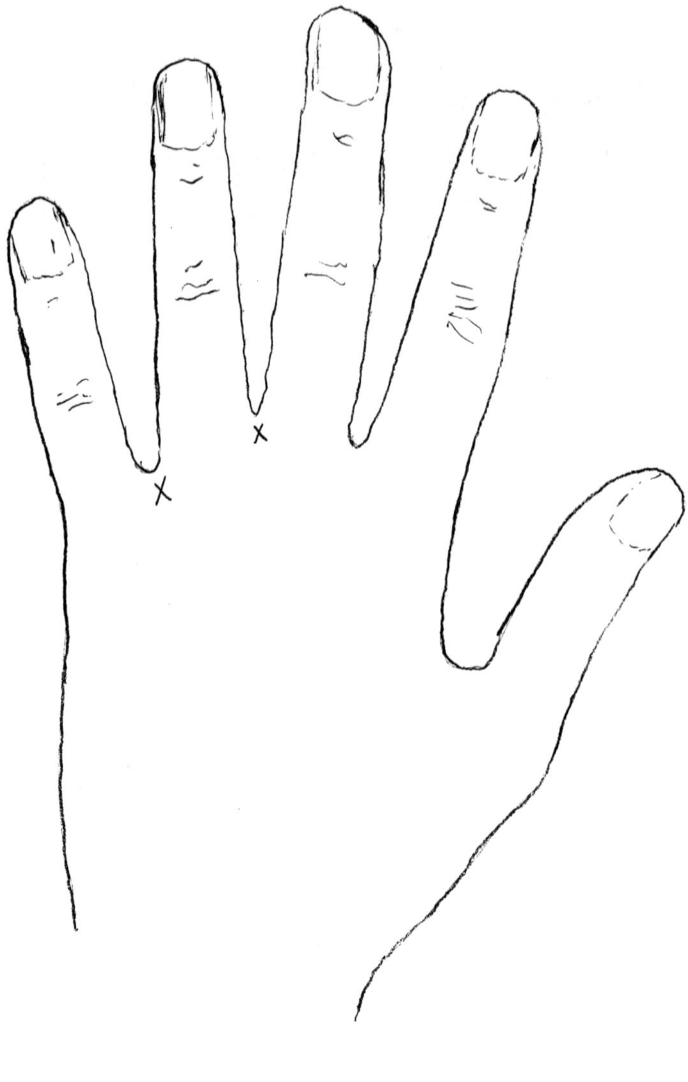

FIGURE 37.2.
Injection sites for digital nerve block.

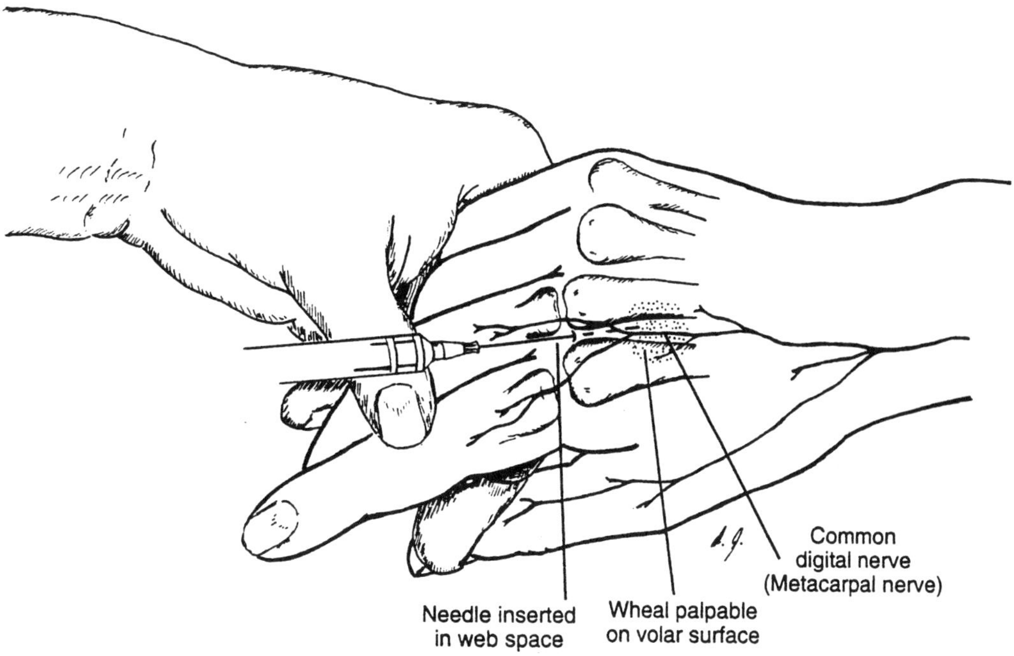

FIGURE 37.3.
Block of the common digital nerve. (Reproduced with permission from Simon RR, Brenner BE. Emergency Procedures and Techniques. *3rd ed. Baltimore: Williams & Wilkins, 1994:113.)*

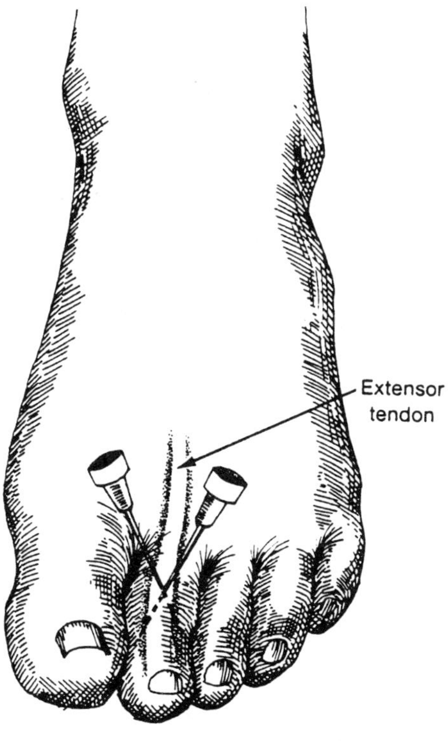

FIGURE 37.4.
Digital block of the toes may be performed with a single needle puncture over the extensor tendon. (Reproduced with permission from Simon RR, Brenner BE. Emergency Procedures and Techniques. *3rd ed. Baltimore: Williams & Wilkins, 1994:118.)*

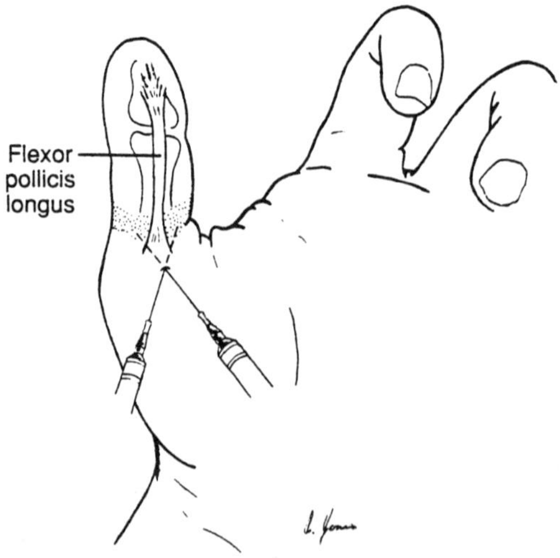

FIGURE 37.5.
Nerve block of the thumb. (Reproduced with permission from Simon RR, Brenner BE. Emergency Procedures and Techniques. *3rd ed. Baltimore: Williams & Wilkins, 1994:113.)*

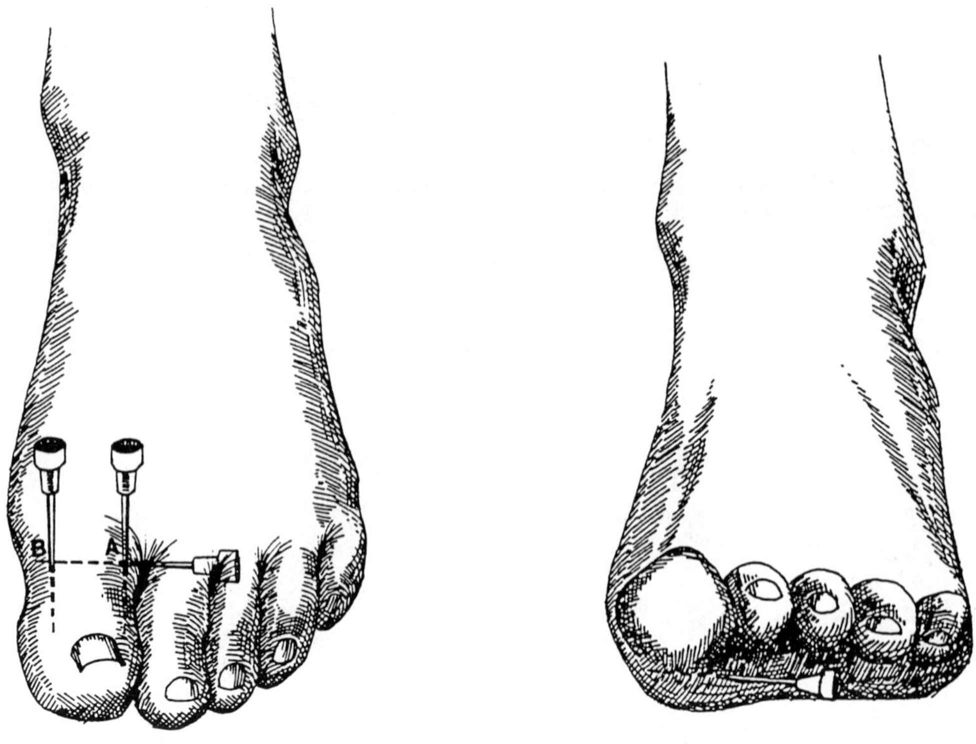

FIGURE 37.6.
Digital block of the great toe requires a circumferential infiltration of local anesthetic. (Reproduced with permission from Simon RR, Brenner BE. Emergency Procedures and Techniques. *3rd ed. Baltimore: Williams & Wilkins, 1994:117–8.)*

To block the thumb or great toe, a slightly different technique must be used. The thumb may be anesthetized by infiltrating local anesthetic adjacent to the readily palpable flexor pollicis longus tendon (Fig. 37.5). Insertion of the needle 2–3 mm in a distal direction and the use of 1–2 mL of anesthetic agent per side provide the best anesthesia. To anesthetize the great toe, a circumferential field block must be established as shown in Figure 37.6.

Special Notes

Epinephrine should never be used in conjunction with digital blocks.

Suggested Readings

Adriani J. Local and regional anesthesia for minor surgery. *Surg Clin North Am* 1951;31:1507.

Covino BG. Local anesthesia. *N Engl J Med* 1972;286:975.

Locke RK, Locke SE. Nerve blocks of the foot. *JACEP* 1976;5:698.

Poulton TJ, Mims GR. Peripheral nerve blocks. *Am Fam Phys* 1977;16:100.

Chapter 38

DRAINAGE OF PARONYCHIA

Paronychia are infections of the proximal and lateral edges of the fingernail or toenail. Redness, swelling, tenderness, and pain are typical.

Equipment

- Sterile gloves, antiseptic solution and sterile cotton balls, or skin preparation swabs
- #11 knife blade
- 5-mL syringe, 25- to 27-gauge needle, and 1% Xylocaine without epinephrine (see technique for digital block in Chapter 37)
- 1/4-inch iodoform gauze (optional)
- Rubber band with hemostat

Training/Credentialing

No special credentialing needed; office procedure only.

Coding

26010 Drainage of finger abscess; simple

Technique

Primary treatment consists of warm soaks and antibiotics. When conservative treatment fails or an abscess forms, the paronychia must be drained.

Incision and drainage of a paronychia are generally done under digital block anesthesia. Once satisfactory anesthesia is accomplished, the skin is cleansed with an appropriate solution or technique. Incision is best made by a simple nick over the most translucent portion of the swelling (Fig. 38.1). Pus should be drained and cultured. A small amount of iodoform gauze may be placed in larger abscess to avoid reformation.

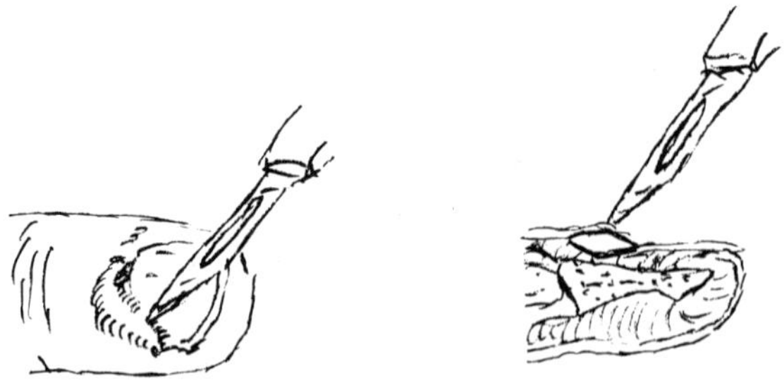

FIGURE 38.1.

Any packing used should be removed after a few days. A rubber band, secured with a hemostat, may be used as a tourniquet if needed.

Special Notes

The incision need only be made deeply enough to provide drainage of the abscess.

Suggested Readings

Black JR. Paronychia. *Clin Podiatr Med Surg* 1995;12:183.
Haneke E, Baran R. Nail surgery. *Clin Dermatol* 1992;10:327.
Hausman MR, Lisser SP. Hand infections. *Orth Clin North Am* 1992;23:171.
Hochman LG. Paronychia: more than just an abscess. *Int J Dermatol* 1995;34:385.
Mack GR. Superficial anatomy and cutaneous surgery of the hand. *Adv Dermatol* 1992;7:315
Moran GJ, Talan DA. Hand infections. *Emerg Med Clin North Am* 1993;11:601.
Murtagh J. Practice tip. Paronychia. *Aust Fam Phys* 1995;24:1506.

Chapter 39

INGROWN NAILS

Ingrown nails cause discomfort and disability. The great toe is almost exclusively involved, but either the medial or lateral edge may be affected. Occasionally, onychomycosis (fungal infection) or a paronychia may require trimming the nail edge in the same way as for an ingrown nail.

Equipment

- Either antiseptic solution and sterile cotton balls or skin preparation swabs
- 5-mL syringe, 25- to 27-gauge needle, and 1% Xylocaine without epinephrine (see technique for digital block in Chapter 37)
- Small nail elevator (periosteal elevator)
- Sterile scissors (straight) or heavy-duty nail clipper
- Small sterile hemostat
- Rubber band with hemostat
- Antibiotic ointment (Mycitracin, Bactroban, Mycolog)
- Tubular gauze or other sterile dressing

Training/Credentialing

No special credentialing needed; office procedure only.

Coding

11730	Avulsion of nail plate, partial or complete, simple, single
11750	Excision of nail and nail matrix, partial or complete (e.g., ingrown or deformed nail), for permanent removal
11755	Biopsy of nail unit, any method (e.g., plate, bed, matrix, hyponychium, proximal and lateral nail folds) (separate procedure)

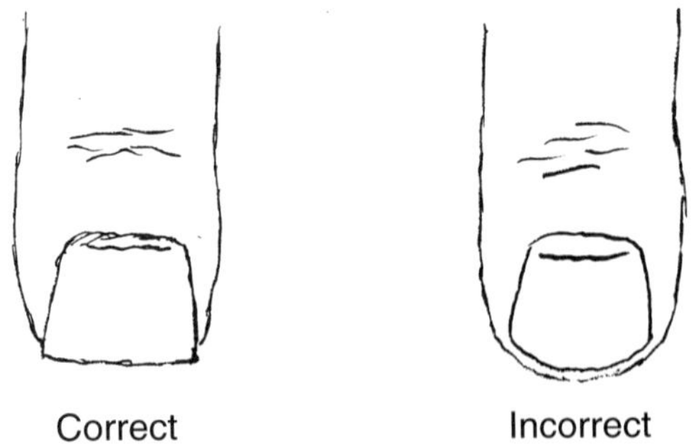

FIGURE 39.1.

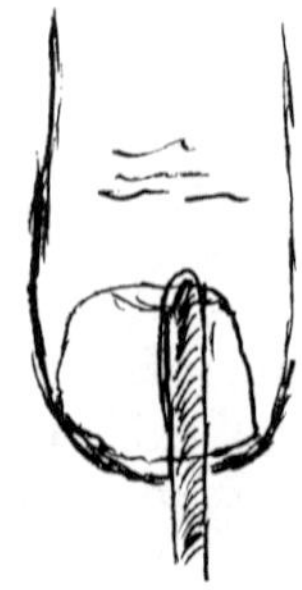

FIGURE 39.2.

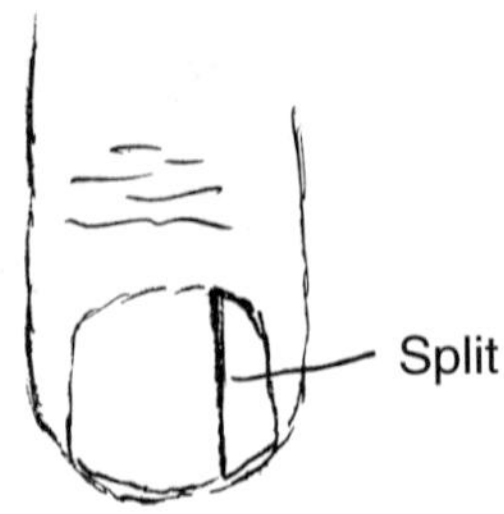

FIGURE 39.3.

Technique

Conservative treatment of an ingrown nail involves placing a small cotton wick under the tip of the nail to help raise the edge and remove pressure. Care must be used to keep the area clean and to avoid excessive pressure. The nail should be trimmed in a square fashion to avoid further ingrowth (Fig. 39.1).

When simple measures are inadequate, a portion of the nail must be excised. To do so, cleanse the affected digit and establish satisfactory digital block anesthesia. The base of the digit should be firmly wrapped with a rubber band and secured with a hemostat to provide a tourniquet. The nail on the affected side must be lifted from the underlying nail bed using a nail elevator, a periosteal elevator, or the tip of a small hemostat. This should include roughly one-quarter of the nail and must extend to the base of the nail at the level of the cuticle (Fig. 39.2).

The nail is now split using scissors or a nail cutter; the split extends to the base of the nail (Fig. 39.3). The now freed portion of the nail on the affected side must be removed by grasping with a hemostat and pulling outward and upward while rotating the fragment toward the affected side and away from the midline. This twisting motion helps free the nail from the affected nail margin.

After the nail edge is removed, antibiotic ointment is applied, the tourniquet is removed, and the digit is dressed appropriately. For ingrown toenails, elevation of the foot with restricted activity for 12 to 24 hours is desirable. Analgesics such as nonsteroidal anti-inflammatory agents are usually sufficient for pain relief. Some authors suggest soaking the digit in warm water twice daily for 4 days. Proper nail hygiene should be stressed.

Special Notes

When the nail is loosened from the underlying bed, force must be directed toward the nail and away from the nail bed. This minimizes injury and bleeding. A sterile exudate from the nail bed is not uncommon in the first few days after resection of part or all of the nail.

Suggested Readings

Anderson JH, Greig JD, Ireland AJ, et al. Randomized prospective study of nailbed ablation for recurrent ingrowing toenails. *J R Coll Surg Edinb* 1990;35:240.

Freiberg A, Dougherty S. A review of management of ingrown toenails and onychogryposis. *Can Fam Phys* 1988;34:2675.

Greig JD, Anderson JH, Ireland AJ, et al. The surgical treatment of ingrowing toenails. *J Bone Joint Surg* 1991;73–B:1, 131.

Haneke E, Baran R. Nail surgery. *Clin Dermatol* 1992;10:327.

VanDerHam AC, Hackeng CA, Tik Len Yo, et al. The treatment of ingrowing toenails. *J Bone Joint Surg* 1990:72–B:3, 507.

Chapter 40

FINGER RING REMOVAL

Swelling of a finger can result in incarceration of a ring and, in turn, circumferential constriction that further aggravates swelling and can lead to neurovascular compromise.

Equipment

- 6- to 9-inch piece of string, umbilical tape, or #1 or 2 suture
- Adhesive tape
- Small hemostat
- Water-based lubricant
- Ring cutter (Beaver) or Steinmann orthopedic pin cutter with small elevator or retractor

Training/Credentialing

No special credentialing needed; office procedure only.

Coding

No specific code for ring removal is used. The inclusion of ring removal may justify or support a higher acuity for the other services rendered.

Technique

The affected finger should be lightly lubricated with water-based lubricant. With the help of a hemostat, a small strip of ¼-inch adhesive tape may be passed under the ring, adhesive side out. Two such strips are passed on the lateral sides of the ring (Fig. 40.1). The tape is folded back and stuck to itself, thereby securing points of traction on the ring at the 3 and 9 o'clock positions. Gentle distal traction on these tapes may be sufficient to free the ring.

String, umbilical tape, or heavy suture may be used to wrap the finger; this reduces swelling and may free the ring. To use this technique, the end of the string is passed beneath the ring with the help of a hemostat. The string is then wound in a single layer, un-

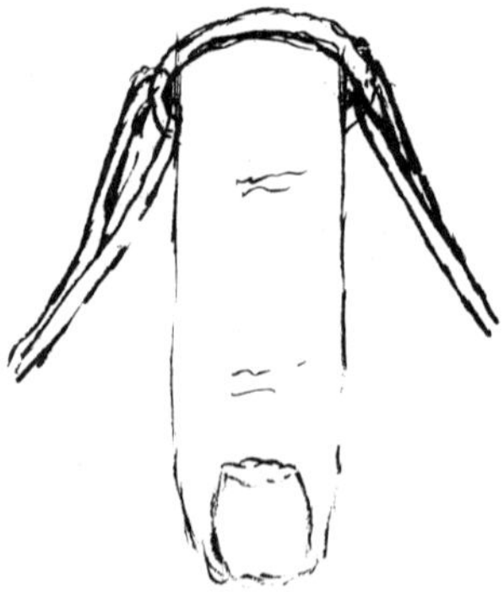

FIGURE 40.1.
Traction applied to tapes passed under the ring at the 3 and 9 o'clock positions may supply adequate traction to allow removal of the ring.

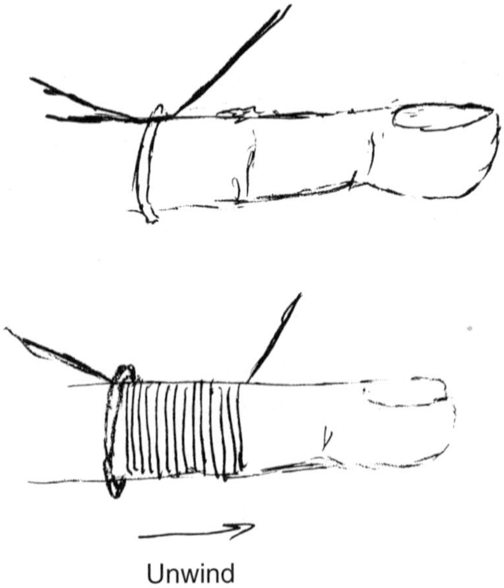

FIGURE 40.2.
Wrapping the finger with string or heavy suture may reduce edema and allow the ring to be moved past the obstruction.

der moderate tension, progressing distally to just beyond the point of obstruction. Traction is placed on the ring while the string is unwound from the proximal end (Fig. 40.2).

If simple techniques do not free the ring, it must be cut. Cutting may be done with specialized ring cutters or an orthopedic pin cutter. The ring cutter hook is inserted under the ring to provide a cutting surface and to protect the tissue of the finger. If a pin cutter is used, a small elevator or retractor should be inserted between the instrument and the skin to provide this protection. Once the ring has been cut, the end may be separated by traction by two heavy hemostats or pliers. Once the ring is removed, attention is directed toward the problem that resulted in entrapping the ring.

Special Notes

If a ring cutter is used, care must be taken to completely remove any metal fragments produced by the process. The easiest way to accomplish this is copious irrigation under moderate pressure. If digital block anesthesia is required, injection should take place proximal to the ring to prevent further tissue swelling.

Suggested Readings

Mizrahi S, Lunski I. A simplified method for ring removal from an edematous finger. *Am J Surg* 1986;151:412.

Chapter 41

SUBUNGUAL HEMATOMA EVACUATION

Trauma to a digit may cause a painful subungual hematoma. The hematoma may be safely drained in the office setting, and the procedure significantly alleviates symptoms.

Equipment

- Alcohol lamp or butane lighter, metal paper clip, hemostat

or

- "Hot" cautery unit (battery- or AC-powered)

or

- Electrosurgery unit with needle electrode

or

- #15 knife blade

Training/Credentialing

No special credentialing needed; office procedure only.

Coding

11740 Subungual hematoma evacuation

Technique

The digit involved should be cleansed thoroughly with antibacterial soap, but surgical antisepsis is not required. The hematoma is decompressed by creating a hole in the overlying nail; the latter is done by using a hot paper clip, "hot" cautery, electrosurgery, or trephinating with a small knife blade.

In the hot paper clip method, a metal paper clip is partially straightened and held in a hemostat; the straight portion is heated in a flame to incandescence. The incandes-

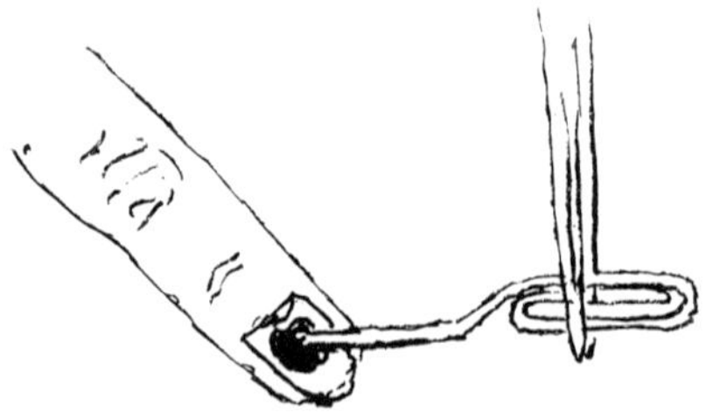

FIGURE 41.1.

cent tip is then quickly pressed against the nail directly over the hematoma (Fig. 41.1). The hot wire produces a hole in the nail and the blood in the hematoma protects the nail bed from thermal damage. The heated wire of a "hot" cautery device may be used in the same way.

An electrosurgical signal generator may also be used to create a hole in the overlying nail. To use this technique, a return electrode should be place on the limb, proximal to the hand or foot and avoiding bony sites. A needle electrode and a relatively low power setting are used and the nail is cauterized. Because of the relatively low water content of the nail, this technique is not as effective as use of a heated paper clip or hot cautery.

A small, #15 scalpel blade may be used to open a hole in the nail. The tip of the blade is placed perpendicular to the nail, and a back and forth drilling motion is used to create the hole. Care must be taken to avoid injuring the underlying nail bed.

Analgesics, a simple dressing, elevation of the injured digit, and cool soaks are all reasonable recommendations for further care.

Special Notes

If the nail is fractured or crushed, the patient should be referred for specialized evaluation and care. Care should be taken to prevent infection of the hematoma after drainage.

Suggested Readings

Van Beek AL. Management of acute fingernail injuries. *Hand Clinics* 1990;1:23.

Wee GC, Shieber W. Painless evacuation of subungual hematoma. *Surg Gynecol Obstet* 1970;131:535.

Zook EG. Nail bed injuries. *Hand Clinics* 1985;1:701.

Chapter 42

EXAMINATION USING A WOOD'S LAMP

The Wood's lamp is a long-wave ultraviolet light source used to facilitate dermatologic evaluations. The invisible ultraviolet light causes characteristic fluorescent light to be emitted from the skin, the color and character of which may be used for diagnosis.

Equipment

- Wood's lamp
- Magnifying lens (optional)

Training/Credentialing

No special credentialing needed; office procedure only.

Coding

No separate CPT code.

Technique

Wood's lamps are available in battery and plug-in configurations (Fig. 42.1). The lamp is turned on and held 6–8 inches above the skin to be examined.

Normal Findings

Normal skin shows little or no fluorescence.

Selected Abnormal Findings

The Wood's lamp may be used to diagnose the following conditions (the color of fluorescence is listed in parentheses): tinea capitis (bright yellow green–pale green); tinea versicolor (golden yellow); *Pseudomonas aeruginosa* infection (aqua green or white green); and erythrasma (coral red–pink).

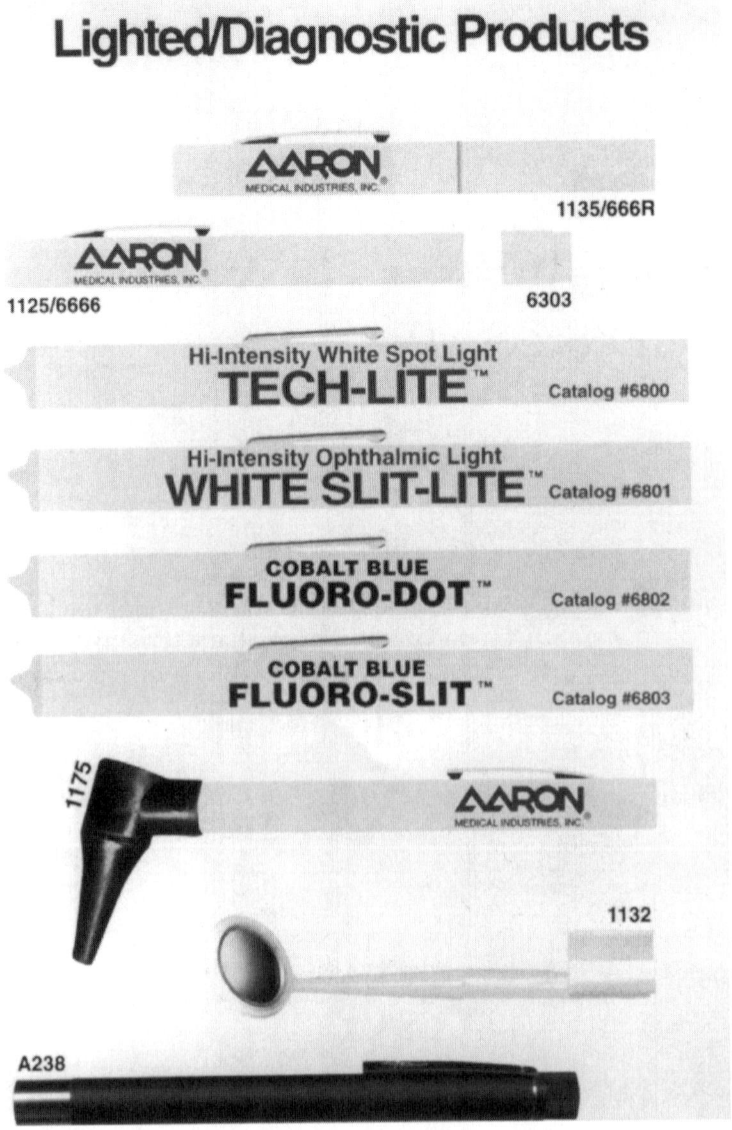

FIGURE 42.1.
Wood's lamps are available as plug-in or portable units such as this one. (Courtesy of Aaron Medical Industries, 7100 30th Avenue North, St. Petersburg, FL 33710.)

Special Notes

Prolonged exposure (especially of the eyes) should be avoided. Tetracycline, fluorescein, and some cosmetics may produce fluorescence in normal skin or such common lesions as acne.

Suggested Readings

Frieden IJ. Diagnosis and management of tinea capitis. *Pediatr Ann* 1987;16:39.

Ginsburg CM. Superficial manifestations of *Corynebacterium* Group JK sepsis. *J Am Acad Dermatol* 1987;16:444.

Pembroke AC. Fungal infections of the skin. *Practitioner* 1986;230:229.

Section V

EAR, NOSE, AND THROAT PROCEDURES

Chapter 43

EAR PIERCING

Piercing of the ears or other body parts is an elective procedure often performed by nonphysicians. Many persons, however, choose to have this procedure performed under more sterile conditions by someone with more skill and knowledge.

Equipment

- Commercial ear piercing guns or disposable devices, as shown in Figure 43.1

or

- One 18- and 21-gauge needle and an earring of the patient's choice (preferably 14-karat gold or surgical stainless steel) for each ear

or

- 20-gauge intravenous needle with plastic cannula (e.g., angiocath) and an earring of the patient's choice for each ear
- Skin preparation materials (e.g., povidone–iodine and 70% isopropyl alcohol)
- Scissors and sterile forceps or hemostat (if a needle technique or patient-supplied earring is used)
- Cold-sterilization solution (if a patient-supplied earring is used)
- Surgical skin-marking pencil (optional but desirable)
- Topical anesthetic spray or ice (optional)

Training/Credentialing

No special credentialing needed; office procedure only.

Coding

69090 Ear piercing

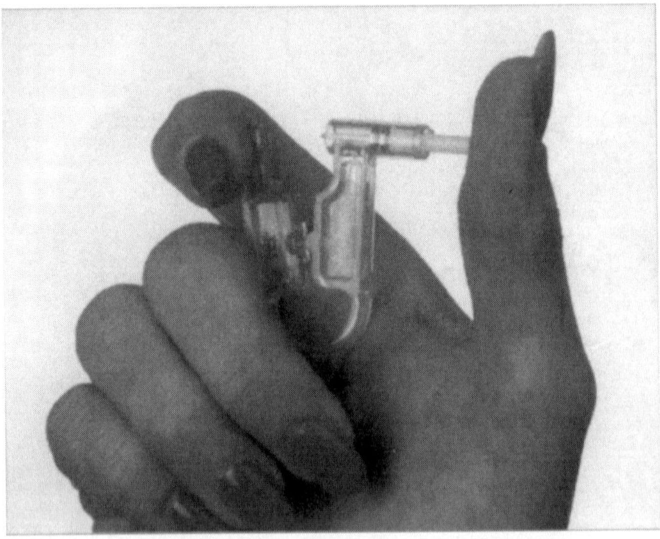

FIGURE 43.1.
Several different makes and types of ear piercing devices are commercially available, ranging from reusable guns that accept a variety of ear studs to disposable units. (Courtesy of Ronile, P.O. Box 1610, Sagamore Beach, MA 02562.)

Technique

Body piercing is a surgical procedure, albeit a minor one. For this reason, informed consent should be obtained and common sense contraindications observed. The procedure should not be performed in the presence of a local infection or significant dermatologic condition, in immunocompromised patients, persons with a coagulation disorder, or anyone deemed incapable of informed consent. (An exception to the latter is the minor for whom a parent or legal guardian provides consent.) Appropriate blood and body fluid precautions should be used.

The technique used varies slightly depending on whether patient-supplied earrings are used and on the site of piercing. A commercially supplied unit may be used for most sites and generally includes an ear piercing needle/stud and backing. When the patient supplies the stud, a needle technique should be used.

PIERCING GUN TECHNIQUE

If the device to be used is not supplied presterilized, the gun, piercing needle and earrings, and backings should be cold-sterilized according to the directions provided with the sterilizing solution. The site to be pierced should be marked by the patient (or family member) so that there is no ambiguity as to the desired placement. (It is recommended that the auricular cartilage be avoided if at all possible.)

Using a sterile technique, the piercing needle should be loaded into the piercing gun. For most guns, the piercing needle is loaded into the proximal portion of the gun with the backing placed in a holder at the tip (Fig. 43.2). If anesthesia is desired, a topical spray, ice held against both sides of the site for a minute or two, or finger compression for 30 seconds provide adequate but brief analgesia.

The site should be disinfected with an antiseptic solution; care should be taken not to obliterate any previously placed skin markings. The piercing gun is applied over the marked site so that the piercing needle will pass from the anterior surface posteriorly. The gun is triggered according to manufacturer's directions and the

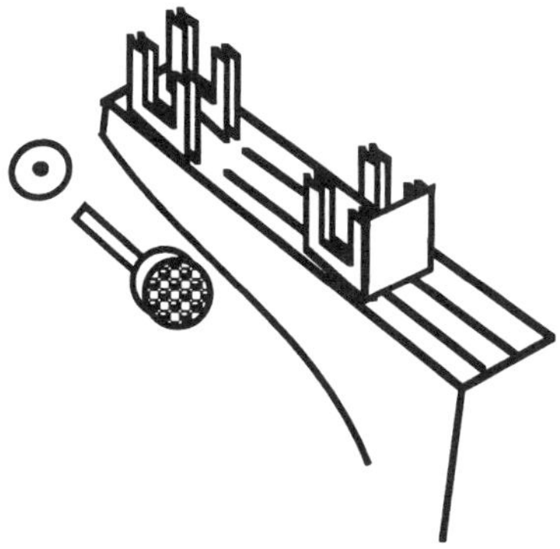

FIGURE 43.2.
By using a sterile technique, the earring and back are placed into the holders of the piercing instrument. The sliding holder for the earring stud is advanced by triggering the device, thereby advancing the shaft through the tissue and into the backing.

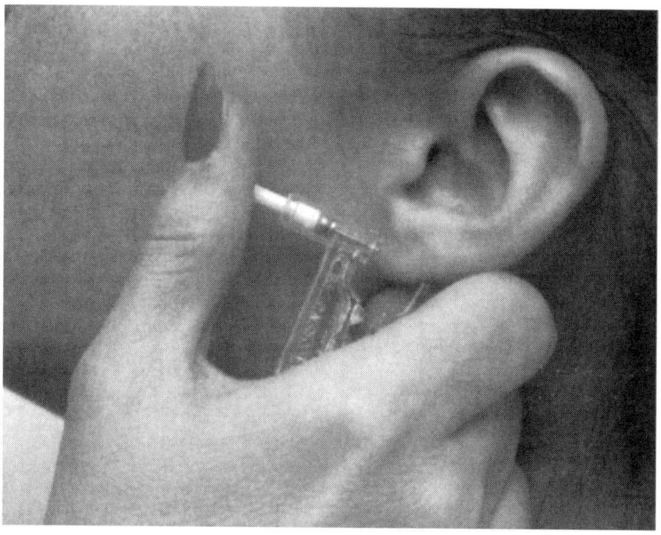

FIGURE 43.3.
Disposable ear piercing guns should be positioned in the same manner as the reusable devices. (Courtesy of Ronile, P.O. Box 1610, Sagamore Beach, MA 02562.)

backing checked for security. The procedure may then be repeated for the opposite side (if desired).

Disposable ear piercing devices integrate the function of the gun into a self-contained unit that comes preloaded with the earring. The device is positioned over the insertion point as shown in Figure 43.3. The jaws of the device are closed, thereby piercing the ear and attaching the clasp. The device is then removed in a downward manner, which releases the clasp.

Needle Technique

The earrings and backings should be cold-sterilized according to the directions supplied with the sterilizing solution. As with gun techniques, the patient should mark the site to be pierced so as to avoid confusion and discord. (With the needle technique, it is also recommended that the auricular cartilage be avoided.) The skin should be prepared and analgesia supplied (if desired) as described above.

If two needles are used, the 21-gauge needle is inserted first, going from anterior to posterior at the chosen site (Fig. 43.4). The 18-gauge needle is placed over the smaller needle (to act as a guide) and is advanced from behind to emerge at the front (Fig. 43.5).

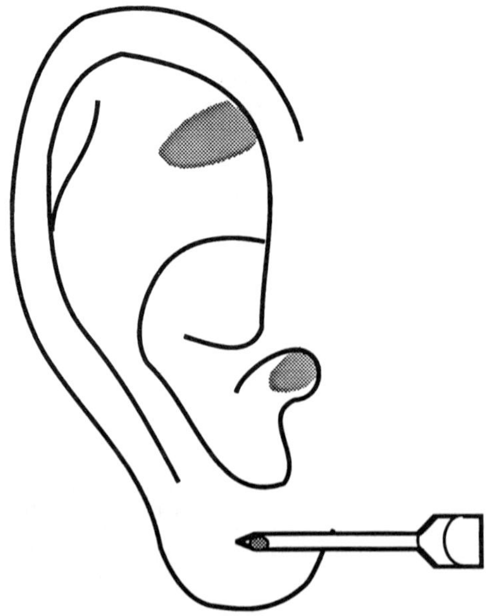

FIGURE 43.4.
The two-needle technique of piercing begins with the passage of the smaller needle (21-gauge) through the tissue from front to back.

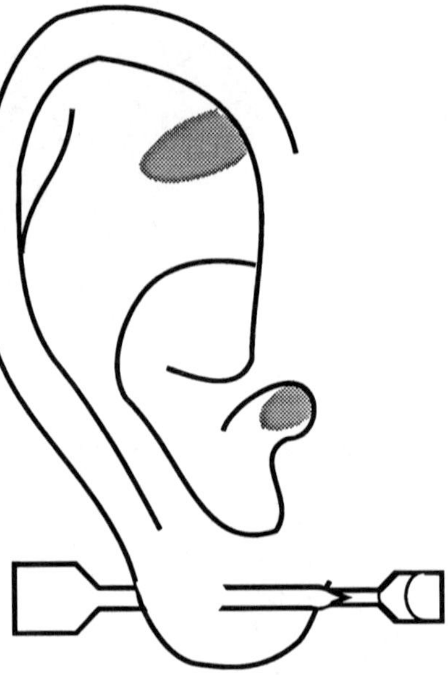

FIGURE 43.5.
Once the smaller needle has been passed from front to back, the larger (18-gauge) needle is threaded over this as a guide and brought to the front.

The smaller needle is removed and the post of the earring is placed (by sterile technique) inside the lumen of the larger needle (Fig. 43.6). The needle is withdrawn and the post is drawn through the tissue. The earring back is then secured.

A single needle pass may be used if an intravenous needle with a plastic sheath is used. With this method, the 20-gauge intravenous needle with sheath is placed from the anterior to posterior location in a single pass (Fig. 43.7). The inner needle is removed and the hub portion of the plastic catheter is cut off using sterile scissors. The sterilized earring post is inserted into the lumen of the plastic sheath using a sterile technique; the sheath is pulled through the tissue, carrying the post at the same time (Fig. 43.8). The sheath is removed and discarded, and the earring back is attached, thereby completing the procedure.

A disposable ear piercing system that integrates the needle and shaft of the earring

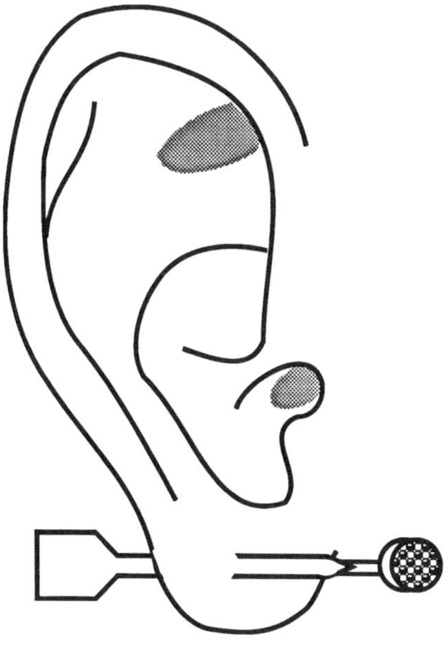

FIGURE 43.6.
Insertion using the two-needle technique is completed by removing the smaller needle and inserting the shaft of the ear stud to be used into the lumen of the large needle. This assembly is then withdrawn as a unit, leaving the stud in place in the tissue. The procedure is completed when the backing is applied to the stud.

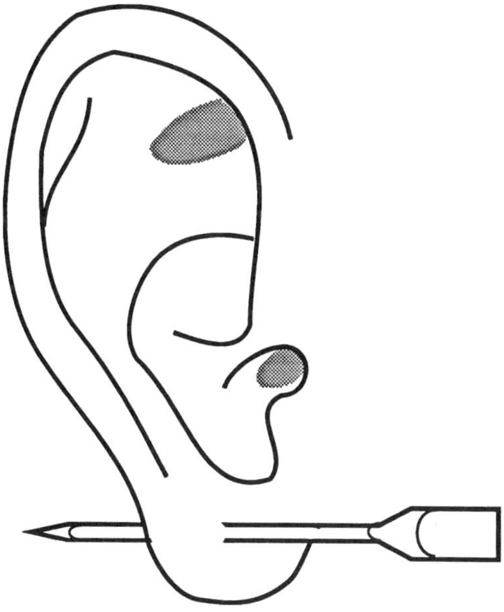

FIGURE 43.7.
Plastic sheathed intravenous needles should be passed from front to back at the desired site; the metal needle is then withdrawn, leaving the plastic canula in place.

is also available (Fig. 43.9). This device combines a 20-gauge injection needle and the shaft of the earring itself. The earring is passed through the tissue (front to back) and into a receiving pad that separates the sharp needle from the normal earring shaft. The earring backing is then applied in a normal manner.

Special Notes

Patients should be instructed to cleanse the site of piercing daily with 70% isopropyl alcohol and to avoiding exposing the area to strong soaps, cosmetics, or hair sprays. The shaft of the earring should be rotated several times a day to reduce the possibility of the post becoming embedded in the tissue. The site should be checked daily for signs

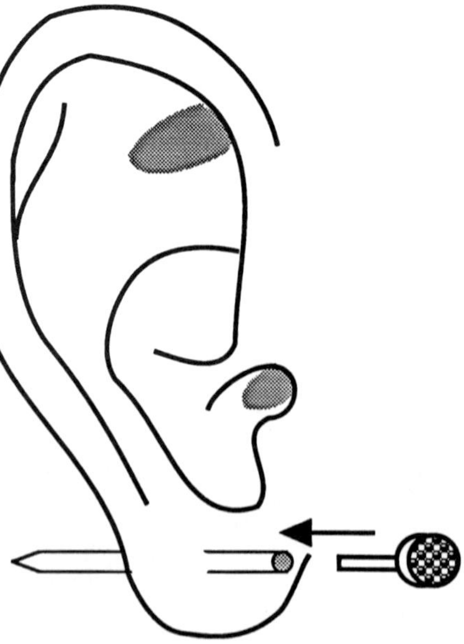

FIGURE 43.8.
The hub of the plastic canula is cut off using sterile scissors, and the shaft of the ear stud is placed in the lumen of the canula. This assembly is then withdrawn through the back of the ear, leaving the stud in place and ready for the attachment of the earring back.

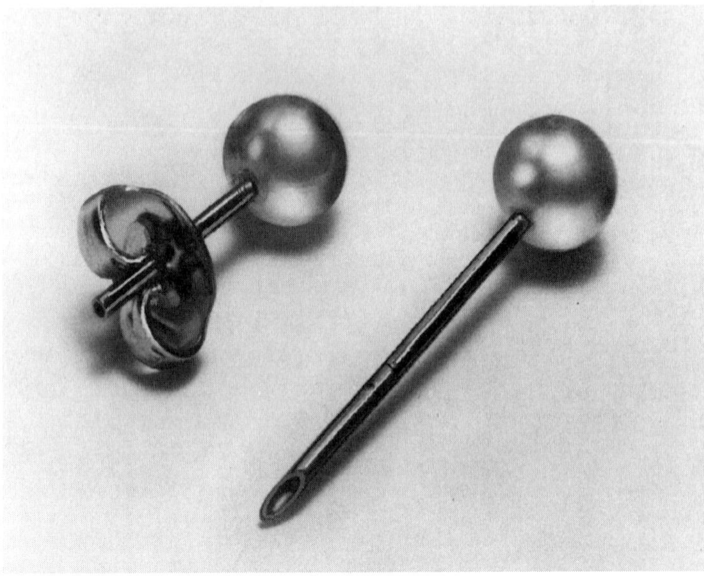

FIGURE 43.9.
An integrated needle and earring allow piercing to be performed in one step. (Courtesy of H & A Enterprises, Inc., 143–19 25th Avenue, Whitestone, NY 11357.)

of inflammation (redness or edema). The earring should be left in place for at least 6 weeks, after which time it may be removed and changed as desired.

Suggested Readings

Cohen HA, Nussinovitch M, Straussberg R. Embedded earrings. *Cutis* 1994;53:82.

Driscoll CE. Procedures for your practice: ear piercing. *Patient Care* 1990;August:194.

Dunlop DG, McCabe M, Evans R, et al. Ear piercing and children's rights. *BMJ* 1994;308:1636.

Fisher AA. Sensitization to nickel from stainless steel ear-piercing kits. *Contact Dermatitis* 1994;30:126.

Inoue T, Kurihara T, Harashina T. Ear-piercing technique by using an eyelet-type Teflon piercer (Eyelet-Piercer). *Ann Plastic Surg* 1993;31:159.

Matarasso SL, Glogau RG. Surgical pearl: ear piercing facilitated by magnetic earrings. *J Am Acad Dermatol* 1994;31:485.

Rasanen L, Lehto M, Mustikka-Maki UP. Sensitization to nickel from stainless steel ear-piercing kits. *Contact Dermatitis* 1993;28:292.

Zachowski DA. An IV cannula stent for ear piercing. *Plast Reconstr Surg* 1987;80:751.

Chapter 44

EXAMINATION OF THE MOUTH AND OROPHARYNX

Several systemic diseases, including many of direct interest to gynecologists (such as sexually transmissible infections), have signs or symptoms that involve the mouth and oropharynx. These structures are often overlooked by physicians, who believe them to be the province of the dental profession. Simple skills and techniques allow this area to be effectively examined.

Equipment

- A good light source or well-functioning flashlight
- A tongue blade
- Gauze sponge(s) (2-inch by 2-inch or 4-inch by 4-inch)
- Examination gloves
- Dental mirror (optional)

Training/Credentialing

No special credentialing needed; office diagnostic procedure only.

Coding

No specific code for examination of the mouth and oropharynx is used. The inclusion of these examinations may justify or support a higher acuity for the other services rendered. If only these examinations are performed, the following code may be considered:

92599 Unlisted otorhinolaryngological service or procedure

Technique

As with most portions of the physical examination, the examination of the mouth and oropharynx begins with inspection. The skin of the lower face, the lips, tongue, cheeks, and posterior oropharynx should be inspected using a good light source. Lesions, discoloration, or asymmetries should be noted.

Sensation and motor function over the lower face and lips should be evaluated to test the function of the facial and trigeminal nerves (Table 44.1). Sensation may be tested using a cotton fluff made by pulling out a few strands of material from the tip of an applicator stick. These strands may be lightly brushed against the skin while the patient closes her eyes and reports the presence and location of touch. Muscle function

TABLE 44.1. Cranial Nerves Represented in the Mouth and Oropharynx

CRANIAL NERVE	MOTOR COMPONENT	SENSORY COMPONENT
Trigeminal (V)	Muscles of mastication (bite)	Facial skin sensation (lower two divisions: V2 and V3)
Facial (VII)	Ability to smile and frown	Taste, anterior two-thirds of tongue
Glossopharyngeal (IX)	Elevation of posterior pharynx and laryngeal muscles (gag reflex)	Taste, posterior one-third of tongue
Vagus (X)	Swallowing, elevation of palate and laryngeal muscles	Gag reflex (afferent loop)
Hypoglossal (XII)	Muscles of the tongue	

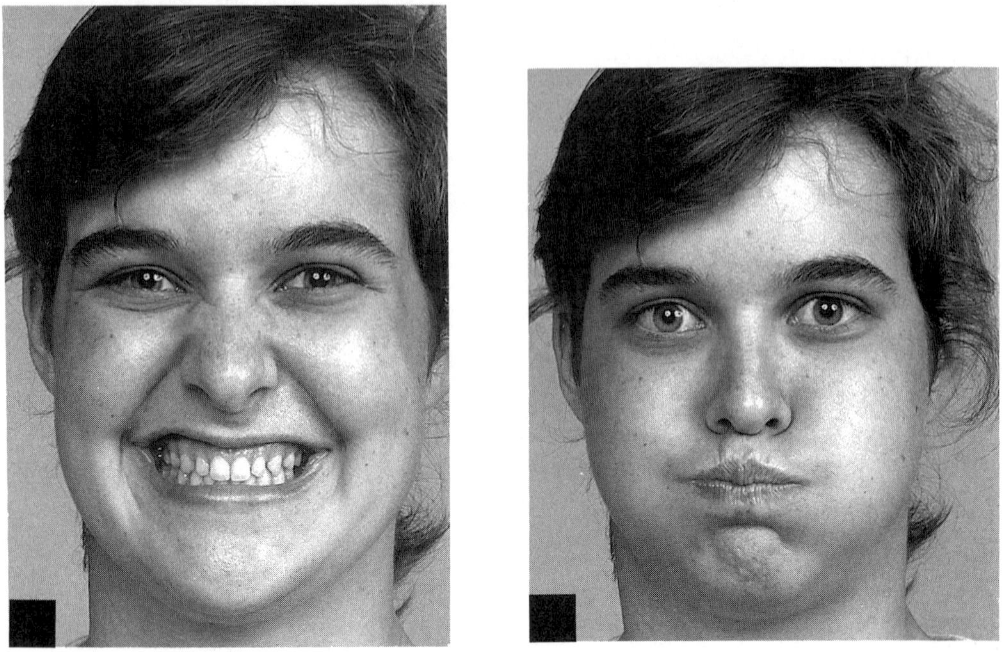

FIGURE 44.1.
The function of the lower portions of the facial nerve (cranial nerve VII) is assessed by asking the patient to smile and puff out the cheeks as shown. (Reproduced with permission from Willms JL, Schneiderman H, Algranati PS. Physical Diagnosis: Bedside Evaluation of Diagnosis and Function. *Baltimore: Williams & Wilkins, 1994:125.)*

may be assessed by asking the patient to smile, puff out her cheeks, open her mouth, and bite down hard (Fig. 44.1). Inspection and palpation during these maneuvers will reveal asymmetry or weakness. The lips should be inspected for color, lesions, and bleeding. The corners of the mouth should be inspected for the integrity of the mucosal junctions.

The patient should be asked to open her mouth widely so that the oral cavity and associated structures can be viewed (Fig. 44.2). A tongue blade may be used to facilitate viewing all quadrants of the oral cavity, tongue (upper and lower surfaces), soft and hard palates, gingival surfaces, and buccal mucosa. Care should be taken to avoid touching the posterior portion of the tongue or the back of the oropharynx with the tongue blade because this will elicit the gag reflex. The gag reflex need not be tested unless cranial nerve damage is very likely. If the base of the mouth is not readily visible, the patient may be asked to tip her head back; the mouth may then be examined from behind the patient (Fig. 44.3).

The general condition of the teeth should be noted. The patient should be asked to stick her tongue out and say "haaatt," which results in elevation of the soft palate (Fig. 44.4). This technique tests the function of cranial nerves X and XII.

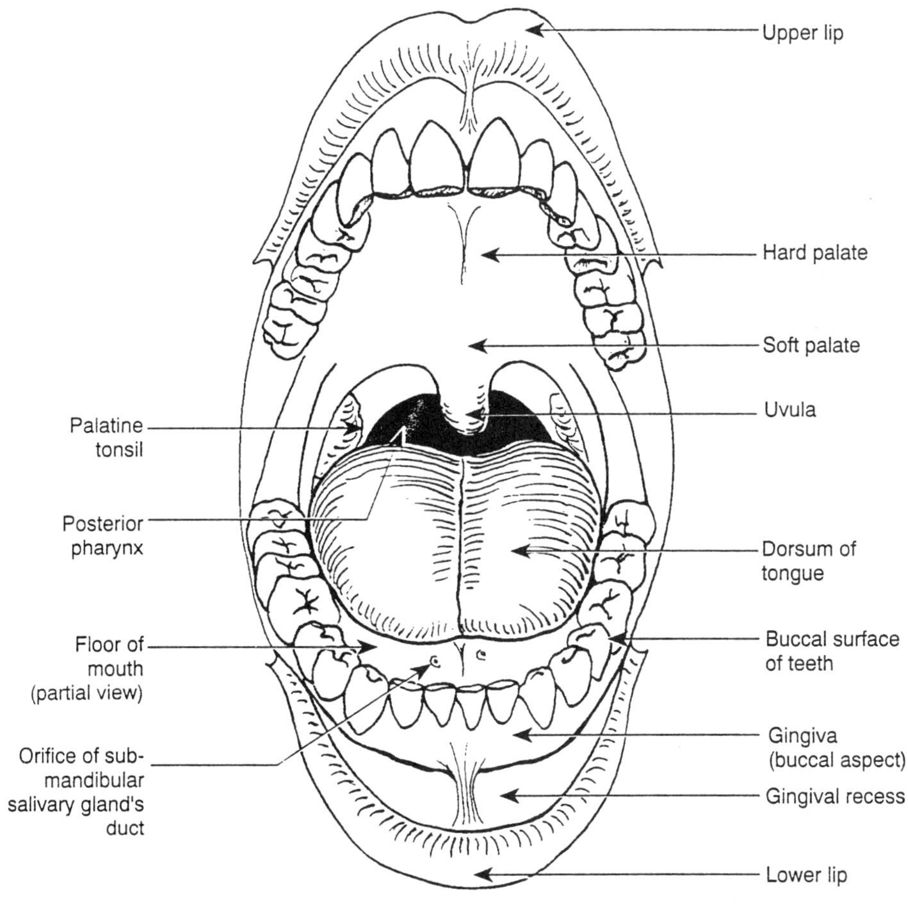

FIGURE 44.2.
Anatomical structures of oral cavity as viewed on inspection. (Reproduced with permission from Willms JL, Schneiderman H, Algranati PS. Physical Diagnosis: Bedside Evaluation of Diagnosis and Function. *Baltimore: Williams & Wilkins, 1994:139.)*

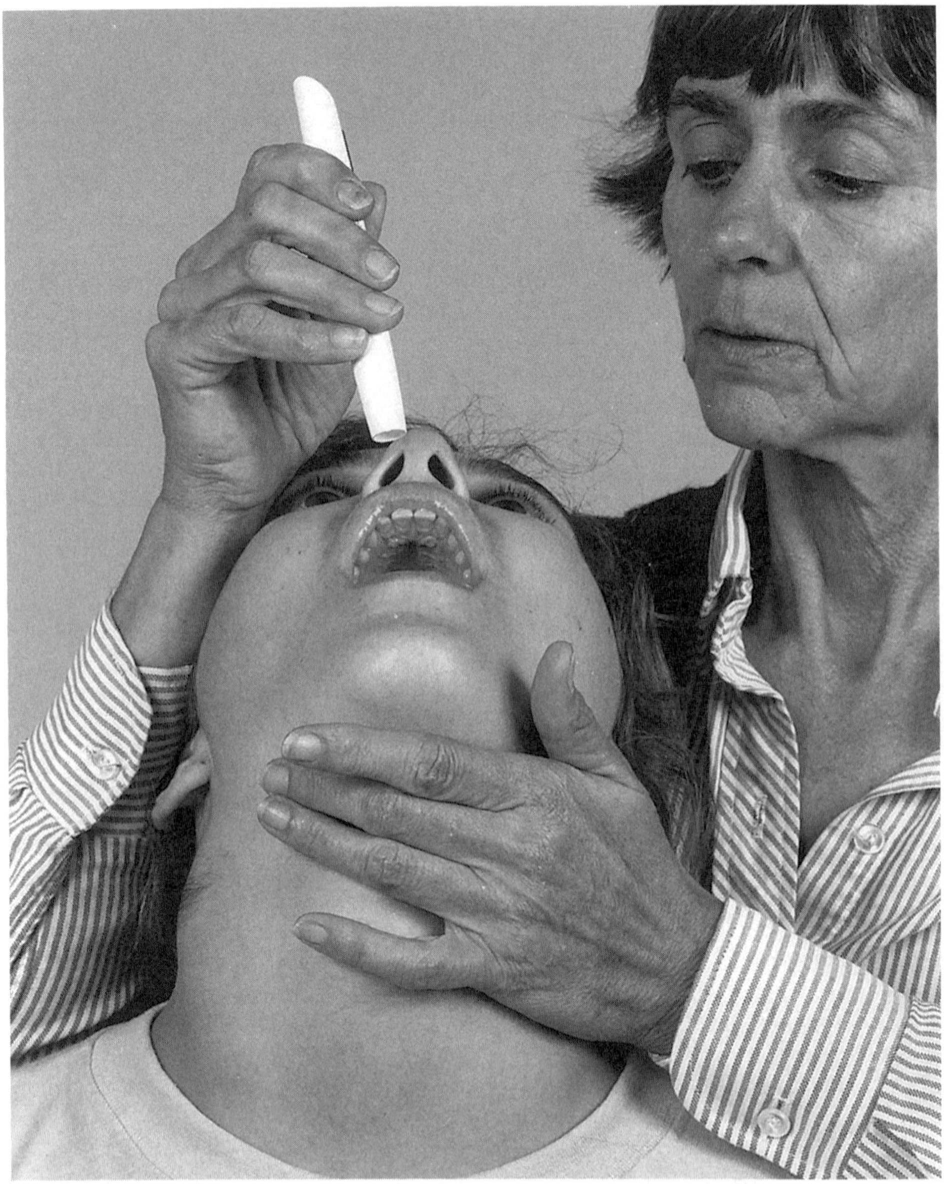

FIGURE 44.3.
Examining the mouth from the back. (Reproduced with permission from Willms JL, Schneiderman H, Algranati PS. Physical Diagnosis: Bedside Evaluation of Diagnosis and Function. *Baltimore: Williams & Wilkins, 1994:166.)*

Examination gloves should be donned and the tongue grasped using the nondominant hand and a gauze pad (Fig. 44.5). The tongue should be moved so that the lateral sides may be inspected. With the tongue alternately elevated and depressed by the patient, the tongue should be gently palpated for masses or tenderness. The buccal groove between the cheek and gum and the line between gingiva and palate should be palpated by gently passing a finger over these areas.

The posterior oropharynx may be further investigated through the use of a dental mirror or laryngoscope (see Chapter 47, Indirect Laryngoscopy).

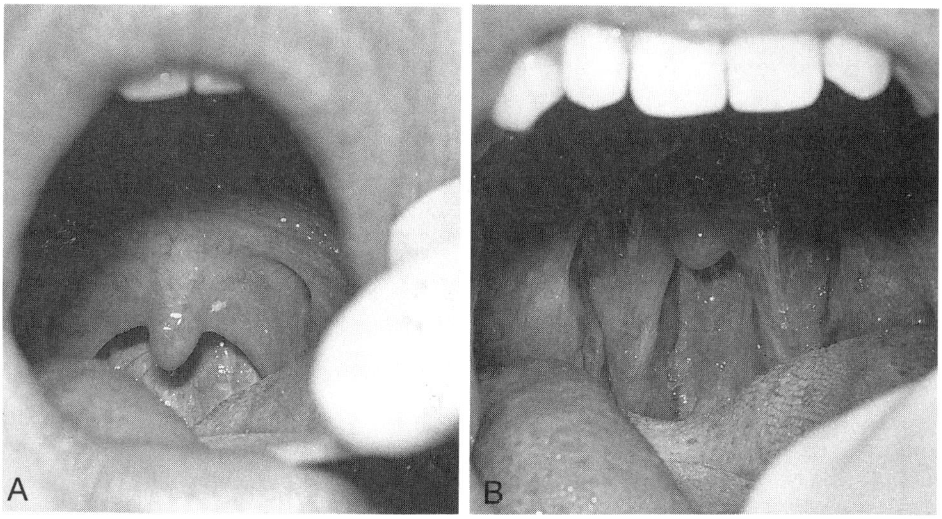

FIGURE 44.4.
The palate is shown in the resting and elevated positions. (Reproduced with permission from Willms JL, Schneiderman H, Algranati PS. Physical Diagnosis: Bedside Evaluation of Diagnosis and Function. *Baltimore: Williams & Wilkins, 1994:140.)*

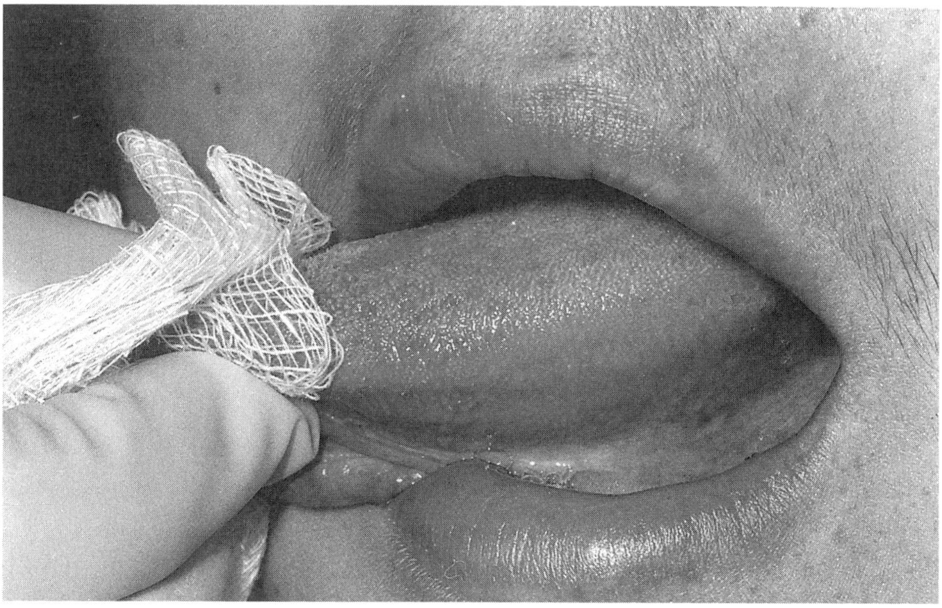

FIGURE 44.5.
Gripping the tongue with a gauze pad. (Reproduced with permission from Willms JL, Schneiderman H, Algranati PS. Physical Diagnosis: Bedside Evaluation of Diagnosis and Function. *Baltimore: Williams & Wilkins, 1994:167.)*

Normal Findings

The oropharynx should appear healthy, smooth, glistening, and pink, with no significant tonsillar or adenoidal tissue visible. No hyperemia or exudate should be present.

Some normal adults retain visible tonsillar tissue that may be seen protruding from behind the tonsillar pillars bilaterally. When present, this tissue may show pitting but should not feature any exudate.

The gag reflex may be absent without disease. Symmetric motion of the posterior oropharynx suggests that the vagus nerve is intact, and taste over the posterior one-third of the tongue indicates the functioning of the glossopharyngeal nerve.

Dark spots on the gingiva are common in dark-pigmented patients and can occur in light-skinned persons with Addison's disease.

Selected Abnormal Findings

If the tongue deviates to one side when extended, it may indicate disease or damage of the hypoglossal nerve (cranial nerve XII) on the side toward which the tongue points. Passive displacement of an otherwise normal tongue may be caused by such factors as partial loss of dentition.

Enlargement of the parotid glands suggests the possibility of starvation (including anorexia and bulimia), Sjögren's syndrome, alcoholism, diabetes mellitus, acute parotitis, or human immunodeficiency virus infection.

Oral candida infections may be suggested by the presence of a white pseudomembranous covering of the tongue, palate, buccal mucosa, or floor of the mouth. Scraping this material away with the side of a tongue blade will reveal a raw, bleeding mucosa below. The white patches found in leukoplakia, early cancer, or hairy leukoplakia do not scrape off.

Herpes gingivostomatitis produces painful vesicles with an erythematous base similar to those found in herpes vulvitis.

Suggested Readings

Ahola SJ. Unexplained parotid enlargement: a clue to occult bulimia. *Conn Med* 1982;46:185.

Anonymous. Orofacial manifestations of HIV infection. *Lancet* 1988;1:976.

Marshberg A, Samit A. Early detection, diagnosis, and management of oral and oropharyngeal cancer. *CA Cancer J Clin* 1989;39:67.

Sapira JD. *The Art and Science of Bedside Diagnosis*. Baltimore: Williams & Wilkins, 1990:221.

Willms JL, Schneiderman H, Algranati PS. *Physical Diagnosis: Bedside Evaluation of Diagnosis and Function*. Baltimore: Williams & Wilkins, 1994:119.

Wood NK, Goaz PW. *Differential Diagnosis of Oral Lesions*. 3rd ed. St. Louis: CV Mosby, 1985.

Chapter 45

REMOVAL OF FOREIGN BODIES FROM THE EAR

Small objects of various sorts may become lodged in the auditory canal. Although this is more common in children and the mentally impaired, any patient may be at risk. To avoid damage or further injury, the object should be promptly removed using the least invasive technique possible.

Equipment

- Operating otoscope or ear speculum and light source
- Topical anesthetic (4% lidocaine or 20% benzocaine)

or

- Local anesthetic (1% lidocaine with epinephrine for the external half of the canal) or 1% lidocaine without epinephrine for subcutaneous injection, with appropriate syringe and needle (22-gauge or finer)

FOR IRRIGATION TECHNIQUE

- Ear syringe, bulb syringe, or 30- to 50-mL hypodermic syringe
- Tubing from a 22-gauge butterfly-type needle (without needle) or the plastic outer canula from an 18-gauge intravenous needle set (e.g., angiocath)
- Body temperature water or saline
- Emesis basin and disposable foam or paper coffee cup
- Towels, sheet, or plastic drape
- Cotton-tipped applicators or small gauze

FOR DIRECT TECHNIQUE

- Ear curette or "scoop"
- Ear forceps or alligator forceps
- 21-gauge 1.5-inch needle with tip bent at right angle
- Small suction tip or plastic intravenous canula and suction source (optional)

Training/Credentialing

No special credentialing needed; generally an office procedure only.

Coding

69200	Removal foreign body from external auditory canal; without general anesthesia
69205	Removal foreign body from external auditory canal; with general anesthesia

Technique

Before any attempt is made to remove a foreign body from the ear, the nature of the object and the status of the patient's ear drum must be known. If there is any possibility that the patient has, or may have sustained, a perforated tympanic membrane, no irrigation or ear drops should be used, and a referral for specialized care is mandated. The type of material involved and the length of time it has been present may also suggest the need for referral. For example, many types of organic materials, such as plant matter, beans, or seeds, may swell with time or if irrigation is used, resulting in further impaction. If simple methods do not dislodge these items, a prompt referral should be made.

Removal begins with direct inspection performed with the aid of an operating otoscopy or an ear speculum and external light. Visualization is facilitated by pulling the auricle upward and backward to straighten the outer portion of the canal. If debris or fluid is present it must be suctioned before a full assessment is possible. When the object is near the opening, an ear curette, alligator forceps, or 22-gauge needle bent to a fine hook on the end may be used to extract the object. For fibrous materials, alligator forceps are the most effective. Care must be used to steady the operating hand by placing the heel of the hand against the patient's head. When a curette or hook is used, the instrument should be passed beyond the object, taking care to avoid the walls of the canal (Fig. 45.1). Gentle traction usually results in the withdrawal of the object. When the object does not occlude the lumen, irrigation with body-temperature water or

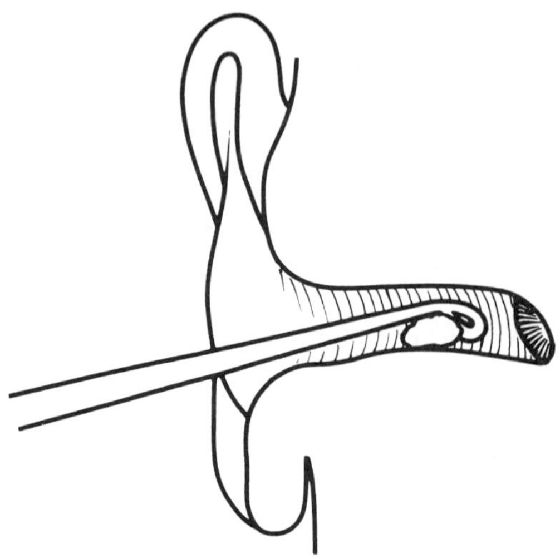

FIGURE 45.1.
Ear curette used to remove a foreign body lodged in the ear canal. (Reproduced with permission from Simon RR, Brenner BE. Emergency Procedures and Techniques. *Baltimore: Williams & Wilkins, 1994:254.)*

saline may be used in a manner similar to that used to remove ear wax (see Chapter 50, Wax [Cerumen] Removal).

When edema is present or examination of the ear is painful, the use of a local anesthetic may be preferable. This may take the form of topical agents instilled into the canal and retained for 10 to 15 minutes or the use of local anesthetics to numb the external ear and the canal. The success of local infiltration depends on an understanding of the nerve supply of the outer ear and distal canal (Fig. 45.2). The distal canal may be anesthetized using a four-quadrant block performed by infiltrating around the opening of the canal, as shown in Figure 45.3. When the helix must also be numbed, infiltration along the sulcus behind the auricle and in a semicircle behind the ear yields good results (Figs. 45.4 and 45.5).

Special Notes

If the foreign body is located in the inner one-third of the canal, referral is preferred. Hearing aid batteries that become trapped in the ear canal must be removed promptly to avoid damaging tissue by the electric current that may be created.

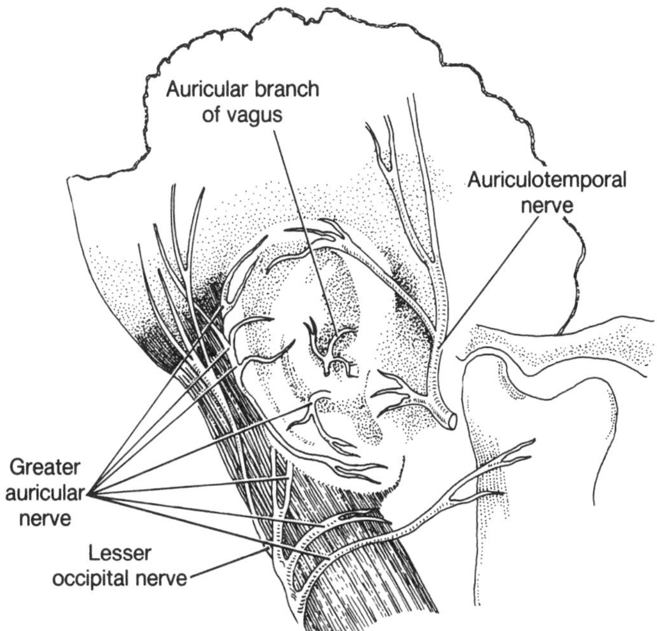

FIGURE 45.2.
The nerves supplying the ear. (Reproduced with permission from Simon RR, Brenner BE. Emergency Procedures and Techniques. *Baltimore: Williams & Wilkins, 1994:103.)*

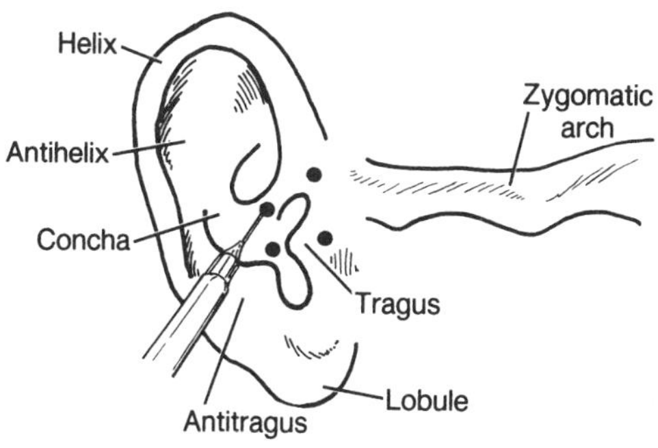

FIGURE 45.3.
The four-quadrant block for anesthetizing the auditory canal. (Reproduced with permission from Simon RR, Brenner BE. Emergency Procedures and Techniques. *Baltimore: Williams & Wilkins, 1994:103.)*

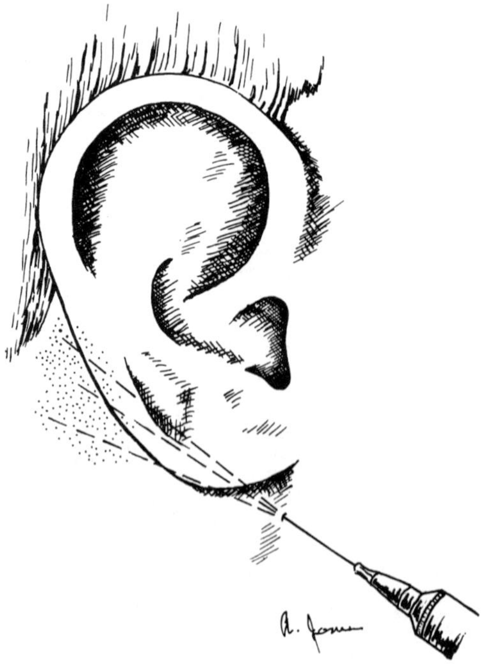

FIGURE 45.4.
Anesthetic solution is deposited in the sulcus behind the auricle. A wheal is raised under the skin that lies over the mastoid process. (Reproduced with permission from Simon RR, Brenner BE. Emergency Procedures and Techniques. *Baltimore: Williams & Wilkins, 1994:104.)*

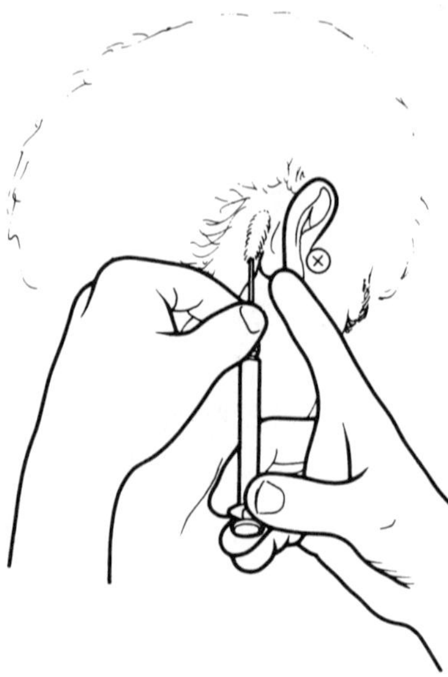

FIGURE 45.5.
Subcutaneous infiltration in a semicircle behind the ear; when accompanied by a block of the auriculotemporal nerve anteriorly, this infiltration provides anesthesia for the auricle. (Reproduced with permission from Simon RR, Brenner BE. Emergency Procedures and Techniques. *Baltimore: Williams & Wilkins, 1994:104.)*

Insects that become trapped in the ear canal should be smothered by instilling lidocaine, benzocaine, or mineral oil before removal is attempted. They may then be grasped with alligator forceps and removed.

Suggested Readings

Anon JB, Pulec JL. Foreign body (tooth) in the external auditory canal. *Ear Nose Throat J* 1994;73:511.

Bessler K, Shelton C. Ear foreign-body removal: a review of 98 consecutive cases. *Laryngoscope* 1993;103:367.

Hanson RM, Stephens M. Cyanoacrylate-assisted foreign body removal from the ear and nose in children. *J Paediatr Child Health* 1994;30:77.

Jensen JH. Technique for removing a spherical foreign body from the nose or ear. *Ear Nose Throat J* 1976;55:46.

Simon RR, Brenner BE. *Emergency Procedures and Techniques*. Baltimore: Williams & Wilkins, 1994:103.

White SJ, Broner S. The use of acetone to dissolve a Styrofoam impaction of the ear. *Ann Emerg Med* 1994;23:580.

Chapter 46

HEARING TESTING (AUDIOMETRY)

Often, an indication of hearing impairment may be noted by the close of the initial medical history. Screening may be used to assess this possibility, detect unilateral loss, or direct the focus of more intensive investigation. Audiometry assesses the patient's ability to hear sound. It may be performed through a formal series of assessments completed over a range of frequencies, or it may be performed as a series of office screening tests used to indicate the need for further testing or referral.

Equipment

- One or more tuning forks tuned to the C-notes of the musical scale; the most common is one tuned to 512 Hz (cycles per second)

or

- Portable or fixed audiometric testing instruments (audioscope)

Training/Credentialing

No special credentialing needed; office procedure only.

Coding

92551	Screening test, pure-tone air only
92552	Pure-tone audiometry (threshold), air only
92553	Pure-tone audiometry, air and bone

Technique

SCREENING

In the simplest form of screening for hearing loss, the investigator rubs his or her thumb and forefinger together at a distance of 10 cm from the patient's ear. This is repeated at approximately 2.5-cm intervals until the patient can no longer detect

TABLE 46.1. Hearing Handicap Inventory for the Elderly—Screening Version

PLEASE CIRCLE THE BEST ANSWER FOR EACH QUESTION

1. Does a hearing problem cause you to feel embarrassed when you meet new people?
   NO SOMETIMES YES
2. Does a hearing problem cause you to feel frustrated when talking to members of your family?
   NO SOMETIMES YES
3. Do you have difficulty hearing when someone speaks in a whisper?
   NO SOMETIMES YES
4. Do you feel handicapped by a hearing problem?
   NO SOMETIMES YES
5. Does a hearing problem cause you difficulty when visiting friends, relatives, or neighbors?
   NO SOMETIMES YES
6. Does a hearing problem cause you to attend religious services less often than you would like?
   NO SOMETIMES YES
7. Does a hearing problem cause you to have arguments with family members?
   NO SOMETIMES YES
8. Does a hearing problem cause you difficulty when listening to television or radio?
   NO SOMETIMES YES
9. Do you feel that any difficulty with your hearing limits or hampers your personal or social life?
   NO SOMETIMES YES
10. Does a hearing problem cause you difficulty when in a restaurant with relatives or friends?
   NO SOMETIMES YES

Reproduced with permission from Williams JL, Schneiderman H, Algranati PS. *Physical diagnosis.* Baltimore: Williams & Wilkins, 1994:158.

the sound. Studies indicate that at 21 cm, this test has a 90% sensitivity for detecting hearing loss. Although the specificity of this test is poor when compared with more formal audiometry, it is superior to whispered voice tests or some tuning-fork testing.

More formal audiometry may be performed using an audioscope to produce pure tones of varying frequency and intensity that may be supplied via air or bone to test the patient's threshold of detection. Diagnostic sensitivity and specificity may be increased by the addition of the Hearing Handicap Inventory for the Elderly—Screening Version (Table 46.1). This scale is scored with 2 points for "sometimes" and 4 points for "yes." No points are scored for "no" answers. A total score greater than 8 indicates probable hearing loss, and a score of 24 or greater demonstrates almost certain loss. When a loss or reduction in hearing acuity is suspected, the Rinne and Weber test should be performed to suggest the type of loss present.

RINNE TEST

The Rinne test is performed using a 512-Hz tuning fork. The tuning fork is set vibrating by gently striking one of its tips against the heal of the investigator's hand or by squeezing the tips together between the thumb and fingers and releasing smartly. The base of the vibrating fork is placed against the mastoid process and the patient is asked to signal when the hum can no longer be heard. At this signal the tuning fork is moved to near the external auditory meatus on the same side, and the patient is asked if the sound can still be detected. In a normal Rinne test result, air conduction should be more sensitive than bone conduction.

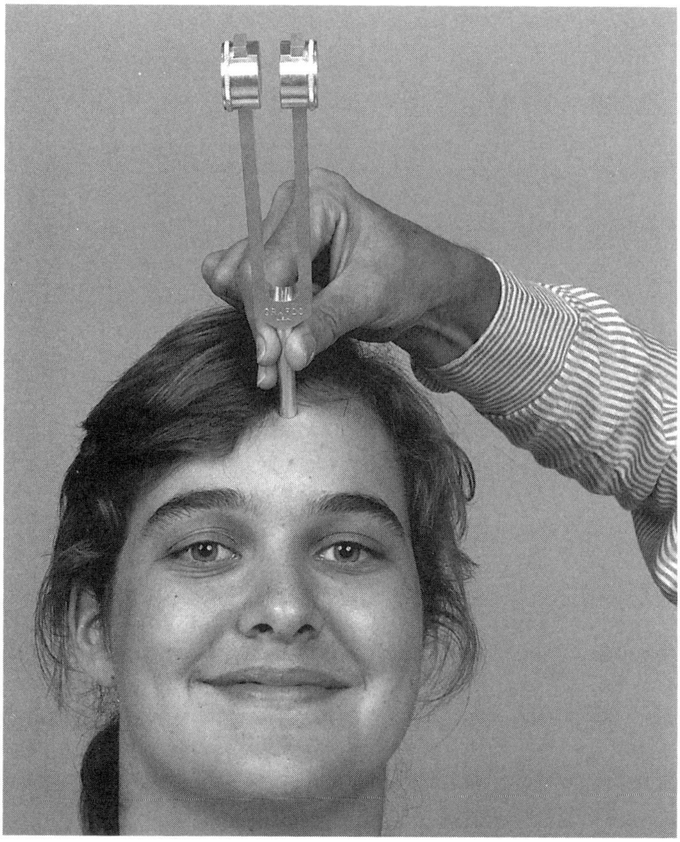

FIGURE 46.1.
Performance of Weber test. (Reproduced with permission from Willms JL, Schneiderman H, Algranati PS. Physical Diagnosis: Bedside Evaluation of Diagnosis and Function. *Baltimore: Williams & Wilkins, 1994:159.)*

WEBER TEST

The Weber test is conducted by holding the base of the vibrating tuning fork on the forehead of the patient in the midline (Fig. 46.1). The patient is asked to indicate where the sound is heard. Patients without hearing loss should hear the sound equally in both ears.

AUDIOMETRY

Audiometric measurement is used to document the patient's ability to hear sound over a range of frequencies and intensities. This is most often performed after the history or physical evaluation has indicated the possibility of a hearing defect. It may also be performed on persons at high risk for hearing loss by virtue of their employment or lifestyle (e.g., exposure to high-intensity sound).

The goal of audiometry is to measure the lowest intensity (in decibels) that can be heard at a given frequency. This threshold of detection is then graphed and compared to standards established by studying a large sample of normal patients.

The audiometer consists of a variable frequency oscillator that can generate pure tones over a range of frequencies and amplitudes, which may be supplied to either headphones or bone vibrator. Formal audiometric measurements generally cover bone and air conduction assessments with and without sound masking. For office screening, air conduction testing without masking is generally sufficient; most nonspecialists refer patients when more extensive testing is indicated.

TABLE 46.2. Symbols Used to Graph Audiometric Findings

	RESPONSE		
MODE (UNMASKED)	RIGHT	UNSPECIFIED	LEFT
Air conduction	O		X
Bone conduction (mastoid)	<	^	>
Bone conduction (forehead)	˥	v	L

The procedure begins with the patient comfortably sitting in a quiet setting, free of distractions and placed so that the patient cannot directly see the examiner or the audiometer. The patient should be acquainted with the test procedure and the need to indicate or signal when a tone is heard. This signal should continue for as long as the sound is heard. For air conduction testing, the headphones are placed comfortably on the patient's head, with care taken to avoid any interference from jewelry, glasses, or hats. The headphones should fit snugly against the ears, although care should be taken that the tragus does not become compressed against the auditory meatus (thereby resulting in obstruction).

Threshold testing is begun using a 2-second 1000-Hz signal at an intensity of 0 dB. The intensity is increased in 10-dB increments until the patient detects the signal. The intensity is then increased by 5 dB to verify the response and then decreased in steps of 10 dB until the sound can no longer be heard. The intensity level at which the tone is heard one-half of the time is the threshold; this value should be plotted on a graph of frequency versus intensity using standard graphing symbols (Table 46.2). This procedure is repeated for tones of 2000 Hz, 4000 Hz, and 8000 Hz, after which the 1000-Hz tone is retested and the frequency is reduced to 500 Hz, ending with a frequency of 250 Hz. Additional frequencies may be used but are generally not required to produce a picture of the patient's hearing abilities.

If bone conduction audiometry is to be performed, the same sequence of testing and threshold determination is carried out.

Normal Findings

Patients without hearing loss will be able to hear the sound of rubbing fingers at a distance of at least 20 cm. The Rinne test should demonstrate a superiority of air conduction over that of bone, and the Weber test should not lateralize to either side. If formal audiometry is performed, threshold detection should generally be below 20 dB at all frequencies (Fig. 46.2).

Selected Abnormal Findings

The Weber and Rinne tests may be used to distinguish between conductive and sensorineural hearing loss (Table 46.3). In general, in sensorineural hearing loss both bone and air conduction are decreased equally on the affected side. Thus, the Rinne test result should be normal (but reduced for both), whereas results of the Weber test should be lateralized away from the affected side. In contrast, conductive deafness produces an abnormal Rinne test result and Weber test results that are lateralize toward the affected ear. Mixed forms of deafness produce an unpredictable pattern of abnormalities that generally show less abnormality than would be expected based on the degree of auditory deficit.

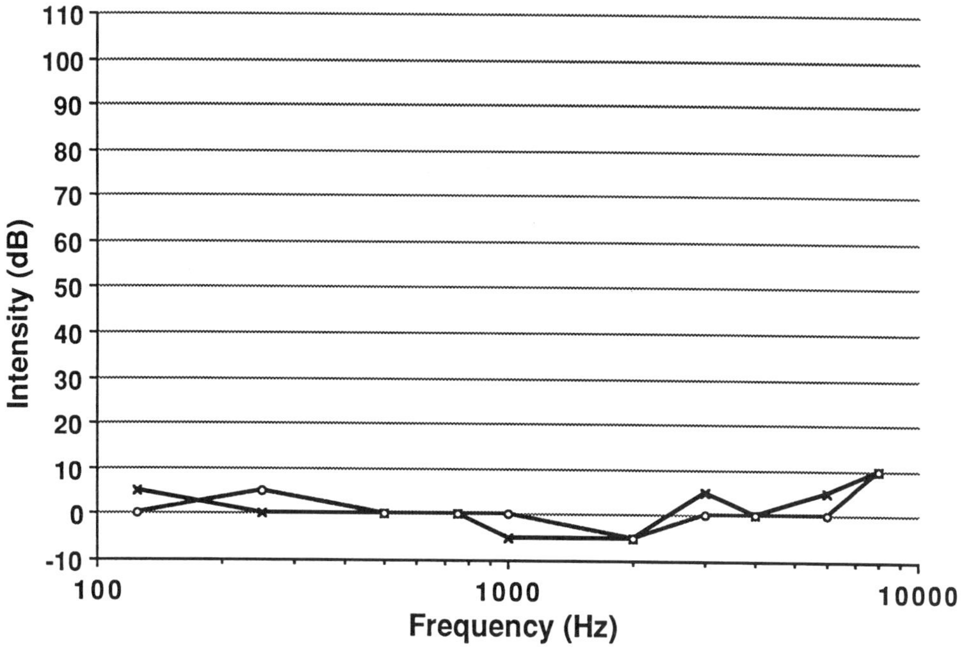

FIGURE 46.2.
Slight variations in threshold intensity are common in patients without hearing loss. A threshold intensity of 0 is defined as normal, although the intensity may be as high as 20 dB without significance. X and O indicate the results of testing from the left and right, respectively.

TABLE 46.3. Interpretation of Rinne and Weber Test Results[a]

DESCRIPTION	RINNE[a]	WEBER
Left ear, pure sensorineural	AC greater than BC	Lateralizes to right
Right ear, normal	AC greater than BC	
Left ear, pure conductive loss	BC greater than AC	Lateralizes to left
Right ear, normal	AC greater than BC	
Left ear, mixed deafness	Cannot predict	Cannot predict
Right ear, normal	AC greater than BC	
Bilateral sensorineural deafness		
Left ear	AC greater than BC	Lateralizes to better (less diseased) ear
Right ear	AC greater than BC	
Bilateral conductive loss		
Left ear	BC greater than AC	Lateralizes to worse (more diseased) ear
Right ear	BC greater than AC	
Bilateral mixed deafness	Cannot predict any test results	

[a]AC, air conduction; BC, bone conduction.
Reproduced with permission from Willms JL, Schneiderman H, Algranati PS.: *Physical Diagnosis.* Baltimore: Williams & Wilkins, 1994:159.)

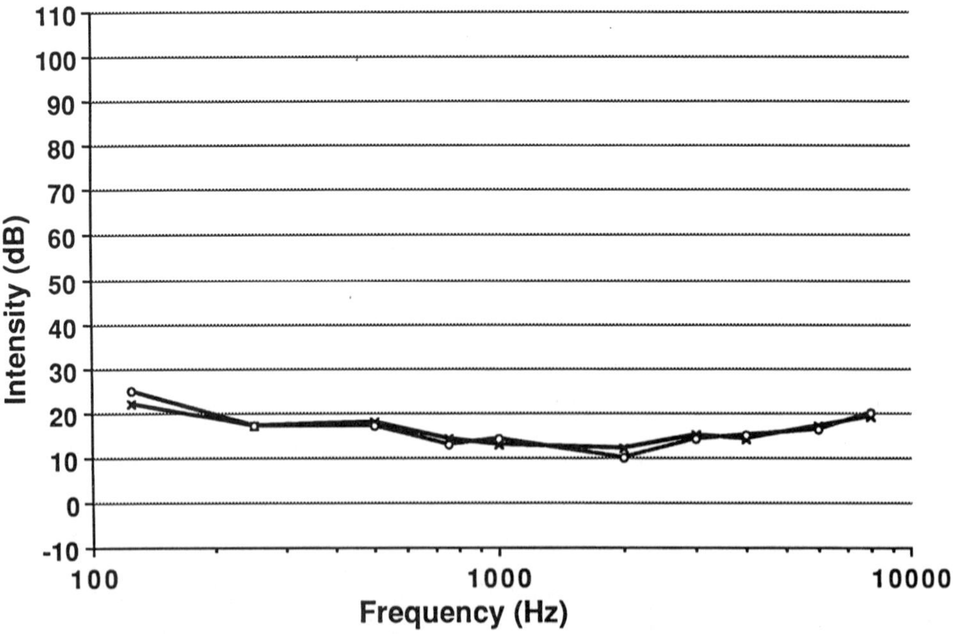

FIGURE 46.3.
An audiogram of a patient with mild presbyacusis. X and O indicate the results of testing from the left and right, respectively.

Slightly elevated audiometric thresholds are seen with presbyacusis (Fig. 46.3). Elevations as high as 20 dB are usually not clinically significant. Thresholds in the range of 21 to 40 dB are classified as mild hearing loss; 41–55 dB, moderate; 56–70 dB, moderately severe; 71–90 dB, severe; and greater than 91 dB, profound. Substantial difference between sides suggests the presence of disease and should prompt a referral for specialized evaluation.

Special Notes

After the initial trial of 1000 Hz, many examiners begin testing of a new frequency with an intensity of 15 to 20 dB below the threshold level found for the previous frequency. This reduces the overall amount of time spent testing without reducing the accuracy of the results.

Suggested Readings

American Speech-Language-Hearing Association. Guidelines for audiometric symbols. *ASHA* 1990;32(Suppl 2):25.

Coren S, Hakstian AR. Predicting speech recognition thresholds from pure tone hearing thresholds. *Perceptual Motor Skills* 1994;79:1003.

Robinson DW. Background noise in rooms used for pure-tone audiometry in disability assessment. *Br J Audiology* 1993;26:43.

Holtby I, Forster DP. Evaluation of pure tone audiometry and impedance screening in infant schoolchildren. *J Epidemiol Community Health* 1992;46:21.

Chapter 47

INDIRECT LARYNGOSCOPY

The availability of small fiberoptic laryngoscopes and bronchoscopes has reduced the use of indirect laryngoscopy by specialists. As an office screening procedure, however, the procedure still has merit. With simple, readily available equipment, indirect laryngoscopy can be a valuable adjunct to the evaluation of the posterior oropharynx and upper airway. With this technique, the upper tracheal rings, vocal cords, epiglottis, larynx, and hypopharynx may be visualized. Because of the minimal equipment and set up required, it is a reasonable procedure to perform in the office setting.

Equipment

- Dental mirror (no. 4 or 5 laryngeal mirror)

and

- Headlight or bright light source and head mirror

or

- Right-angle direct laryngoscope
- 4-inch by 4-inch gauze sponges
- Goggles or face-shield type surgical mask
- Topical anesthetic (lidocaine 10% spray, benzocaine 14% spray) (optional)
- Alcohol lamp or antifog agent (optional)

Training/Credentialing

No special credentialing needed; office procedure only.

Coding

31505	Laryngoscopy, indirect (separate procedure); diagnostic
31510	with biopsy

31511	with removal of foreign body
31512	with removal of lesion
31513	with vocal cord injection

Technique

The patient should be seated comfortably, facing the examiner and at an appropriate height for the examiner. The procedure should be explained to the patient and the patient reassured that the procedure should be painless and that every effort will be made to avoid the gag reflex. Dentures should be removed before the procedure.

If anesthesia is desired, the posterior oropharynx should be sprayed with a topical anesthetic such as lidocaine (10%) or benzocaine (14%). This should be done several minutes before beginning the procedure to allow time for full anesthesia to be accomplished. With care, the procedure may be performed equally well without anesthesia, although more skill and experience are required.

The examiner should position the headlight so that the axis of illumination is parallel to the axis of vision. If a head mirror is used, the examiner should seat himself or herself slightly to the side of the patient, with a bright light positioned behind the patient and shining into the mirror. The mirror is then adjusted to provide illumination in the same manner as with a head lamp. The dental mirror to be used should be the largest that can be accommodated in the back of the throat. The mirror should be warmed over an alcohol flame, in the examiner's hand, or inside the patient's cheek. If an external heat source is used, the temperature must be checked for safety before the mirror is introduced into the patient's mouth.

The patient should be requested to lean slightly forward and protrude the tongue. The head and jaw should protrude somewhat. The tongue is then gently grasped using a gauze sponge to allow it to be retracted and manipulated. The upper lip may be protected and retracted using the index or middle finger of the same hand. The patient should be asked to breathe in and out through the mouth in a panting-like manner, allowing the posterior oropharynx to open maximally. The back of the mirror should be applied to the roof of the mouth and used to gently lift the uvula out of the way (Fig. 47.1). Care should be used to avoid touching either the base of the tongue or the posterior pharyngeal wall; touching either of these produces a strong gag reflex. The gag reflex need only be tested when there is a strong possibility of cranial nerve damage (cranial nerves IX and X).

With the mirror in this position, it may be gently tilted to allow the larynx, hypopharynx, anterior oropharynx, and the base of the tongue to be inspected. The action of the vocal cords should be assessed at rest and by having the patient produce a high pitched "eee" sound.

An alternative method of performing laryngoscopy uses a right-angle laryngoscope (Fig. 47.2). As with the mirror technique, the tongue is gently retracted and the laryngoscope inserted behind the base of the tongue (Fig. 47.3). This allows a view of structures in the posterior oropharynx that is not reversed (as with the mirror) and is potentially larger and more detailed.

Normal Findings

The tissues of the oropharynx should be pink and moist, without lesions or asymmetry. Erythema and exudates should not be present. The vocal cords should be smooth and symmetric while at rest and vibrate evenly when phonation is attempted.

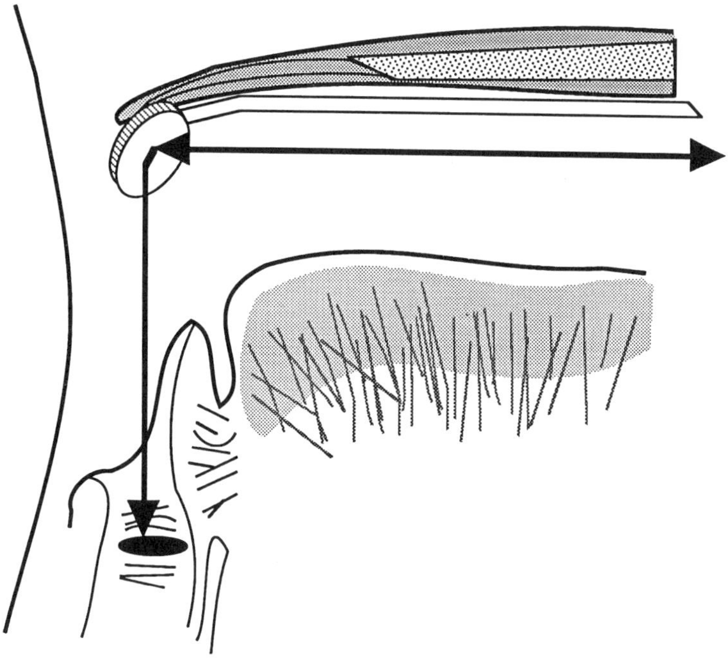

FIGURE 47.1.
The dental mirror is inserted into the posterior oropharynx, lifting the uvula and avoiding contact with the pharyngeal wall and the base of the tongue.

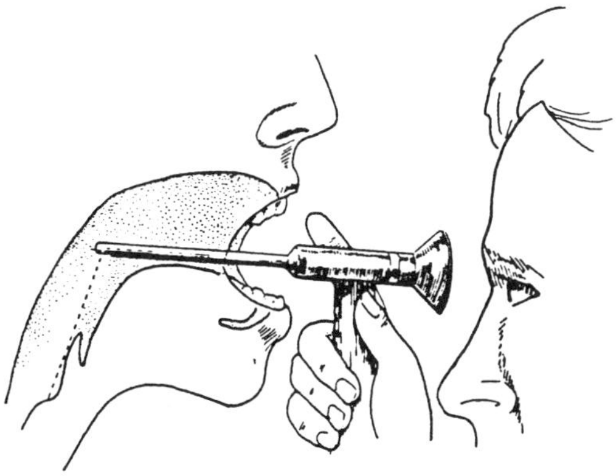

FIGURE 47.2.
The right-angle laryngoscope permits visualization at an angle that is perpendicular to the tip. (Reproduced with permission from Simon RR, Brenner BE. Emergency Procedures and Techniques. *Baltimore: Williams & Wilkins, 1994:270.)*

Selected Abnormal Findings

Telangiectases are sometimes found in the posterior oropharynx. These may be manifestations of hereditary hemorrhagic telangiectasia (Osler-Weber-Rendu syndrome) or cirrhosis. Telangiectases may be mistaken for evidence of pharyngitis. When there is doubt, a culture is indicated.

If the gag reflex is tested, the examiner must appreciate that some otherwise normal patients will have an absent gag reflex on one or both sides. It may be also suppressed or absent in the face of acute illness. An absent gag reflex is a poor predictor of risk for aspiration, just as an intact reflex provides only partial protection.

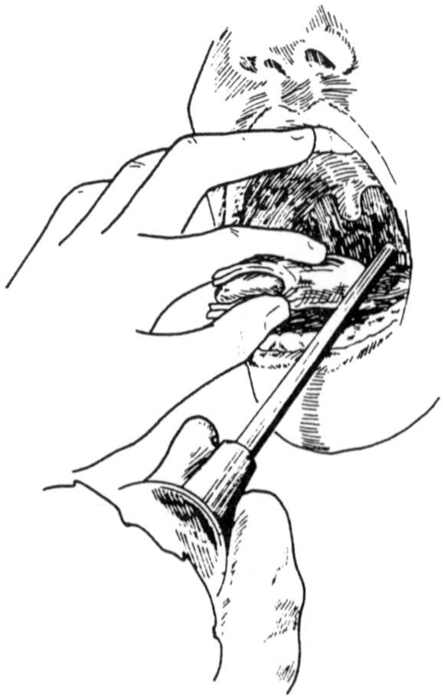

FIGURE 47.3.
In performing laryngoscopy with this instrument, a 4-inch by 4-inch piece of gauze is wrapped around the tip of the tongue and the tongue is grasped by the thumb and index finger. The tongue is pulled forward, and the laryngoscope is inserted so that the tip of the instrument is in the posterior pharynx behind the base of the tongue. This permits adequate visualization of the entire glottic area and supraglottic region. (Reproduced with permission from Simon RR, Brenner BE. Emergency Procedures and Techniques. *Baltimore: Williams & Wilkins, 1994:270.)*

Special Notes

Indirect laryngoscopy should not be performed in patients with acute epiglottitis. Attempting laryngoscopy under these conditions may precipitate reactive airway spasm and complete obstruction.

Suggested Readings

Abramson AL, Gilberto E, Mullooly V, et al. Microbial adherence to and disinfection of laryngoscopes used in office practice *Laryngoscope* 1993;103:503.

Foweraker JE. The laryngoscope as a potential source of cross-infection. *J Hosp Infect* 1995;29:315.

Saunders WH. Indirect mirror laryngoscopy: the larynx. *Clin Symp* 1964;16:67.

Simon RR, Brenner BE. *Emergency Procedures and Techniques.* Baltimore: Williams & Wilkins, 1994:270.

Chapter 48

NASAL EXAMINATION

Although proper examination of the nose and paranasal sinuses is simple, it is often overlooked in the course of routine examination. As primary care and triage occupy a greater proportion of office practice, gynecologists must be able to correctly perform this examination when patients present with nasal symptoms.

Equipment

- A good light source or well-functioning flashlight
- Nasal speculum
- Examination gloves
- Dental mirror (optional)

Training/Credentialing

No special credentialing needed; office diagnostic procedure only.

Coding

No specific code for nasal examination is used. The inclusion of this examination may justify or support a higher acuity for the other services rendered. If only this examination is performed, the following code may be considered:

92599 Unlisted otorhinolaryngological service or procedure

Technique

The landmarks and structures that are a part of examination of the nose and paranasal sinuses are shown in Figure 48.1. Examination of the nose begins with inspection of the external nares and philtrum. The nose should be centrally and symmetrically located, although mild deviation from the midline is common. If there is concern that the septum is substantially deviated, compression of each side of the nose while having the patient sniff allows assessment of patency and function.

The interior of the nose and the distal portion of the nasal passages, including portions of the turbinates, may be seen by gently compressing the tip of the nose upward

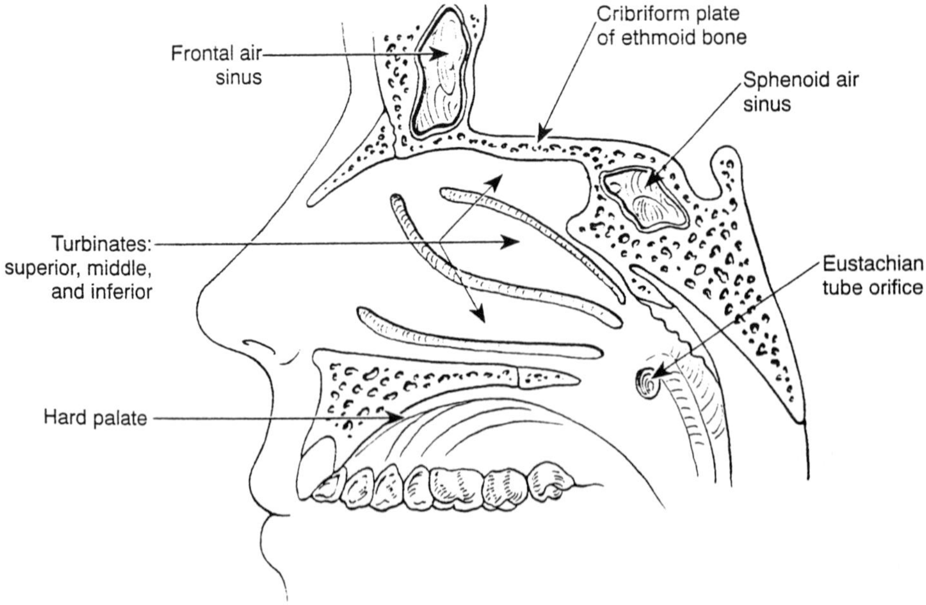

FIGURE 48.1.
Lateral wall of right naris showing nasal and related structures. (Reproduced with permission from Willms JL, Schneiderman H, Algranati PS. Physical Diagnosis: Bedside Evaluation of Diagnosis and Function. *Baltimore: Williams & Wilkins, 1994:137.)*

with the patient's head tipped slightly backward. The resulting flair of the alae and nares allows the septum and nasal mucosa to be seen. The inferior and middle turbinates are generally visible. A nasal speculum may be inserted to further facilitate inspection. An otoscope with disposable cover may also be used.

The sense of smell may be tested (when indicated by the patient's symptoms) by using small amounts of tobacco and ground coffee contained in small pill bottles. The patient is instructed to close her eyes and obstruct one nostril. The patient then sniffs one of these samples and is asked to identify the substance. If the patient can identify the substance or indicate that she can smell something but not identify it, olfaction is considered intact.

The maxillary and frontal sinuses may be assessed by gentle pressure and transillumination. Palpation and percussion over the area of the sinuses should not elicit pain. Transillumination may be attempted using a strong penlight or sinus illuminator (Fig. 48.2). To perform transillumination, the patient should be seated in a completely darkened room. The tip of the illuminator is placed just under the rim of the inferior orbit (Fig. 48.3). The degree of light transmission to the antrum is noted and compared with that seen on the other side. The frontal sinuses are examined in a similar way (Fig. 48.4).

Normal Findings

The nasal mucosa should be pink and moist, without discharge or bleeding sites. Mucus, if present, should be thin and clear. The septum should be central, although deviation is acceptable unless it compromises ventilatory function or is of cosmetic concern.

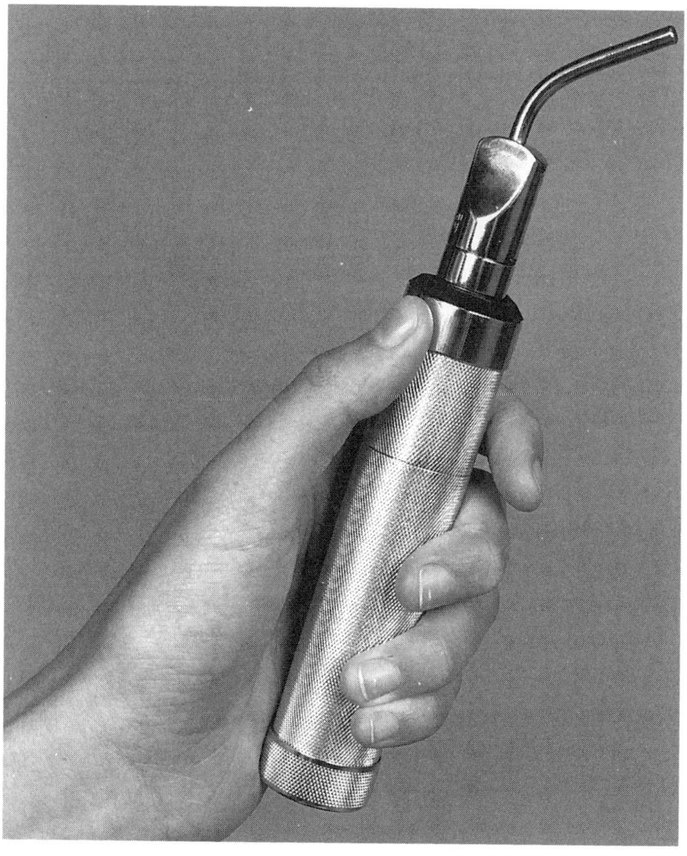

FIGURE 48.2.
Sinus transilluminator. (Reproduced with permission from Willms JL, Schneiderman H, Algranati PS. Physical Diagnosis: Bedside Evaluation of Diagnosis and Function. *Baltimore: Williams & Wilkins, 1994:162.)*

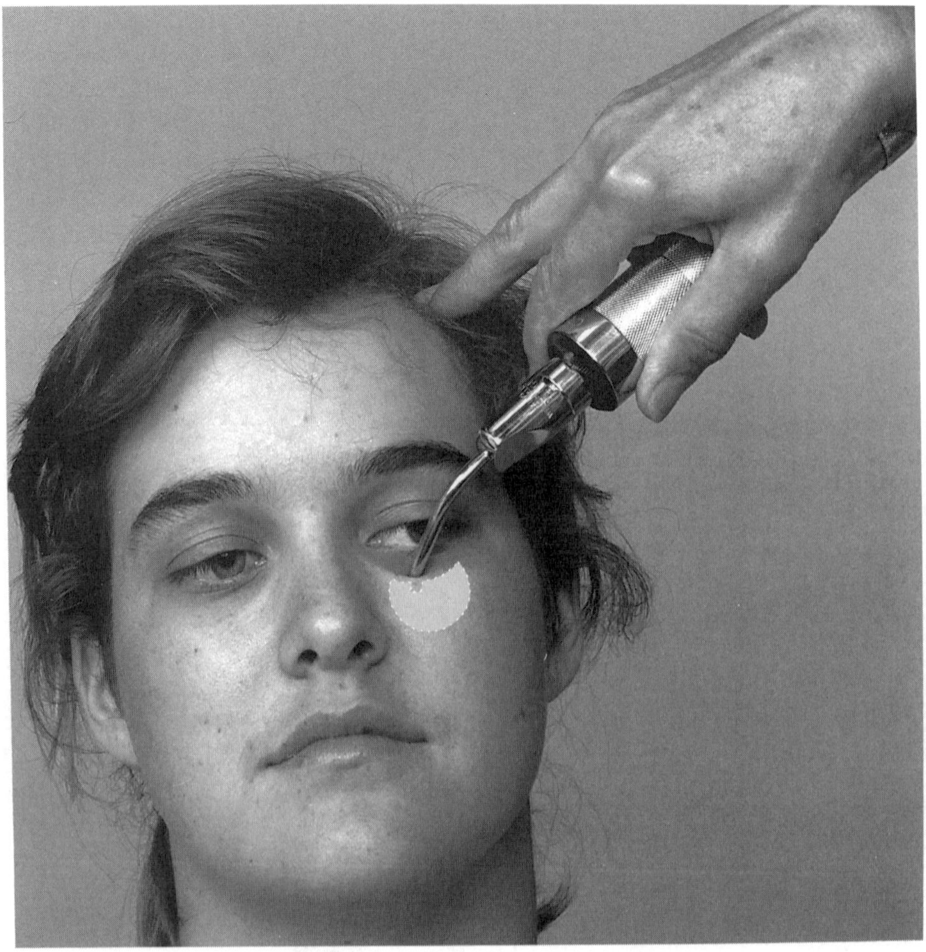

FIGURE 48.3.
Sinus transilluminator held to inferior orbit to assess maxillary sinus.(Reproduced with permission from Willms JL, Schneiderman H, Algranati PS. Physical Diagnosis: Bedside Evaluation of Diagnosis and Function. *Baltimore: Williams & Wilkins, 1994:163.)*

Selected Abnormal Findings

During upper respiratory infection, the nasal mucosa may be swollen and inflamed, with yellow mucus present in both sides. Allergic rhinitis, in contrast, produces a pale (occasionally bluish) and boggy mucosa with a watery discharge. A purulent discharge seen on only side of the nose should suggest a sinus infection.

The nasal septum may become perforated as the result of infections (syphilis and tuberculosis), immune disorders (systemic lupus erythematosus and Wegener's granulomatosis), and behavior (cocaine abuse and excessive nose picking).

Nasal polyps generally appear as small intranasal balloons and are most often associated with long-standing nasal allergy. They are generally edematous, gray-blue to yellow-tan, soft, and insensitive to touch. Edema of the turbinate may be confused with a polyp but may be differentiated by the exquisite sensitivity of the turbinate when touched with any instrument.

Bilateral anosmia may be found in patients with Parkinson's disease and Kallmann's syndrome.

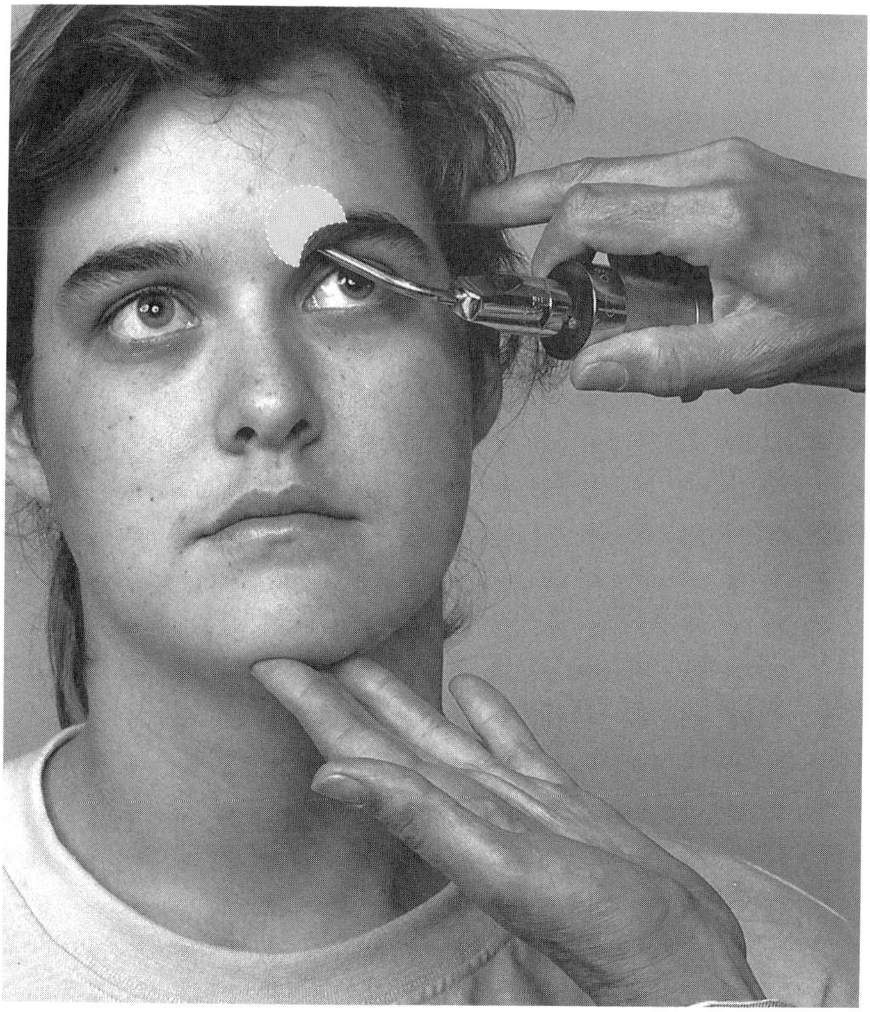

FIGURE 48.4.
Sinus transilluminator under superior orbital rim to assess frontal sinus. (Reproduced with permission from Willms JL, Schneiderman H, Algranati PS. Physical Diagnosis: Bedside Evaluation of Diagnosis and Function. *Baltimore: Williams & Wilkins, 1994:164.)*

Suggested Readings

Sapira JD. *The Art and Science of Bedside Diagnosis*. Baltimore: Williams & Wilkins, 1990:215.

Willms JL, Schneiderman H, Algranati PS. *Physical Diagnosis: Bedside Evaluation of Diagnosis and Function*. Baltimore: Williams & Wilkins, 1994:119.

Chapter 49

OTOSCOPY

From ear aches to the possibility of ear wax build-up, the otoscope is invaluable for addressing commonly encountered primary care concerns because it allows careful inspection of the auditory canal and tympanic membrane. A familiarity with the use of this instrument and the likely findings it may reveal will facilitate caring for patients with otologic problems.

Equipment

- Otoscope with otic speculum (disposable preferred) (an ear speculum with head mirror or good light may also be used but is generally less satisfactory)

Training/Credentialing

No special credentialing needed; office diagnostic procedure only.

Coding

No specific code for otoscopic examination of the ear is used. The inclusion of this examination may justify or support a higher acuity for the other services rendered. If only this examination is performed, the following code may be considered:

92599 Unlisted otorhinolaryngological service or procedure

Technique

Before otoscopy, all surfaces of the external ear should be inspected for signs of lesions, discoloration, excoriation, erythema, or edema. Palpation of the auricle should seek signs of tenderness, nodules, or discomfort during manipulation. The area behind and below the auricle should be palpated for signs of enlarged lymph nodes. Once these evaluations have been completed, the otoscopic examination may proceed.

An otic speculum should be placed over the tip of the otoscope, and the quality of the light supplied by the otoscope should be checked. The patient is instructed to remain still but report any significant discomfort. The helix of the auricle is gently grasped and drawn backward and upward. This movement straightens the outer portion of the auditory canal (Fig. 49.1). The speculum is directed at an angle of approxi-

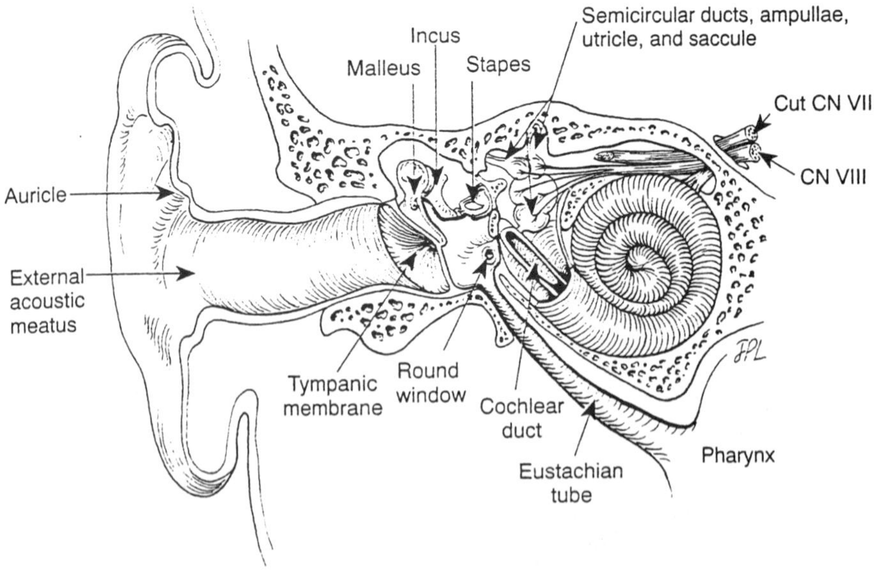

FIGURE 49.1.
The relationship among the outer portions of the ear, the auditory canal, the tympanic membrane, and inner ear structures is shown. (Reproduced with permission from Willms JL, Schneiderman H, Algranati PS. Physical Diagnosis: Bedside Evaluation of Diagnosis and Function. *Baltimore: Williams & Wilkins, 1994:135.)*

mately 10° to the posterior and gently inserted under direct vision through the external opening of the auditory canal (Fig. 49.2). The initial direction of the speculum toward the back makes it easier to pass the soft tissues of the external ear and anterior canal.

As the external auditory canal is traversed, it should be inspected for scaling, erythema, or discharge. Any cerumen obstructing the view of the inner canal and tympanic membrane should be gently removed (see Chapter 50, Wax [Cerumen] Removal).

Once the ear speculum has been fully and painlessly inserted, the tympanic membrane may be inspected. The membrane should be translucent, gray-tan to pink-white, with the head of the malleus (umbo) visible in the center (Fig. 49.3). Radiating out, down, and anteriorly from the umbo, the conical light reflex indicates a healthy drum. The flaccid portion of the membrane is located anterosuperior and the pars tensa lies posterior to the handle of the malleus.

Normal Findings

The external auditory canal is normally about 2.5 cm long. It should be free of scaling, bleeding, and edema.

Selected Abnormal Findings

Tophi (nodules of uric acid) may be found under the skin of the external ear. These are generally associated with inflammation and scarring and are seen with chronic gout. Preauricular lymph node enlargement suggests otitis external or adenoviral conjunctivitis. Visible vessels over the surface of the tympanic membrane indicate inflammation.

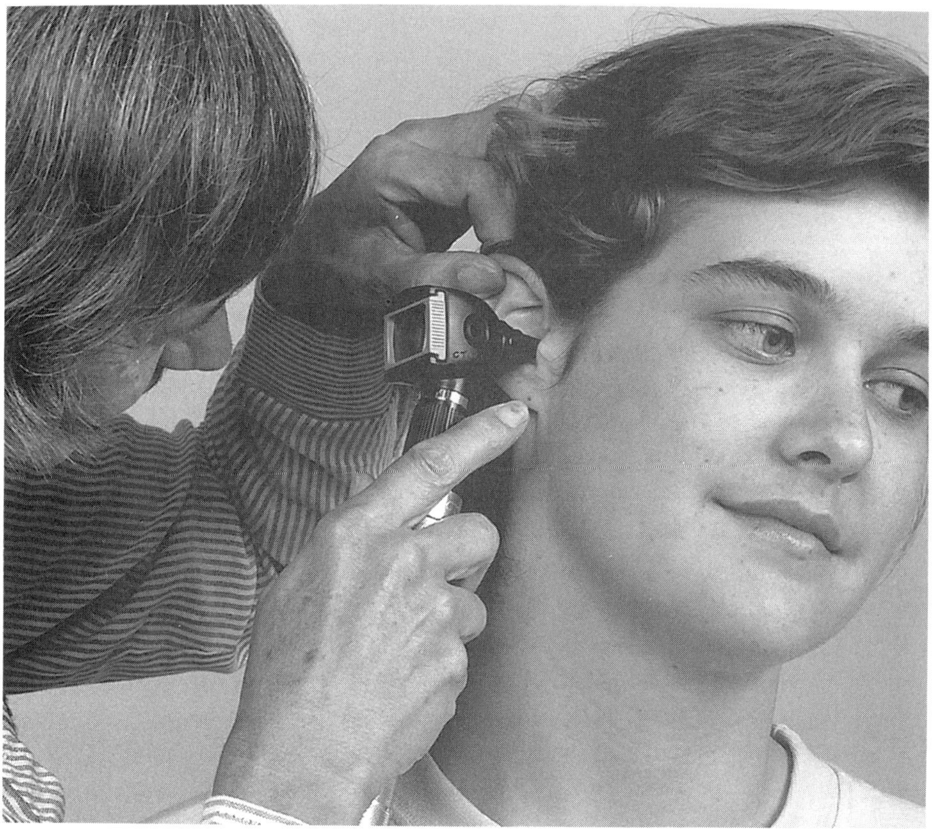

FIGURE 49.2.
Positioning of otoscope for ear inspection; note upward and backward traction on the auricle to facilitate insertion of the speculum into the external auditory canal. (Reproduced with permission from Willms JL, Schneiderman H, Algranati PS. Physical Diagnosis: Bedside Evaluation of Diagnosis and Function. *Baltimore: Williams & Wilkins, 1994:136.)*

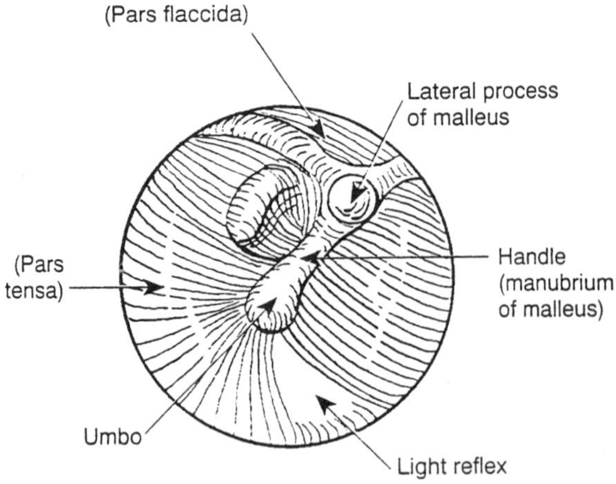

FIGURE 49.3.
The appearance of the right tympic membrane is shown. (Reproduced with permission from Willms JL, Schneiderman H, Algranati PS. Physical Diagnosis: Bedside Evaluation of Diagnosis and Function. *Baltimore: Williams & Wilkins, 1994:135.)*

A reddened tympanic membrane is the hallmark of acute otitis media. Additional signs include the loss of the light reflection and shininess of the membrane (early), redness, bulging with loss of landmarks (late), and perforation with drainage. When otitis media is present, traction on the external ear does not cause pain because inflammation is limited to the middle ear.

Special Notes

Otoscopy should not cause pain. If the examination is painful, either the technique is flawed or a pathologic condition is present. Testing the motion of the tympanic membrane by insufflation has limited indications and is best reserved for the specialist.

Suggested Readings

Bennett JD. The value of otoscopy. *J Accident Emerg Med* 1994;11:209.
Sapira JD. *The Art and Science of Bedside Diagnosis.* Baltimore: Williams & Wilkins, 1990:207.
Willms JL, Schneiderman H, Algranati PS. *Physical Diagnosis: Bedside Evaluation of Diagnosis and Function.* Baltimore: Williams & Wilkins, 1994:119.

Chapter 50

WAX (CERUMEN) REMOVAL

Ear wax (cerumen) is a protectant and lubricant for the ear canal. When this wax hardens it can form a thick, sticky material that may build up and eventually obstruct the ear canal. This build-up can result in hearing loss, a sense of ringing in the ear (tinnitus), or pressure. Infection or vertigo may also occur. Obstruction of the ear canal is the most common cause of hearing loss in young, healthy adults. Over-the-counter wax removal or softening agents may be effective, but most patients attempt removal without these agents and succeed only in further impacting the wax, damaging the external ear canal, or both.

Equipment

- Operating otoscope or ear speculum and light source
- Cerumen-softening agent (mineral oil, 3% hydrogen peroxide, triethanolamine (Cerumenex)), carbamide peroxide (Debrox), or cresyl acetate (Cresylate)

FOR IRRIGATION TECHNIQUE

- Ear syringe, bulb syringe, or 30- to 50-mL hypodermic syringe
- Tubing from a 22-gauge butterfly-type needle (without needle) or the plastic outer canula from an 18-gauge intravenous needle set (e.g., angiocath)
- Body temperature water or saline
- Emesis basin and disposable foam or paper coffee cup
- Towels, sheet, or plastic drape
- Cotton-tipped applicators or small gauze

FOR DIRECT TECHNIQUE

- Ear curette or "scoop"
- Ear forceps
- Small suction tip or plastic intravenous canula and suction source (optional)

Training/Credentialing

No special credentialing needed; office procedure only.

Coding

69210 Removal impacted cerumen (separate procedure), one or both ears

Technique

Removal of ear wax should not be attempted until the diagnosis has been confirmed. The ear should be directly inspected with the aid of an operating otoscopy or an ear speculum and external light. Visualization is facilitated by pulling the auricle upward and backward to straighten the outer portion of the canal. When the wax is soft, initially or after the use of a softening agent, it may be extracted by gently inserting a cotton-tipped applicator under direct vision.

If the wax completely obstructs the canal, preliminary softening (in the office or at home) should be undertaken before removal is attempted. Several commercial products for softening ear wax are available; a 10% solution of sodium bicarbonate in glycerol may also be used for this purpose. To use softening agents, the patient's head should be tipped so that the affected ear is uppermost. Several drops of the solution to be used are placed in the external canal and allowed to run inward by gravity. If both ears are to be treated, a cotton pledget should be placed in the external ear to prevent the loss of softening agent while solution is placed in the other ear (Fig. 50.1). Reinspection in 24–48 hours generally finds that the wax has softened and drained on its own.

Tenacious wax may be removed using a direct technique with a curette or suction, or it may be removed by irrigation. The irrigation technique takes more time and is undeniably more messy, but it rarely fails. With care, it is also less likely to damage the ear canal.

IRRIGATION TECHNIQUES

The patient should be protected from the spill of irrigation solution by appropriate draping or the use of a disposable coffee cup. A portion of the cup may be cut or torn away to allow the ear to be placed over the edge, allowing most of the fluid to be caught. The head should be tipped toward the side to be treated, further facilitating the flushing action of the irrigation and reducing spill.

A plastic intravenous catheter or short length of small intravenous tubing should be attached to a large-capacity syringe filled with body temperature water or saline. An ear or bulb syringe may also be used. The tip of the chosen device should be inserted into the external auditory canal and a stream of liquid should be directed superiorly and slightly posteriorly (Fig. 50.2). The catheter or syringe tip must be placed in such a way that fluid may exit unimpeded.

Often, one or more large pieces of wax will be flushed out of the ear with the first few milliliters of fluid. When this occurs, irrigation should be suspended and the canal should be inspected. Occasionally, several pulses of irrigation or a more vigorous stream may be required, but care must be taken to avoid forces that could rupture the tympanic membrane. If an intravenous catheter or tubing is used, attaching it to a large-capacity syringe (30–50 mL or greater) prevents the development of high pressures at the catheter tip.

If the obstructing wax is not promptly dislodged by irrigation, a softening agent

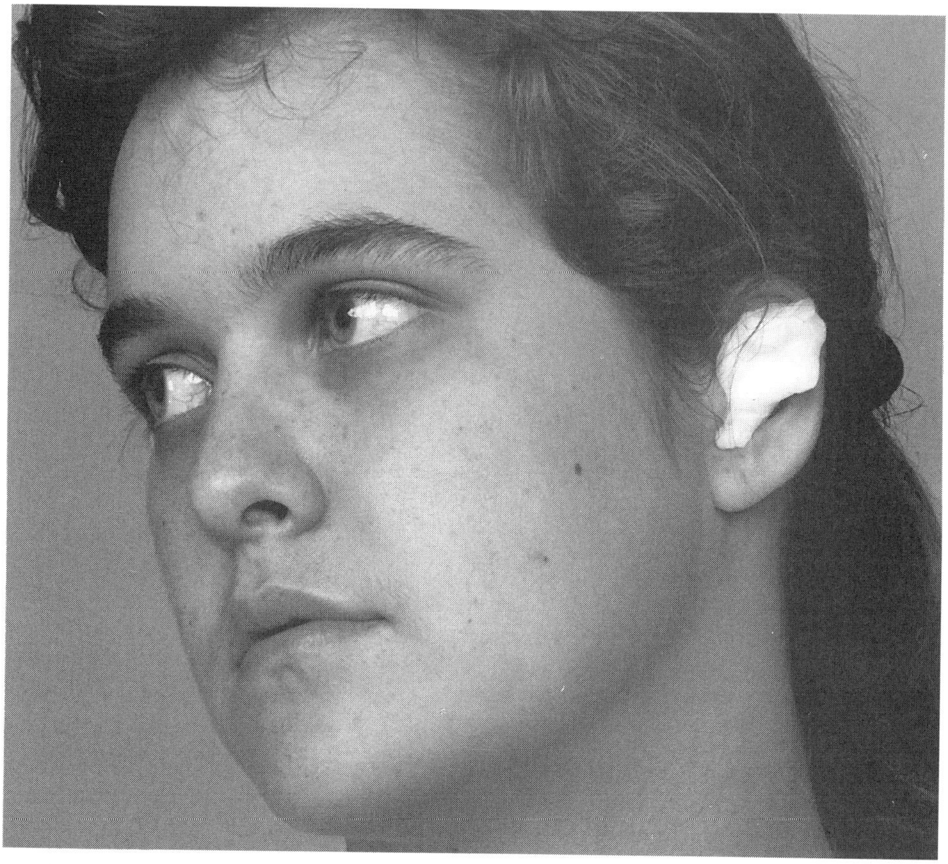

FIGURE 50.1.
Pledget at external auditory meatus to keep ceruminolytic agent in place. (Reproduced with permission from Willms JL, Schneiderman H, Algranati PS. Physical Diagnosis: Bedside Evaluation of Diagnosis and Function. *Baltimore: Williams & Wilkins, 1994:161.)*

should be used for 1 or 2 days; at that time, the patient should be re-evaluated or referral to a specialist should be considered.

DIRECT TECHNIQUES

Obstructing wax may be directly removed in much the same way as is a foreign body (see Chapter 45, Removal of Foreign Bodies from the Ear). A small suction tip or an ear curette is used under direct vision through the operating otoscope or speculum. These methods are inherently more dangerous and carry a greater risk for epithelial trauma or perforation. For this reason, many physicians believe that referral is preferable if simpler methods of wax removal are not successful.

Special Notes

Removal of ear wax should only be attempted if the patient is willing to be fully cooperative. Wax removal should not be attempted in patients who have had a perforated ear drum or previous ear surgery that may have resulted in distortion or increased risk for perforation. These patients should be referred to a specialist for evaluation. Patients who have only one hearing ear should also be evaluated by a specialist.

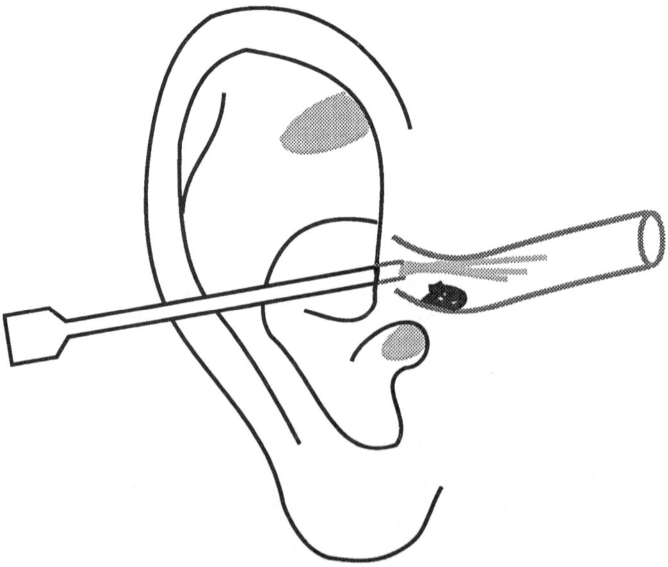

FIGURE 50.2.
Irrigating solution should be directed toward the superior position of the auditory canal while space is allowed for the effluent to pass freely.

If the irrigation technique is chosen, care must be taken that the liquid used is body temperature. Failure to do so may induce substantial vertigo, nausea, or pain. A jet irrigator (e.g., Water-Pik) has been advocated as an irrigation source for wax removal. Such an irrigator is often not readily available in a gynecologic office and carries a greater risk for perforation. If the instrument is used, only the lowest possible setting should be used.

If any trauma has occurred in the wall of the auditory canal or the epithelium has been frankly disrupted, a topical otic antibiotic should be prescribed.

After the wax has been removed (by any technique), the patient should be instructed to seek care if vertigo, pain, dizziness, a discharge, or decrease in hearing are noted.

Patients should be advised to periodically cleanse the ears using a bulb syringe or wax softener, but they should avoid placing any object into the ear canal itself (e.g., applicator sticks, tissues).

Suggested Readings

Larsen G. Removing cerumen with a water pick. *Am J Nurs* 1976;70:264.

Lyndon S, Roy P, Grillage MG, et al. A comparison of the efficacy of two ear drop preparations ('Audax' and 'Earex') in the softening and removal of impacted ear wax. *Curr Med Res Opin* 1992;13:21.

Macknin ML, Talo H, Medendrop SV. Effect of cotton-tipped swab use on ear-wax occlusion. *Clin Pediatr* 1994;33:14.

Meador JA. Cerumen impaction in the elderly. *J Gerontol Nurs* 1995;21:43.

Zivic RC, King S. Cerumen-impaction management for clients of all ages. *Nurse Practitioner* 1993;18:29.

Section VI

NEUROLOGIC EVALUATIONS

Chapter 51

USEFUL REFLEXES

An important part of screening for neurologic disease is the performance of muscle stretch reflexes (also known as deep tendon reflexes). Although the equipment required is minimal, some skill and attention to technique are required to avoid inaccurate result that can lead to expensive, invasive, and unnecessary further testing.

Equipment

- Reflex hammer (various styles are available and are a matter of personal choice).

Training/Credentialing

No special credentialing needed.

Coding

No specific code for reflex testing is used. The inclusion of reflex testing may justify or support a higher acuity for the other services rendered. If only reflex testing is performed, the following code may be considered:

95999 Unlisted neurological or neurovascular diagnostic procedure

Technique

GENERAL CONSIDERATIONS

A successful muscle stretch reflex (MSR) requires fulfillment of five conditions: 1) the muscle group must be well relaxed, 2) the patient must not watch the testing (by averting or closing the eyes) so that anticipatory muscle tensing does not occur, 3) a reflex hammer of appropriate size and weight must be used, 4) the tendon of the muscle group to be tested must be accurately located, and 5) the reflex hammer must be used with a loose swinging motion that produces a sharp displacement and bouncing rebound from the stimulated tendon. Most of these requirements are easily met, but several require special approaches. Asking the patient to "relax" a given muscle group is almost always futile. Instructions that are specific and result in relaxation are more successful. Examples of such instructions are "let me support your arm and just let me do all the work" (triceps reflex) or "let your legs swing loosely" (patellar reflex).

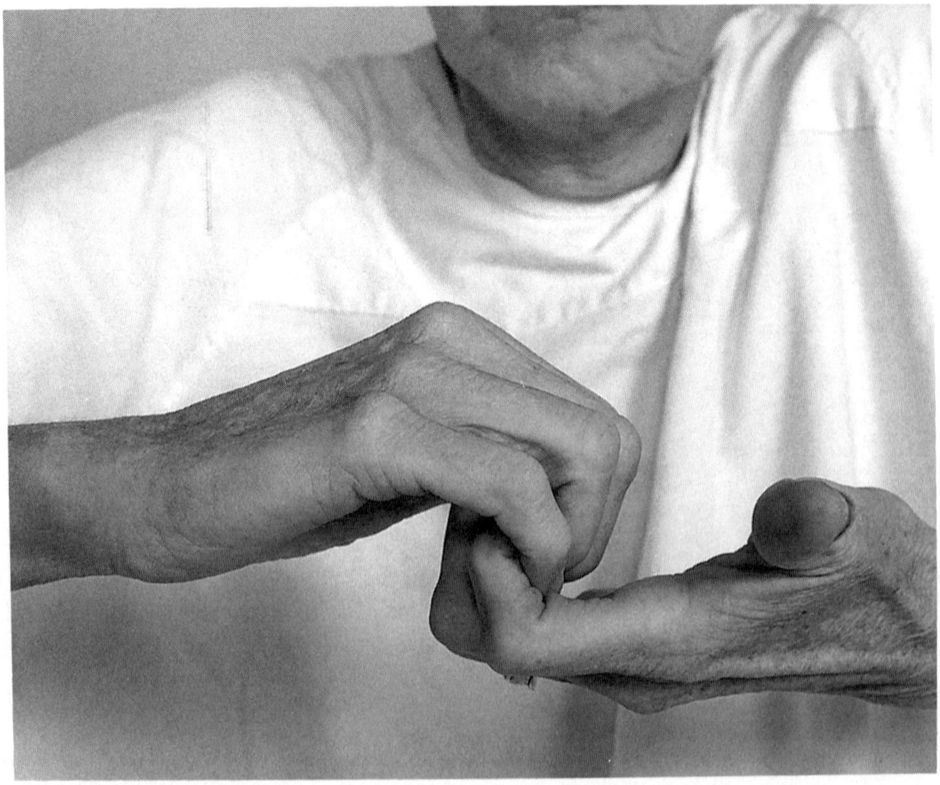

FIGURE 51.1.
Lower limb reflexes may be reinforced by having the patient grasp her hands as shown and tugging outward as the reflex is tested. (Reproduced with permission from Willms JL, Schneiderman H, Algranati PS. Physical Diagnosis: Bedside Evaluation of Diagnosis and Function. *Baltimore: Williams & Wilkins, 1994:474.)*

When an MSR is unexpectedly absent, the test should be repeated using reinforcement. This technique is based on creating a diversionary spinal arc at a level above that being tested. This arc acts to inhibit cortical suppression coming from above. For lower extremity MSRs, reinforcement may be accomplished by asking the patient to clasp the hands in front of the chest and pull one against the other at the time the reflex is tested. This is referred to as the Jendrassik maneuver (Fig. 51.1). Upper limb reflexes may be reinforced by asking the patient to clench her teeth as the reflex is stimulated.

TRICEPS REFLEX

The triceps reflex tests the integrity of the C6–C8 level of the spinal cord. To test the triceps reflex, the patient's forearm should be support by the examiner's nondominant hand so that the arm swings loosely with the elbow bent at roughly a 90° angle and the upper arm is slightly hyperadducted toward the chest (Fig. 51.2). The triceps tendon is identified near its insertion to the olecranon on the extensor surface of the distal (upper) arm. The tendon should be struck sharply using the broad side of the reflex hammer (if a triangular hammer is used). The triceps muscle should visibly contract in response to the impact, and slight extension of the elbow may be felt.

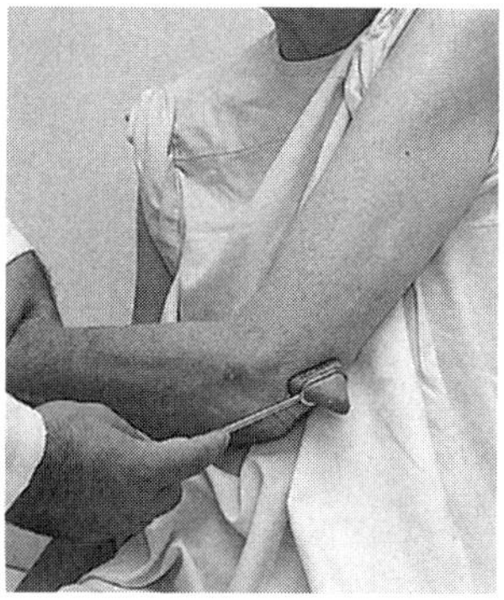

FIGURE 51.2.
The triceps reflex is tested with the forearm supported by the examiner and maintained with the elbow flexed to approximately 90° and the upper arm hyperadducted. The triceps tendon is then identified and stimulated. (Reproduced with permission from Willms JL, Schneiderman H, Algranati PS. Physical Diagnosis: Bedside Evaluation of Diagnosis and Function. *Baltimore: Williams & Wilkins, 1994:476.)*

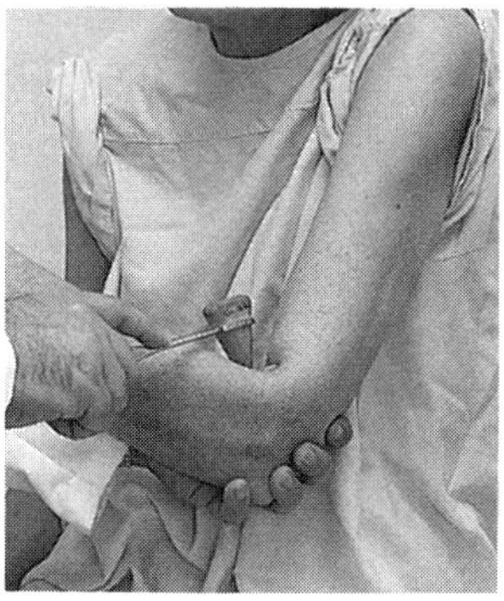

FIGURE 51.3.
The biceps tendon is stimulated indirectly by striking the examiner's thumb, which palpates the tendon. (Reproduced with permission from Willms JL, Schneiderman H, Algranati PS. Physical Diagnosis: Bedside Evaluation of Diagnosis and Function. *Baltimore: Williams & Wilkins, 1994:476.)*

BICEPS REFLEX

To test the biceps reflex, the patient is asked to rest the forearm in her lap while the elbow is grasped by the examiner's nondominant hand; the examiner's thumb is placed over the biceps tendon and the remainder of the fingers encircle the elbow, as shown in Figure 51.3. The biceps tendon is stimulated indirectly by striking the examiner's thumb with the reflex hammer. The biceps muscle should be seen to contract briefly and may be evidenced by further flexion of the forearm. The biceps reflex tests the function of the C5–C6 spinal level.

BRACHIORADIALIS REFLEX

The brachioradialis reflex is less frequently performed than other MSRs. This reflex tests the integrity of the C5–C6 level of the spinal cord. To test this reflex, the patient should place her arm in the same position as used for the biceps reflex (Fig. 51.3). The brachioradialis muscle is identified on the radial surface of the mid–upper forearm. The muscle tendon is struck lightly along the course of the radius until a radial deviation of the wrist or extension of the wrist or index or middle finger is elicited (Fig. 51.4).

PATELLAR (KNEE JERK) REFLEX

The patellar reflex is tested with the patient sitting on the edge of the examination table and the legs dangling freely. The tendon distal to the patella is struck sharply (using the narrow portion of the reflex hammer) and the quadriceps muscle is observed for contraction. Extension of the knee is common in a +3 response. Weak responses may be detected by resting the nondominant hand on the body of the muscle. The patellar reflex may also be tested with the patient supine and the knee gently supported (Fig. 51.5). Patellar clonus may be stimulated by sharply moving the patella distally. The patellar reflex tests the L2–L4 spinal levels.

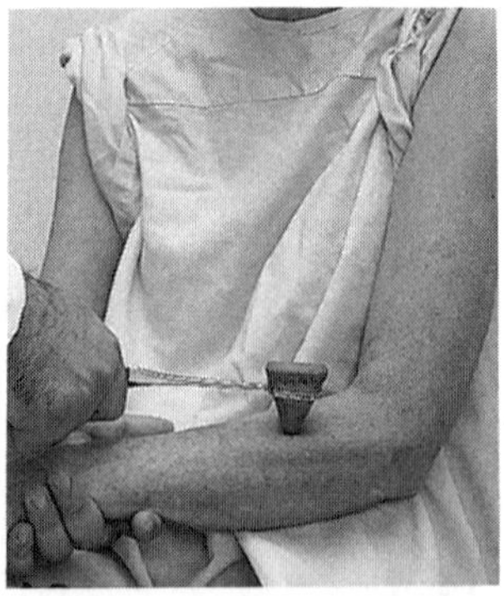

FIGURE 51.4.
The brachioradialis reflex is stimulated by lightly tapping along the course of the brachioradialis tendon as it courses over the radius. (Reproduced with permission from Willms JL, Schneiderman H, Algranati PS. Physical Diagnosis: Bedside Evaluation of Diagnosis and Function. *Baltimore: Williams & Wilkins, 1994:476.)*

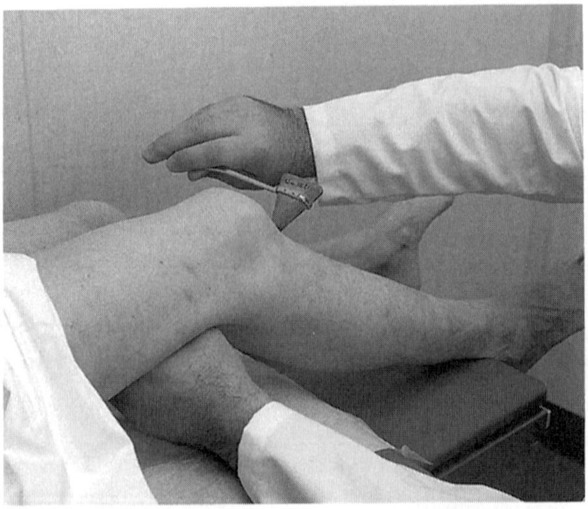

FIGURE 51.5.
The patellar reflex may be elicited with the knee flexed and supported by the examiner's hand. (Reproduced with permission from Willms JL, Schneiderman H, Algranati PS. Physical Diagnosis: Bedside Evaluation of Diagnosis and Function. *Baltimore: Williams & Wilkins, 1994:477.)*

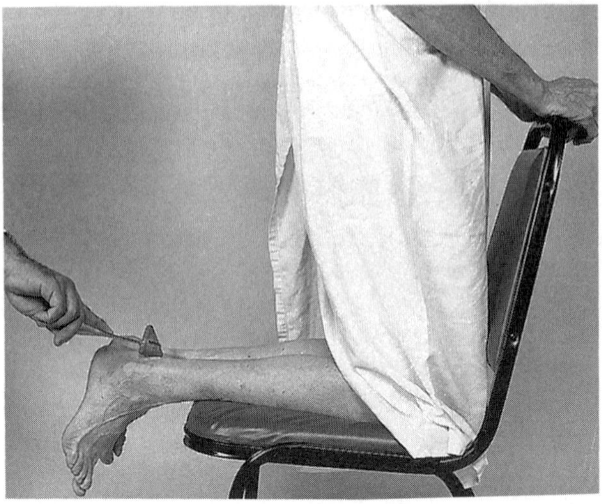

FIGURE 51.6.
When the Achilles reflex is difficult to demonstrate, it may be tested with the patient kneeling on a chair and grasping the chair back with her hands. This provides reinforcement and muscle relaxation that may allow a weak reflex to be demonstrated. (Reproduced with permission from Willms JL, Schneiderman H, Algranati PS. Physical Diagnosis: Bedside Evaluation of Diagnosis and Function. *Baltimore: Williams & Wilkins, 1994:477.)*

ACHILLES (ANKLE JERK) REFLEX

The Achilles reflex is often the most difficult to elicit. For testing of this reflex, the patient should be positioned with the legs and feet hanging freely as for the patellar reflex. The Achilles tendon should be located at the level of the metatarsals. The foot should be rested in the examiner's palm with slight upward pressure. This slightly tenses the tendon and allows flexion of the foot in response to striking the tendon with the broad portion of the reflex hammer. If no reflex is seen, reinforcement should be attempted or the patient should be examined while kneeling on a chair seat (Fig. 51.6). If clonus is not shown by striking the tendon, it may be sought by sharp dorsiflexion of the ankle. The Achilles reflex tests the S1–S2 spinal levels.

PLANTAR REFLEX

The plantar reflex (often called the Babinski test) tests the range of spinal function from L4 to S2. With the patient resting comfortably, the sole of the foot is stroked with a pointed object (such as a key, the handle of the reflex hammer, or the shaft of an applicator stick). The stroke should begin near the heal and cross to the ball of the foot, ending at the base of the great toe (Fig. 51.7). This motion should be firm and continuous, producing a noxious but not painful stimulus. The toes are observed for any response; the initial motion is the most important. After the age of 2 years, flexion is considered normal. Dorsiflexion or the great toe with flaring of the other toes is the so-called Babinski response and is considered abnormal (Fig. 51.8). The absence of toe motion is, by itself, not abnormal.

When no response is generated, the Chaddock maneuver (stroking the superolateral side of the foot (Fig. 51.9)), or the Oppenheim maneuver (pressure from the thumb and index finger swept down the tibia) may be used to induce the same responses. These maneuvers are less reliable in their ability to produce a response. When the Babinski sign is present, no further confirmation is needed.

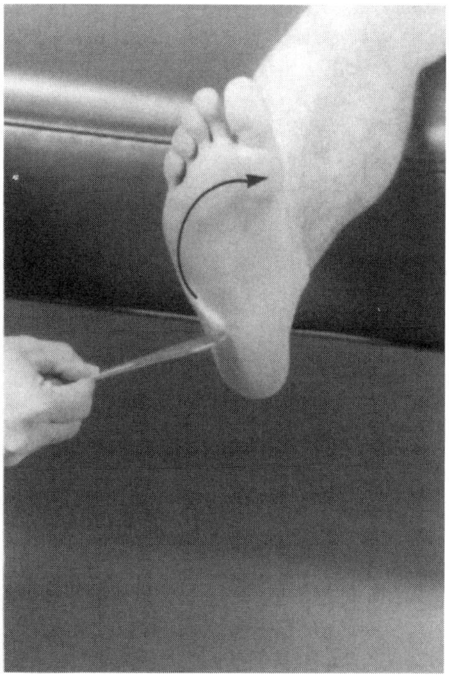

FIGURE 51.7.
The plantar reflex is tested by stroking the sole of the foot along the path shown. (Reproduced with permission from Cipriano JJ. Photographic Manual of Regional Orthopaedic and Neurological Testing. *Baltimore: Williams & Wilkins, 1991:251.)*

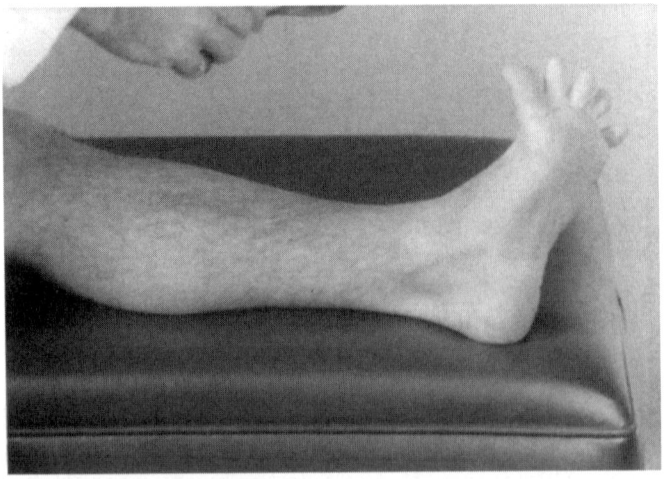

FIGURE 51.8.
Upward motion of the great toe and flaring of the other toes constitute the Babinski sign; these findings are always considered abnormal. (Reproduced with permission from Cipriano JJ. Photographic Manual of Regional Orthopaedic and Neurological Testing. *Baltimore: Williams & Wilkins, 1991:251.)*

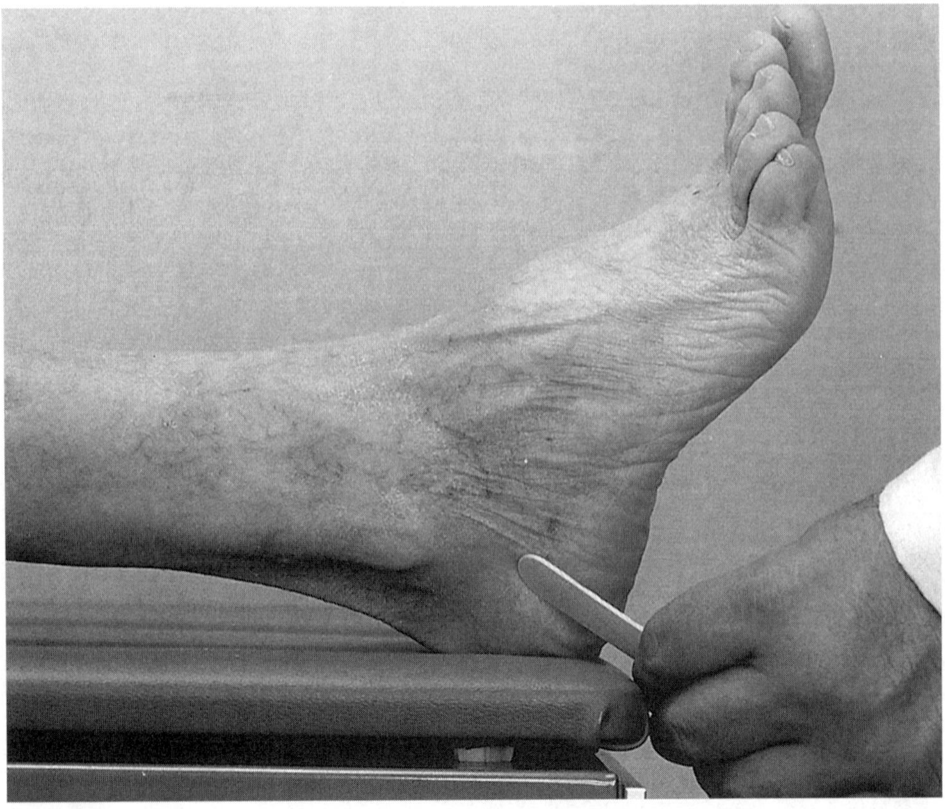

FIGURE 51.9.
The Chaddock test may be performed to test the plantar reflex by firmly stroking the superolateral side of the foot from the ankle to toe. (Reproduced with permission from Willms JL, Schneiderman H, Algranati PS. Physical Diagnosis: Bedside Evaluation of Diagnosis and Function. *Baltimore: Williams & Wilkins, 1994:487.)*

SUPERFICIAL REFLEXES

Superficial reflexes (abdominal and cremasteric reflexes) are generally only tested when there is a question about a lesion affecting specific spinal cord levels or certain types of corticospinal or cortical lesions.

Abdominal Reflex

While the patient is in a relaxed supine position, the four quadrants of the abdominal wall are stroked with the handle of a reflex hammer or other suitable object. The normal reflex contraction of the abdominal wall caused by this stimulation results in a slight movement of the umbilicus toward the quadrant being studied. The upper quadrants of the abdominal wall reflect the function of spinal levels T7–T9, whereas the lower quadrants test the T11–L1 levels.

Cremasteric Reflex

The cremasteric reflex is generally associated with male patients but may also be used to test the integrity of the L1–L2 spinal function of women. While the patient is positioned as for a gynecologic examination, the inner thigh is stroked lightly. The labia on the simulated side should contract slightly in a cephalad direction.

Normal Findings

Muscle stretch reflexes are graded on a scale of 0–4 (Table 51.1). The results of muscle stretch reflex testing is often recorded in tabular form, as shown in Table 51.2. Bilateral symmetry of the tested reflexes is of greater significance than the absolute magnitude of the response elicited, but reflexes graded as +4 are always considered abnormal.

Selected Abnormal Findings

As patients age, it is not uncommon for muscle stretch reflexes to be diminished or absent. This is especially true of such distal reflexes as the Achilles or plantar reflexes. When bilateral symmetry is preserved, absent reflexes are probably normal and should not prompt undue concern.

TABLE 51.1. Rating of Muscle Stretch Reflex Responses

GRADE	RESPONSE
0	No response, even with reinforcement
+1	Response only with reinforcement
+2	Moderate response without reinforcement
+3[a]	Brisk response, clonus with 1–3 beats
+4	Exaggerated response with sustained clonus

[a]Some authors separate +3 and +4 grades into three grades ending with +5: +3, hyperreflexia; +4, hyperreflexia with transient clonus; and +5, hyperreflexia with sustained clonus.

TABLE 51.2. Example of Reflex Recording in Tabular Form

SIDE	BICEPS	TRICEPS	BRACHIORADIALIS	PATELLAR	ACHILLES	PLANTAR
Right	+2	+2	+2	+2	+1	Normal
Left	+2	+2	+2	+2	+1	Normal

TABLE 51.3. Differences between Upper and Lower Motor Neuronal Disease

VARIABLE	UPPER MOTOR LESION	LOWER MOTOR LESION
Muscle tone	Spastic, greatest in upper flexors and lower extensors	Flaccid
Reflexes	Accentuated	Variable
Clonus	Present	Absent
Fasciculations	Absent	Present
Muscle bulk	Atrophy, late	Substantial atrophy, early
Babinski response	Present	Absent

Reflex testing can be an important part of evaluating patients for possible upper and lower motor neuronal disease. Findings in these two conditions are summarized in Table 51.3.

Suggested Readings

Chimowitz MI, Logigian EL, Caplan LR. The accuracy of bedside neurologic diagnoses. *Ann Neurol* 1990;28:78.

Cipriano JJ. *Photographic Manual of Regional Orthopaedic and Neurological Tests.* Baltimore: Williams & Wilkins, 1991:245.

Gray CS, Walker A. The plantar response: caution in the elderly. *Br J Hosp Med* 1989;42:105.

Landau WM. Strategy, tactics, and accuracy in neurological evaluation. *Ann Neurol* 1990;28:86.

Maher J, Reilly M, Daly L, et al. Plantar power: reproducibility of the plantar response. *BMJ* 1992;304:482.

O'Brien MD. Ankle jerk assessment. *Lancet* 1995;345:331.

O'Keeffe ST, Smith T, Valacio R, et al. A comparison of two techniques for ankle jerk assessment in elderly subjects. *Lancet* 1994;344:1619.

Pryor JP. Ankle jerk assessment. *Lancet* 1995;345:331.

Sapira JD. *The Art and Science of Bedside Diagnosis*. Baltimore: Williams & Wilkins, 1990:474.

Schwartz RS, Morris JGL, Crimmins D, et al. A comparison of two methods of eliciting the ankle jerk. *Aust N Z J Med* 1990;20:116.

van Gijn J. The Babinski reflex. *Postgrad Med J* 1995;71:645.

Walshe TM. Neurologic examination of the elderly patient: signs of normal aging. *Postgrad Med J* 1987;81:375.

Ziegler DK. Is the neurologic examination becoming obsolete? *Neurology* 1985;35:559.

Chapter 52

SCREENING TESTS FOR BALANCE

Maintaining balance or equilibrium requires the combined function of the cerebellum, the motor system, the middle ear, and proprioception. All these may be tested by simple office tests of balance.

Equipment

No special equipment is rcquired.

Training/Credentialing

No special credentialing is needed.

Coding

No specific code for balance testing is used. The inclusion of balance testing may justify or support a higher acuity for the other services rendered. If only balance testing is performed, the following code may be considered:

95999 Unlisted neurological or neurovascular diagnostic procedure

Technique

The standard test of balance is the Romberg test (Fig. 52.1). To perform this test, the patient is asked to stand erect with her feet together, arms extended forward. The examiner should stand in a position to stabilize the patient should balance be lost. The patient first stands with her eyes open then with the eyes closed. When the eyes are open cerebral and visual inputs are tested, and when the eyes are closed proprioception must take the place of visual cues.

Once the Romberg test has been successfully "passed," the patient should be asked to turn her palms upward, close her eyes, and maintain this position. A downward drift or pronation (a palm-down rotation) is abnormal and should be noted (Fig. 52.2).

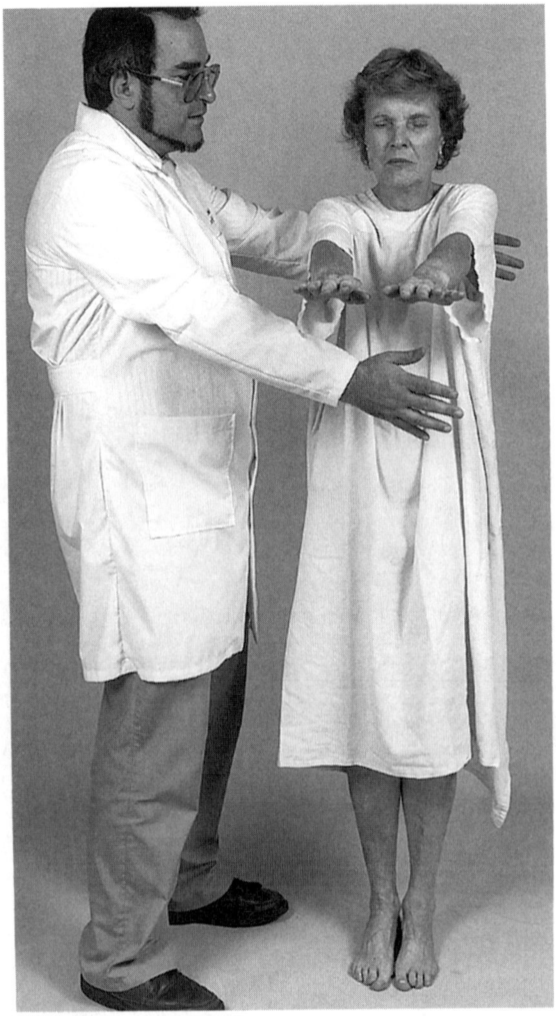

FIGURE 52.1.
Romberg test. The examiner stands ready to catch the patient should she fall. (Reproduced with permission from Willms JL, Schneiderman H, Algranati PS. Physical Diagnosis: Bedside Evaluation of Diagnosis and Function. *Baltimore: Williams & Wilkins, 1994:484.)*

Normal Findings

Neurologically intact patients should be able to stand in the Romberg position for more than 15 seconds without loosing their balance, swaying substantially, or having to reposition their feet. Extended and pronated arm positions should be maintained for a similar period.

Special Notes

Should the patient be unable to safely stand with her eyes open, the test should not be performed with the eyes closed.

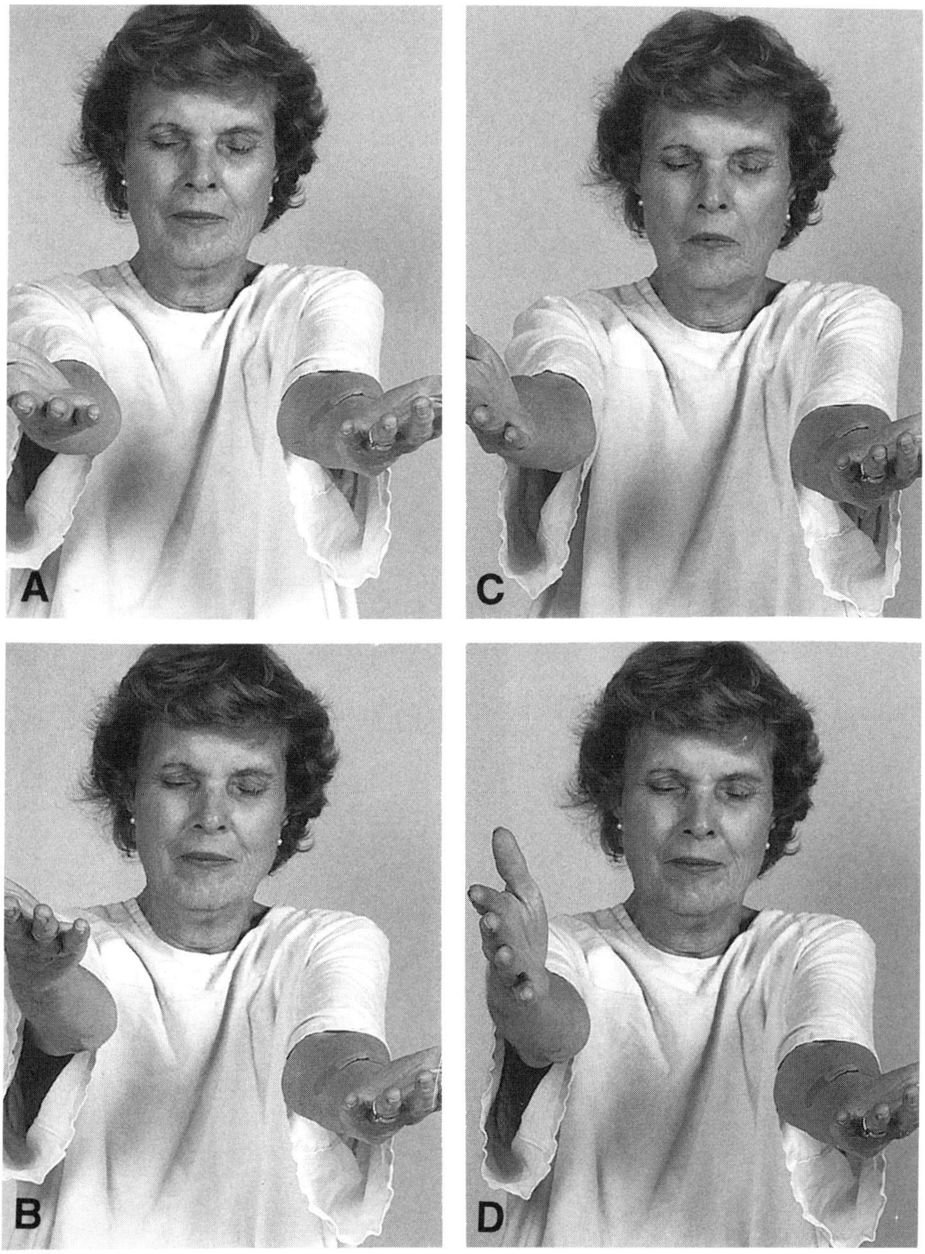

FIGURE 52.2.
Test for pronator drift. ***A.*** *Patient is instructed to maintain arm and hand position as placed at start, with eyes closed.* ***B.*** *Abnormal test result: the right arm has pronated.* ***C.*** *Abnormal test result: the right arm has drifted upward.* ***D.*** *Abnormal test result: the right arm has drifted upward, and the right hand has pronated. (Reproduced with permission from Willms JL, Schneiderman H, Algranati PS.* Physical Diagnosis: Bedside Evaluation of Diagnosis and Function. *Baltimore: Williams & Wilkins, 1994:485.)*

Suggested Readings

Cipriano JJ. *Photographic Manual of Regional Orthopaedic and Neurological Tests.* Baltimore: Williams & Wilkins, 1991:263.

Fife TD, Baloh RW. Disequilibrium of unknown cause in older people. *Ann Neurol* 1993:34:694.

Harburn KL, Hill KM, Kramer JF, et al. Clinical applicability and test-retest reliability of an external perturbation test of balance in stroke subjects. *Arch Phys Med Rehab* 1995;76:317.

Judge JO, King MB, Whipple R, et al. Dynamic balance in older persons: effects of reduced visual and proprioceptive input. *J Gerontol* 1995;50M:263–270.

Maki BE, Holliday PJ, Topper AK. A prospective study of postural balance and risk of falling in an ambulatory and independent elderly population. *J Gerontol* 1994; 49:M72.

Roland NJ, Smith CA, Miller IW, et al. A simple technique to measure body sway in normal subjects and patients with dizziness. *J Laryngol Otol* 1995;109:189.

Sapira JD. *The Art and Science of Bedside Diagnosis*. Baltimore: Williams & Wilkins, 1990:477.

Willms JL, Schneiderman H, Algranati PS. *Physical Diagnosis: Bedside Evaluation of Diagnosis and Function*. Baltimore: Williams & Wilkins, 1994:484.

Chapter 53

SCREENING TESTS FOR SENSATION

Sensation testing involves the evaluation of the integrity of the patient's major sensory modalities, peripheral nerves, and spinal cord tracts. These tests are an important part of the neurologic examination.

Equipment

- Tuning fork, low frequency (128 Hz)
- Cotton ball or cotton-tipped swab, teased into a wisp or soft point
- Pointed object such as broken wooden swab or broken tongue blade

Training/Credentialing

No special credentialing is needed.

Coding

No specific code for sensation testing is used. The inclusion of sensation testing may justify or support a higher acuity for the other services rendered. If only sensation testing is performed, the following code may be considered:

95999 Unlisted neurological or neurovascular diagnostic procedure

Technique

Evaluation of sensation involves four characteristics: light touch, superficial pain, vibration, and joint position sensation. Successful evaluation requires that "three Cs" be present: concentration, comprehension, and cooperation. Any patient incapable or unwilling to supply each of these is not a candidate for sensation testing. All sensory tests should be performed with the patient's eyes closed.

LIGHT TOUCH

Light touch is tested by gently touching the skin with a wisp of cotton or the tip of a finger. The investigator demonstrates the sensation with the patient's eyes open and asks the patient to "tell me each time you feel this and where you feel it." The patient should be asked to close her eyes; tests of various dermatomes then begins. It is best to avoid a predictable pattern of testing (e.g., alternating sides with each touch) so that the patient must respond to the sensation of touch and not the pattern or rhythm.

SUPERFICIAL PAIN

The capacity tested by superficial pain sensation is typified by the ability to distinguish between sharp and dull. The easiest tool for this testing is the broken shaft of an applicator stick or a broken tongue blade. Whatever tool is chosen, the material used for both sharp and dull testing should be the same so that the correct answer is not indicated through other clues such as temperature or texture.

To test superficial pain sensation, the patient is again instructed about the nature of the test. Both sensations should be demonstrated and confirmed to be different while the patient watches. The patient is again instructed to close her eyes; the testing is done in a manner similar to that used for light touch. The important difference is that the patient is to report the character (sharp or dull) of the sensation as well as the occurrence and location.

VIBRATION

To test vibratory sensation, a low-frequency (128 Hz) tuning fork is used. When vibration is tested, the patient is asked to report the character of the sensation, its location, and when the sensation stops. The tuning fork should be set vibrating by gently tapping it on the heel of the examiner's hand or by strongly pinching the tines between the thumb and base of the first finger and sharply releasing them. The vibrating tuning fork should then be placed against the bony prominence to be assessed (Fig. 53.1). Once the patient reports that the vibrations have ceased, the tuning fork should be placed on the examiner, who acts as a control. If vibration is still perceived by the examiner, diminished vibratory sensation may be present and should be further tested.

JOINT POSITION SENSATION

To check for joint position sensation, the tested joint is passively moved through a few degrees of its range. This is done by grasping the medial and lateral surfaces to avoid pressure cueing as the joint is moved (Fig. 53.2). The patient is asked to close her eyes and to indicate whether the joint is moved upward or downward. This testing is usually performed on the great toe and the index finger on each side. If sensation is normal at this level, proximal position sensation is also presumed to be normal.

Normal Findings

Results of all sensation testing should be evaluated for symmetry, consistency, and the ability of the patient to correctly identify the side and site of the body that has been stimulated.

Testing of the ability to sense vibration and joint position should start in the periphery and progress proximally until normal sensation is demonstrated. When the sensation is intact at the most distal point tested, no further testing for that ability need be done on that extremity.

Selected Abnormal Findings

A deficit in sensory perception must be carefully related to the specific dermatome responsible and judged against the response elicited from the same dermatome on the

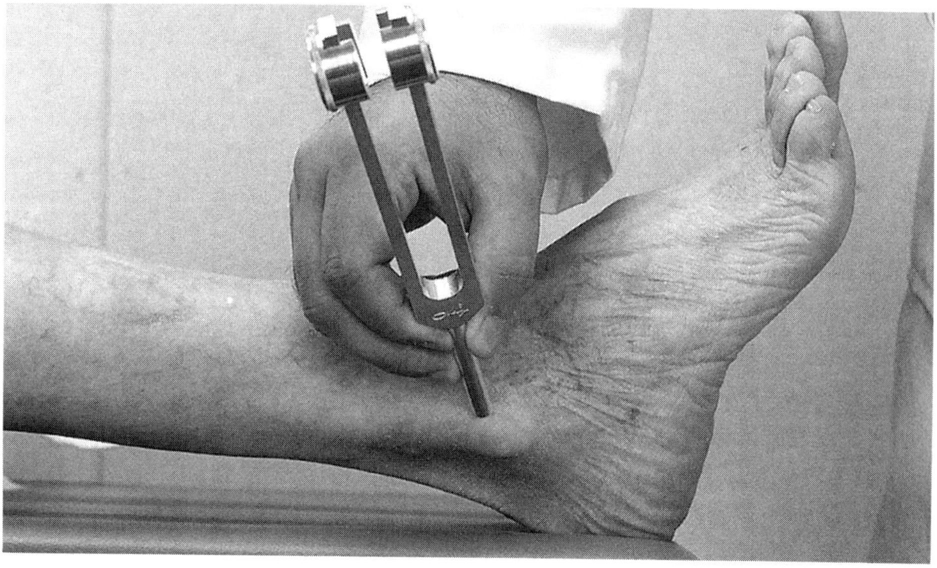

FIGURE 53.1.
Vibration testing is done over a bony prominence such as the lateral malleolus or wrist. The proximal phalanx of the great toe or the base of the thumb may also be used. (Reproduced with permission from Willms JL, Schneiderman H, Algranati PS. Physical Diagnosis: Bedside Evaluation of Diagnosis and Function. *Baltimore: Williams & Wilkins, 1994:481.)*

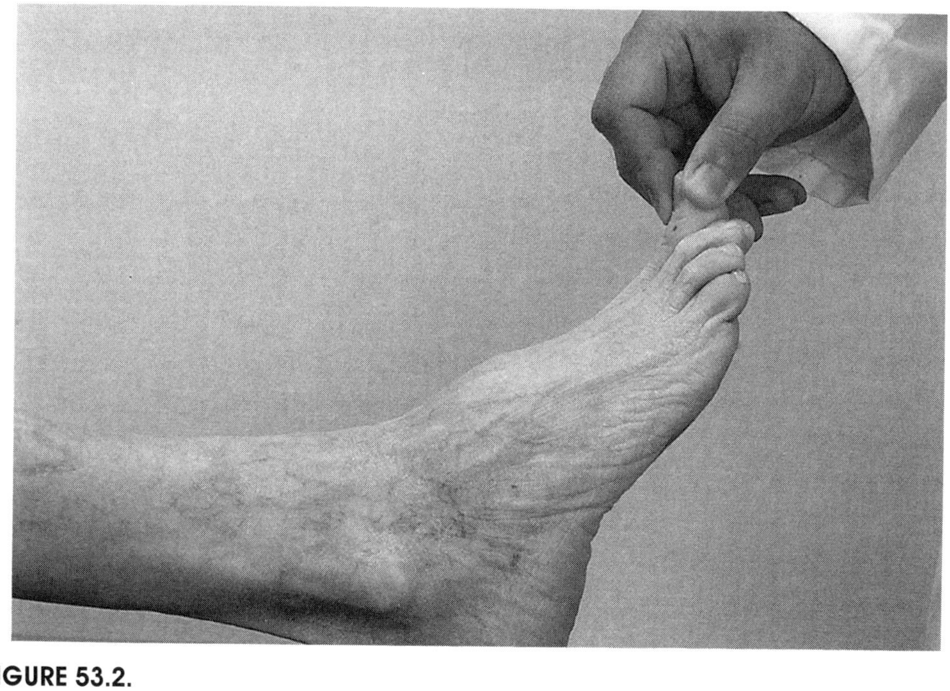

FIGURE 53.2.
Joint position sensation is tested by grasping the joint on the medial and lateral sides and gently moving the joint through a portion of its range. (Reproduced with permission from Willms JL, Schneiderman H, Algranati PS. Physical Diagnosis: Bedside Evaluation of Diagnosis and Function. *Baltimore: Williams & Wilkins, 1994:481.)*

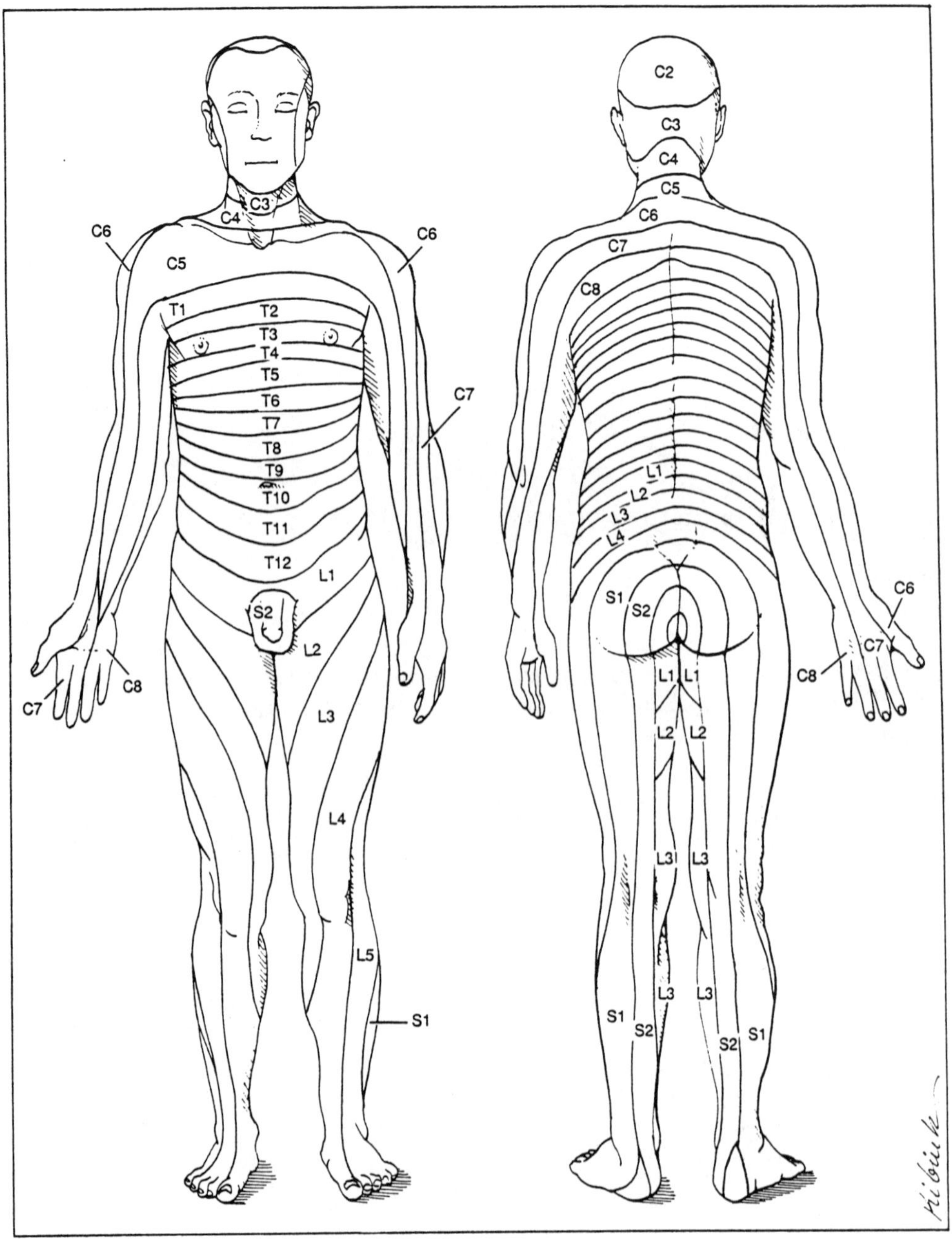

FIGURE 53.3.
The sensory distributions relating to spinal cord level are shown. In women, the vulva and perineum are served by nerves from the levels of S2 downward. (Reproduced with permission from Cipriano JJ. Photographic Manual of Regional Orthopaedics and Neurological Testing. *2nd ed. Baltimore: Williams & Wilkins, 1991:222.)*

opposite side of the body. (Dermatome distributions are shown in Figure 53.3.) In addition, the specifically involved test should be repeated, either immediately or after other tests are performed. Confusion or inattention may have caused a falsely absent finding, which will be corrected on retesting.

Care must be taken in the interpretation of absent sensation. Any stimulus must be adequate to be perceived, and this will vary by body site. Sensation over areas of callus (such as the heel) or of decreased sensory nerve density (the buttocks) is diminished compared with more richly innervated area such as the lips.

An area of diminished sensation should be mapped by moving the stimulus from the area of reduced sensation to normal touch. The point of transition should be marked and the procedure repeated until the affected area has been outlined.

The ability to sense vibration is often reduced in elderly patients, but joint position sensation does not undergo the same age-related change. Because both sensations are transmitted by the posterior columns of the spinal cord, preservation of joint position sense implies integrity of these structures even in the absence of vibrator sense.

Suggested Readings

Nelson KR. Use new pins for each neurologic examination. *N Engl J Med* 1986; 314:581.

Sapira JD. *The Art and Science of Bedside Diagnosis*. Baltimore: Williams & Wilkins, 1990:508.

Willms JL, Schneiderman H, Algranati PS. *Physical Diagnosis: Bedside Evaluation of Diagnosis and Function*. Baltimore: Williams & Wilkins, 1994:482.

Chapter 54

SCREENING TESTS FOR GAIT

As with balance, a functional gait requires the coordinated functions of bones, muscles, joints, and tendons, in addition to the neurologic functions of the motor, sensory, vestibular, and cerebellar systems.

Equipment

No special equipment is required.

Training/Credentialing

No special credentialing is needed.

Coding

No specific code for gait testing is used. The inclusion of gait testing may justify or support a higher acuity for the other services rendered. If only gait testing is performed, the following code may be considered:

95999 Unlisted neurological or neurovascular diagnostic procedure

Technique

Any patient who is not bed- or wheelchair-bound may undergo gait testing. If needed, gait may be tested with assist devices, such as a cane, crutches, or walker. The patient is asked to walk a few paces away from the observer, turn, and return. This may be repeated using a heel–toe (tandem) gait or by walking only on the heels or on the balls of the feet (Fig. 54.1). These tests should be reserved for patients who can safely attempt them with a low probability of an unanticipated fall.

Normal Findings

The normal patient should be able to walk in a smooth, confident manner without requiring exaggerated foot placement (broad-based gait), excessive arm swing, shortened

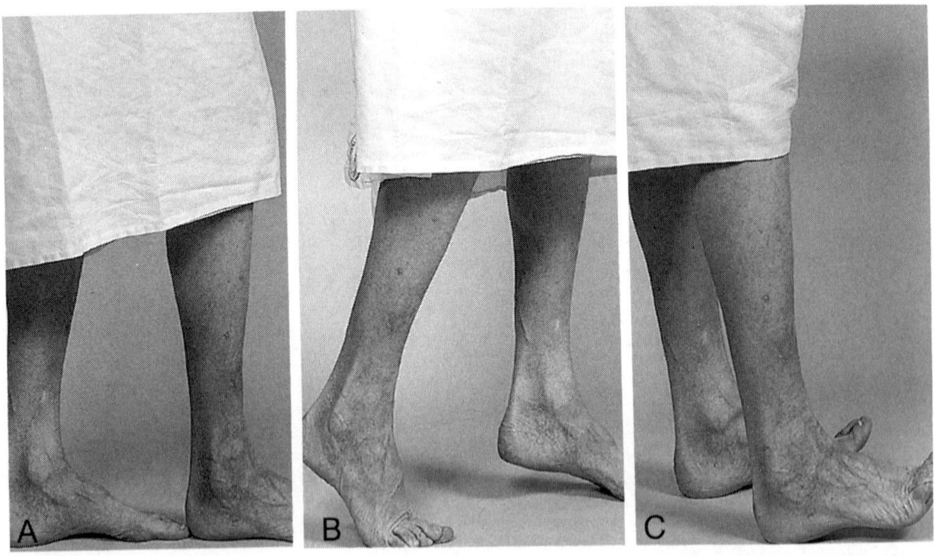

FIGURE 54.1.
Gait evaluation. ***A****. Tandem gait.* ***B****. Walking on toes.* ***C****. Walking on heels. (Reproduced with permission from Willms JL, Schneiderman H, Algranati PS.* Physical Diagnosis: Bedside Evaluation of Diagnosis and Function. *Baltimore: Williams & Wilkins, 1994:486.)*

stride, or unusual step height (steppage gait). All movements should be symmetrical. The turn should be smooth, with few extra steps. Most patients can walk on the heels or toes for at least short distances, but not all can perform these gaits for extended distances.

Special Notes

Gait should be tested with the patient in bare or stocking feet, with appropriate attention to safe footing to prevent a fall. The patient's clothing should allow the actions of the legs, hips, and spine to be observed or inferred.

Suggested Readings

Bohannon RW, Walsh S. Nature, reliability, and predictive value of muscle performance measures in patients with hemiparesis following stroke. *Arch Phys Med Rehab* 1992;73:721.

Cavanagh PR, Derr JA, Ulbrecht JS, et al. Problems with gait and posture in neuropathic patients with insulin-dependent diabetes mellitus. *Diabetic Med* 1992; 9:469.

Quane T, Chambers CV, Snyderman D. Conversion disorder presenting as gait disturbance in an adolescent. *Arch Fam Med* 1995;4:805.

Sapira JD. *The Art and Science of Bedside Diagnosis.* Baltimore: Williams & Wilkins, 1990:471.

Waters RL, Yakura JS, Adkins RH. Gait performance after spinal cord injury. *Clin Orthopaed Related Res* 1993;288:87.

Willms JL, Schneiderman H, Algranati PS. *Physical Diagnosis: Bedside Evaluation of Diagnosis and Function.* Baltimore: Williams & Wilkins, 1994:484.

Chapter 55

SPINAL PUNCTURE

From the staging of syphilis to the evaluation of neurologic disease, the lumbar puncture is an important skill that may be required for the primary care of women (Table 55.1).

Equipment

- Sterile gloves, antiseptic solution and sterile cotton balls, or skin preparation swabs
- Sterile draping material
- Commercially available spinal tap kit

or

- 25-gauge 2.5-inch spinal needle, 22-gauge 1.5-inch needle, 25-gauge 5/8-inch needle for local anesthesia, 3- or 5-mL syringe, 1% lidocaine with epinephrine 1:100,000, three-way stopcock, four specimen collection tubes, 2-inch by 2-inch or 4-inch by 4-inch gauze sponges, and manometer
- Self-adherent bandage

Training/Credentialing

No special credentialing needed; office procedure only.

Coding

62270 Spinal puncture, lumbar, diagnostic (procedure only)

62272 Spinal puncture, therapeutic, for drainage of spinal fluid

Technique

PATIENT PREPARATION

Proper positioning of the patient is essential to ensure successful lumbar puncture. The patient should be placed in the lateral decubitus position; the back should be par-

TABLE 55.1. Common Indications and Contraindications for Lumbar Puncture

TYPE	CONDITION
Diagnostic	Known or suspected infection or inflammation Acute bacterial or viral Subacute caused by tuberculosis, syphilis, fungi, neoplasm Chronic because of syphilis, tuberculosis, neoplasm Suspected hemorrhage—intracranial or intraspinal (generally replaced by computed tomography or magnetic resonance imaging) Suspected metastatic carcinoma or demyelinating conditions Selected imaging procedures (superseded in many cases by newer technologies)
Adjunctive	Acute polyneuropathy Intracranial hypertension Multiple sclerosis Systemic lupus erythematosus
Therapeutic	Antimicrobial Chemotherapy Reduction of intracranial hypertension (e.g., pseudotumor cerebri)
Contraindicated	Anticoagulation Local skin infection Noninfectious, undiagnosed increased intracranial pressure Suspected epidural infection Suspected intracranial mass Thrombocytopenia (<50,000 platelets/mm^3) Unevaluated papilledema

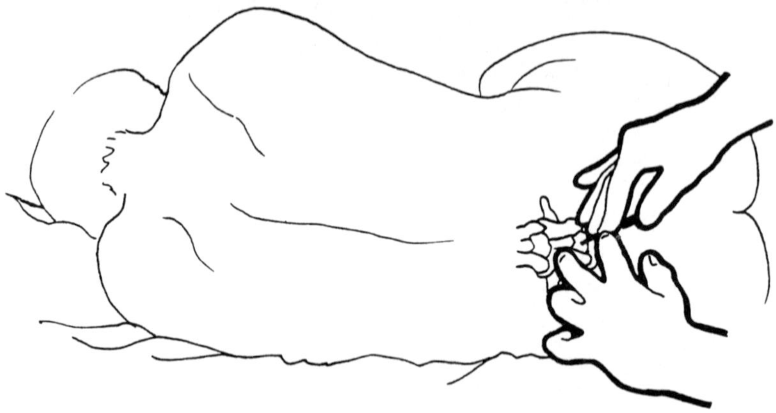

FIGURE 55.1.
Proper positioning of the patient is essential for a successful lumbar puncture. The ideal position is with the spine maximally flexed and the hips and shoulders perpendicular to the examining table. In this position, the interspinous space may be more easily palpated and the needle passed. Note that the needle remains parallel to the surface of the examination table. (Reproduced with permission from Simon RR, Brenner BE. Emergency Procedures and Techniques. *3rd ed. Baltimore: Williams & Wilkins, 1994:169.)*

allel to the edge of the examining table and maximally flexed (Fig. 55.1). The neck, knees, and hips should be flexed and the shoulders and pelvis should be perpendicular to the examining table. The head should be supported on a small pillow to allow the shoulders to be maintained in this perpendicular position. In this position the lumbar spinous processes are slightly "opened" or "separated" by the flexion, giving a larger area through which to pass the needle without impinging on the periosteum or nerve roots.

When the spinous processes are hard to palpate, as in obese patients, or when scoliosis or ankylosing spondylitis is present, the patient may be positioned in a slumped sitting position. For this technique, the patient should be situated with her buttocks at the near edge of the examination table. The patient should slump forward, supporting the upper body by bracing her arms on her knees or by leaning onto a Mayo stand padded with a pillow. The back must be kept straight, with no rotation of the shoulders. The back should be arched or "pushed" toward the examiner to maximize the extension of the back in the area of the needle passage.

Once the patient has been positioned in a satisfactory manner, the skin over the L4–L5 or L5–S1 interspace and the adjacent area are cleansed and prepared as for surgery. This preparation should include the skin over one additional interspace cephalad and caudad so that these interspaces may be used should the need arise. Sterile drapes should be applied to ensure a sterile field in which to work.

PERFORMING THE PROCEDURE

The chosen interspace should be repalpated, and a small skin weal of local anesthetic should placed in the skin and superficial subcutaneous tissues. No more than 3 mL of anesthetic solution should be used so that the palpable landmarks are not obscured. The spinal needle is next introduced through this weal, in the midline, with the bevel directed parallel to the axis of the spinal collum (horizontally for the patient in the lateral position). The needle should be directed toward the umbilicus (approximately 10–15° cephalad) and maintained in the midline horizontal plane when the lateral position is used (or the vertical plane when the patient is sitting).

Some physicians prefer to use a 22-gauge needle as a guide for the finer, more flexible 25-gauge spinal needle. If this is the case, the needle should be placed first, to the level of the interspinous ligament, using the same technique noted above. The spinal needle itself is then introduced through this guide needle and advanced toward the spinal canal. If bone is encountered, the needle should be withdrawn to the level of the subcutaneous tissue, realigned with the midline, and readvanced.

As the covering dural layer is punctured, a loss of resistance (or "pop") may be experienced. When this is felt, or the spinal needle has been advanced to a depth of 3–4 cm, the needle stylet is removed and the hub of the needle inspected for signs of cerebrospinal fluid. When fluid is noted, a three-way stopclock and manometer should be attached and a reading of fluid pressure obtained. The hub of the needle is used as the zero point of the reading, and the height of the meniscus of fluid is measured to establish the pressure. The most accurate readings are obtained when the patient straightens her legs, which reduces intra-abdominal pressure.

After manometric readings, samples may be obtained as needed (Fig. 55.2). Four samples are usually obtained: 1–2 mL for a Gram stain, culture, and sensitivity testing; 0.5–1 mL for glucose and protein determinations; 2 mL for antibody, antigen, or cytologic testing as needed; and 1 mL for a cell count. After completion of sampling, the stylet is reinserted into the needle, the needle is gently withdrawn, and a self-adherent bandage is applied.

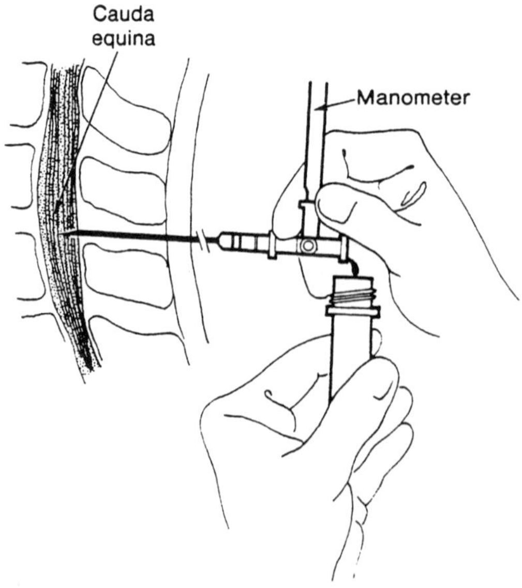

FIGURE 55.2.
Once manometric readings have been obtained, samples may be collected. (Reproduced with permission from Simon RR, Brenner BE. Emergency Procedures and Techniques. *3rd ed. Baltimore: Williams & Wilkins, 1994:172.)*

TABLE 55.2. Normal Values for Cerebrospinal Fluid

PHYSICOCHEMICAL PROPERTY	NORMAL VALUE
Appearance	Water-white, clear
Pressure	6–20 cm H_2O
	4.5–15 mm Hg
Number of cells	0–3 cells/mm^3
Specific gravity	1.005–1.009
pH value	7.32 ± 0.09 (range, 7.14–7.50)
Proteins	
Total	20–40 mg/dL
Albumin: globulin ratio	4:1
Urea	10–30 mg/dL
Creatinine	0.54–1.91 mg/dL
Glucose	45–80 mg/dL (60–70% of blood value)

Normal Findings

Normal cerebrospinal fluid pressures range from 60 to 200 mm H_2O. Normal values for the laboratory analysis of cerebrospinal fluid are shown in Table 55.2.

Selected Abnormal Findings

Bloody fluid may indicate either intracranial bleeding or a bloody tap. Distinguishing between these two possibilities is very important. If the fluid clears as more fluid is obtained, a bloody tap is most likely. A cell count of the first and last samples obtained may be able to make this distinction when it is not apparent to the unaided eye. The sample may be centrifuged and the supernatant inspected. Clear supernatant suggests that the blood has been present for less than 2 hours. Xanthochromic fluid may be present when the patient is jaundiced or if the cerebrospinal fluid protein level is greater than 150 mg/dL.

Special Notes

The use of a 25-gauge spinal needle reduces the incidence of headache while allowing rapid, relatively painless insertion. A line drawn between the iliac crests intersects the spinous process of L4. Lumbar puncture should only be performed below the level of L3.

Because a "pop" is not always felt as the needle punctures the dura, there is a risk for inserting the needle too far and entering the anterior epidural space, which has a rich vascular supply. To reduce this risk, the stylet should be removed from the needle to check for cerebrospinal fluid with every 1–2 mm of advancement. An alternative technique is to place a drop of saline at the needle hub once the interspinous ligament is encountered. As the needle is advanced to the dura, a slight negative pressure in the epidural space is created, displacing the drop inward and indicating impending dural puncture.

Forced deep breathing or rapid shallow breathing should be discouraged because they may result in hypocapnia, which, in turn, induces a falsely low cerebrospinal fluid pressure reading.

Because cerebrospinal fluid pressure reading may change rapidly after placement of the spinal needle, manometric readings should always be taken as soon as possible, and always before specimens are removed.

If the flow of cerebrospinal fluid decreases while samples are being taken, the needle should be rotated 180° to move the bevel away from any nerve roots that may be impinging on the needle opening.

Rapid withdrawal of the spinal needle, even with the obturator in place, may result in herniation of part of the nerve root into the needle tack. Spinal headaches are reported to occur in 10–15% of patients, although the use of a 25-gauge needle should reduce this number substantially. Some studies suggest that having the patient lie in the prone position for 3 hours before ambulation significantly reduces the risk for headache. When possible, this is not unreasonable advice, but it is difficult to accomplish in the office setting. These headaches are usually self-limited, resolve in a few days, and require only mild analgesics.

Suggested Readings

Bocker RJ. Technique to avoid spinal tap headache. *JAMA* 1958;168:261.

Brown JK. Lumbar puncture and its hazards. *Dev Med Child Neurol* 1976;18:803.

Livingstone KE. Technique of lumbar puncture [Letter]. *N Engl J Med* 1974;287:724.

Marton KI, Gean AD. The spinal tap: a new look at an old test. *Ann Intern Med* 1986;104:840.

Petito F, Plum F. The lumbar puncture [Letter]. *N Engl J Med* 1974;290:225.

Raskin NK. Lumbar puncture headache: a review. *Headache* 1990;30:197.

Wetchler BV, Brace DE. A technique to minimize the occurrence of headache after lumbar puncture by use of small bore spinal needles. *Anesthesiology* 1955;16:270.

Section VII

OPHTHALMOLOGIC EVALUATIONS

Chapter 56

CORNEAL EXAMINATION

Foreign bodies and corneal abrasions are not infrequent problems seen in primary care settings. With a passing familiarity with the technique of corneal examination, the gynecologist will be better able to diagnose and treat these problems.

In its simplest form, the examination of the cornea is performed without special equipment or skills. When the possibility of corneal abrasion or foreign body is raised, a more thorough evaluation is required. This includes the eversion of the eyelid so that the entire cornea may be seen and the use of local anesthetics, staining agents, special light sources, and magnification.

Equipment

- Topical ophthalmic anesthetic agent (proparacaine 0.5% or benoxinate 0.4%)
- Fluorescein sodium strips or drops
- Bright white light source (penlight is sufficient)
- Cobalt-blue light source (Wood's lamp may be used)
- Magnifying loop (8× to 10×), ophthalmoscope, or colposcope
- Sterile cotton-tipped applicator sticks
- Sterile saline irrigation fluid
- Snellen visual acuity chart or equivalent
- Sterile eye patch or gauze pads
- Ophthalmic antibiotic (tobramycin ointment, 3 mg/g, or sulfacetamide ointment, 10%)
- Cycloplegic drops (cyclopentolate HCl, 1–2%)
- Slit lamp (optional)

Training/Credentialing

No special credentialing needed; office procedure only.

Coding

65205	Removal of foreign body, external eye; conjunctival superficial (surgical procedure only)
65210	conjunctival embedded (includes concretions), subconjunctival, or scleral nonperforating
65220	corneal, without slit lamp
65222	corneal, with slit lamp
99070	Material and supplies provided by physician beyond that normally used with office visit

Technique

Before formal corneal examination, the visual acuity of the patient should be assessed by using a Snellen chart or equivalent or by having the patient read magazine print held at arm's length. If the patient cannot read print at this distance, she should bring the print closer; the distance at which the characters may be distinguished should be noted.

A cursory examination of the conjunctiva and cornea may be done with the patient either upright or supine. If anesthetic drops, fluorescein, or irrigation may be required, the supine position is more convenient. If the examination is being performed to evaluate the possibility of an abrasion or foreign body, a local anesthetic should be used. One or two drops of proparacaine (0.5%) or benoxinate (0.4%) may be used for this purpose.

While the anesthetic drops take effect, each eye should be inspected under white light. This inspection should include the sclera, interior chamber, iris, and pupil. The size, shape, and reactivity of the pupil should be noted. The upper lid should be everted over the tip of a cotton-tipped applicator to allow inspection of the hidden portions of the conjunctiva (Fig. 56.1). The inner aspect of the lid should also be inspected for the presence of a foreign body, hordeolum, or inverted eyelash.

A fluorescein strip should be moistened with a single drop of sterile saline or local anesthetic; the strip is then applied to the lower conjunctival sac for 3–5 seconds. If too much solution is used to wet the fluorescein strip, excess staining of the entire sclera may result. If this happens, the eye should be irrigated with a small amount of sterile saline. When this is done, only defects or abrasions should show the stain.

By using magnification and a blue light source, the entire cornea is inspected for signs of staining that may indicate a defect or abrasion. The lesions appear as bright yellow or white areas on the relatively dark blue background of the normal sclera. Any abnormalities found should be recorded in an appropriate note to be placed in the patient's record. If no lesions are found to account for the patient's symptoms, the possibility of an embedded foreign body should be suspected. The eye should be examined by using a slit lamp, or the patient should be referred for further evaluation.

TREATMENT OF UNCOMPLICATED CORNEAL ABRASIONS

The patient should be placed in the supine position with the head turned toward the affected side. The eye is irrigated with sterile saline, and one or two drops of topical anesthetic should be applied. The use of cycloplegic drops lessens the patient's discomfort. An antibiotic ointment should be applied and the eye patched. If commercially available patches are used, two should be used; the first is folded in half and placed under the brow, and the second is secured over the first. Paper tape should be used when possible, and the tape should be applied in a diagonal fashion, running from the middle of the

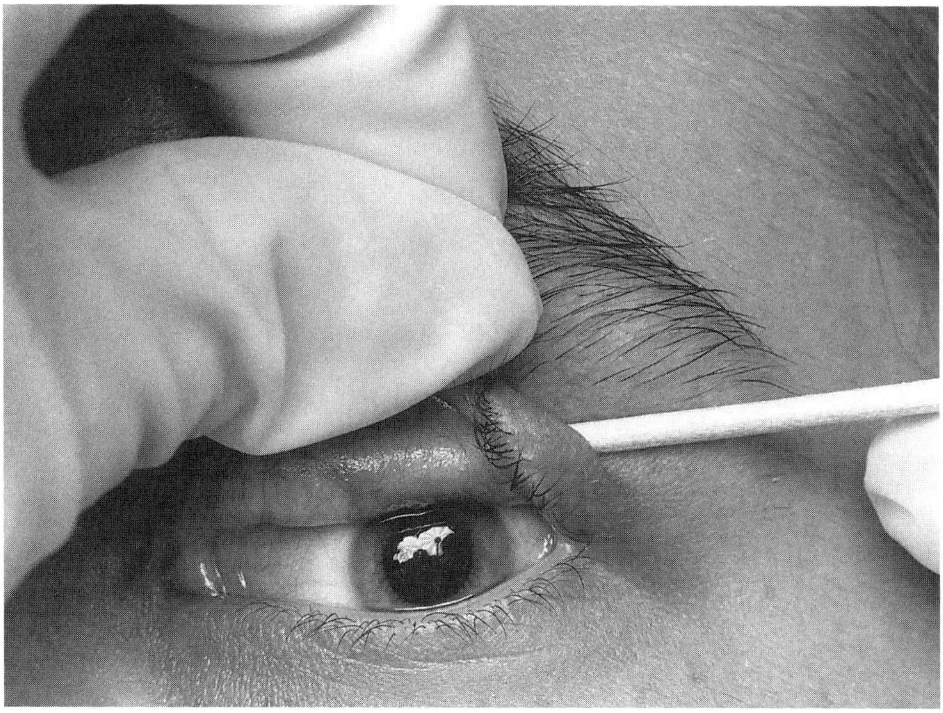

FIGURE 56.1.
The upper lid may be everted over the tip of an applicator stick by grasping the lashes and gently pulling outward and upward. (Reproduced with permission from Willms JL, Schneiderman H, Algranati PS. Physical Diagnosis: Bedside Evaluation of Diagnosis and Function. *Baltimore: Williams & Wilkins, 1994:154.)*

forehead toward the base of the ear. The eye should be reevaluated in 24 hours. Analgesics may be prescribed if needed. Antibiotic ointment treatment should be continued for at least 72 hours. The eye patch should remain in place until discomfort abates.

REMOVAL OF FOREIGN BODY

When a foreign body is suspected, documentation of the patient's visual acuity is especially important. Once this has been accomplished, the patient is placed in a position that permits the best access to the eye and foreign body. For cooperative patients this may be upright; younger patients and those with substantial pain or tearing are best examined in the supine position.

The lids should be gently separated by using the thumb and index finger. The head may be repositioned as needed to make the foreign body most accessible. The patient must be instructed to remain motionless and fix his or her gaze on one point. One to two drops of topical anesthetic should be instilled and allowed to act. If the foreign body is readily visible, it may often be removed by touching it with a cotton-tipped applicator moistened with sterile saline or local anesthetic. The upper lid may be inverted as described above to gain access to the entire conjunctiva. The tip of a sterile hypodermic needle may also be used to lift the object away from the cornea or conjunctiva. If this method is used, the needle should be stabilized on the end of a syringe and should only be applied to the sclera in a tangential, bevel-up manner.

Once the foreign object has been removed, the eye should be treated as for an abrasion. Follow-up evaluation and a second examination of visual acuity should be scheduled before the patient departs.

Normal Findings

When viewed in white light, the sclera should be intact, the anterior chamber should be free of blood and pus, and the size and shape of the iris should be normal.

Selected Abnormal Findings

Clouding of the cornea, edema, the presence of a purulent discharge, deep ulcerations, central lesions, and dendritic lesions all suggest the need for ophthalmologic consultation.

Abrasions that consist of linear scratches or lines are typical of those found with direct trauma or a foreign body. Foreign bodies trapped under the lid produce a series of "spotty" or "blotchy" lesions in a roughly parallel pattern. Circular or well-inscribed lesions may result from use of contact lenses. Deep or dendritic lesions suggest infection.

Special Notes

Local anesthetics are contraindicated if rupture of the eye globe is possible.

Fluorescein strips are preferred to drops because of the possibility of contamination with *Pseudomonas* organisms when multidose bottles are used.

Continued use of local anesthetics to treat the pain of a corneal abrasion should be avoided because it will retard the healing process.

Contact lenses should always be removed before fluorescein is used.

Metallic foreign bodies may swiftly lead to rust staining of the cornea even if rapidly removed. Complete removal of the object combined with chemical treatment with agents such as Desferal (deferoxamine mesylate) may also be advisable. Early consultation is suggested in these cases.

Suggested Readings

Aquavella JV, Eiferman RA, Sher NA. Treating superficial corneal injuries. *Patient Care* 1985;19:27.

Bertolini J, Pelucio M. The red eye. *Emerg Med Clin North Am* 1995;13:561.

Connenfeld ED, Selkin BA, Perry HD, et al. Controlled evaluation of a bandage contact lens and a topical nonsteroidal anti-inflammatory drug in treating traumatic corneal abrasions. *Ophthalmology* 1995;102:979.

Patterson J, Fetzer D, Krall J, et al. Eye patch treatment for the pain of corneal abrasions. *So Med J* 1996;89:227.

Schein OD. Contact lens abrasions and the nonophthalmologist. *Am J Emerg Med* 1993;11:606.

Willms JL, Schneiderman H, Algranati PS. *Physical Diagnosis: Bedside Evaluation of Diagnosis and Function*. Baltimore: Williams & Wilkins, 1994:119.

Chapter 57

FUNDUSCOPIC EXAMINATION

Although the funduscopic examination is an often-bypassed portion of the physical examination, facility with this diagnostic procedure is important in evaluating many conditions seen in day-to-day gynecologic practice. As with most diagnostic techniques, the value gained is in direct proportion to the skill and facility of the examiner. When performed correctly, this brief examination will pay dividends in excess of the time required to perform the test.

Equipment

- Ophthalmoscope
- Bright white light source (pen light)

Training/Credentialing

No special credentialing needed; office procedure only.

Coding

The funduscopic examination cannot be billed as a separate item. It is considered a part of an office examination.

Technique

The funduscopic examination must be preceded by an inspection of the external portions of the globe and the cornea (see Chapter 56, Corneal Examination). To obtain the best ophthalmoscopic examination, the pupil should be dilated using a drop of a mydriatic agent such as tropicamide (0.5 or 1% ophthalmic solution). Because there is a small chance of precipitating an acute attack of glaucoma or displacing an implanted lens, the physician should be aware of contraindications to the routine use of mydriatic agents (Table 57.1). It is probably safe to use a mydriatic agent if, in the past 2 years, the patient has undergone routine refraction in which drops were used that made the vision blurry without complication. The use of a mydriatic agent requires

TABLE 57.1. Contraindications to the Use of Mydriatic Agents

Acute angle-closure glaucoma
Eye pain that occurs only at night or in the dark
Implanted lens
Positive nipple test result (see Chapter 58, Tonometry)

roughly 30 minutes to take effect and results in blurred vision and photophobia for an hour or two thereafter. These effects must be considered in making the decision to dilate the pupil.

If a mydriatic agent is to be used, the patient should incline her head backward with the eyes directed upward. The lower lid may be retracted slightly to form a sac to receive the drops. The dropper should be held no closer than 1 inch from the eye so that it does not touch either the globe or eyelashes. A single drop of agent in the conjunctival sac of each eye is sufficient; additional drops do not increase efficacy. These drops may cause a slight stinging, which will pass in a few moments. To prevent confusion about the patient's fixed pupil or pupils, the fact that a mydriatic agent has been used should be noted in the patient's chart; as an alternative, other personnel may be notified.

The ophthalmoscope should be checked for functionality before the examination begins. The light should be bright and white, the filters and slits should allow free interposition, and the lens contained in the lens wheel should be clean and clear. The magnification should be set for +8 to +10 to begin the examination.

With the ophthalmoscope held close to the examiner's eye, the examination begins approximately 30 cm from the patient's eye with an evaluation of the red reflex. (In all cases, the eye used by the examiner is the same as the eye to be examined; right eye for right eye and left for left.) The clarity of the lens and the presence of any black spots apparent in front of the dull red reflex should be noted. The location of these spots may be assessed by having the patient look upward and noting the relative movement of the spot (Fig. 57.1). The relative clarity of the cornea and lens should also be noted.

The ophthalmoscope is then moved toward the patient's eye while observation of the red reflex continues. The lens diopters are turned downward (toward 0) as the retina comes into view and a sharp focus on the vessels of the retina is obtained (Fig. 57.2). For most patients and examiners, the final position of the ophthalmoscope will be within a few centimeters of the front of the eye. Once a clear image is obtained, the retina should be systematically evaluated by quadrants. Five key elements should be evaluated: the lens, the optic disc, the arteries and veins of the retina, the retina itself, and the macula. Expected findings are reviewed below. Once inspection of one eye is complete, the procedure is repeated for the other eye.

Normal Findings

THE LENS

The lens should be clear and central, with few or no spots or opacities.

OPTIC DISC

The optic disc should be butter-yellow and slightly elliptical, with the ellipse oriented horizontally (Fig. 57.3). In the center of the disc is a pale white area representing the physiologic cup, which is devoid of nerve fibers. Vessels should be seen emerging from

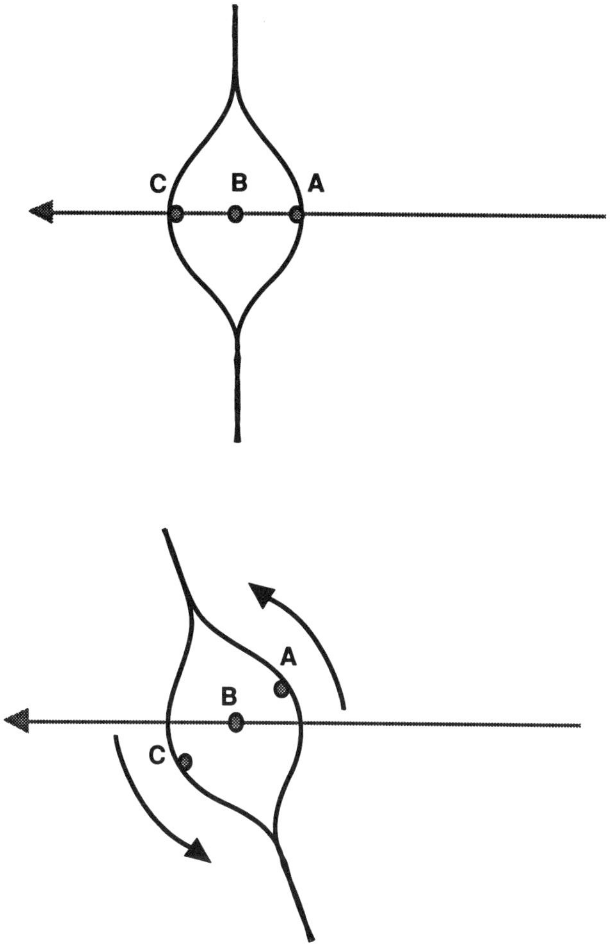

FIGURE 57.1.
Objects on the front of the lens or on the cornea appear to move in the direction of movement of the eye, whereas objects on the back side of the lens or in the vitreous appear to move in the opposite direction. Mid-lens opacities appear to be stationary.

the center, and the margins of the disc should be crisp; however, some blurring on the nasal side may be present in normal patients. The disc and margins should be in focus at the same time, indicating that they occupy the same plane. Some normal patients, especially those with myopia, may have a crescent of dark pigmented dots at the temporal border of the disc.

ARTERIES AND VEINS

The four sets of vessels of the optic disc emerge and spread over the retina in pairs to serve each quadrant. The arteries appear brighter red, with a white strip along the center. A slight pulsation may be noted in the veins but not in the arteries. Points at which the arteries and veins cross should not show any obscuring of the vein (Fig. 57.4).

RETINA

The retina should be uniform in color and free of discoloration, lesions, and exudates.

MACULA

The macula or fovea is more darkly pigmented than the surrounding retina. It is roughly one-fourth the size of the optic disc and is located approximately two to three disc diameters from the temporal margin of the disc. The macula is devoid of vessels and has a central dark spot, the fovea centralis. The macula can be seen if the patient

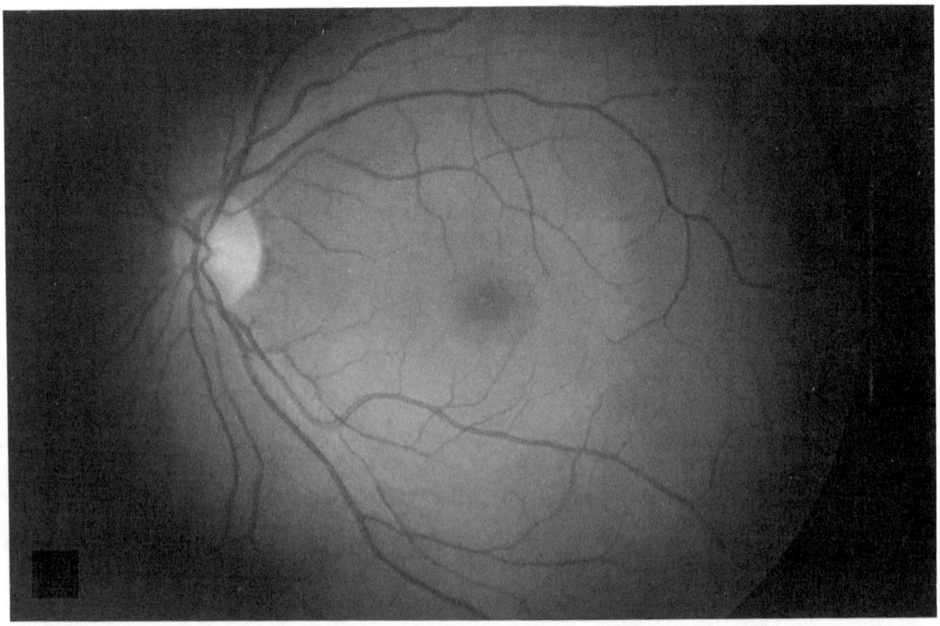

FIGURE 57.2.
Panoramic view of left retina. The optic disc is at left edge, and the macula is the darker area without vessels at the center of the photograph. (Reproduced with permission from Willms JL, Schneiderman H, Algranati PS. Physical Diagnosis: Bedside Evaluation of Diagnosis and Function. *Baltimore: Williams & Wilkins, 1994:157.)*

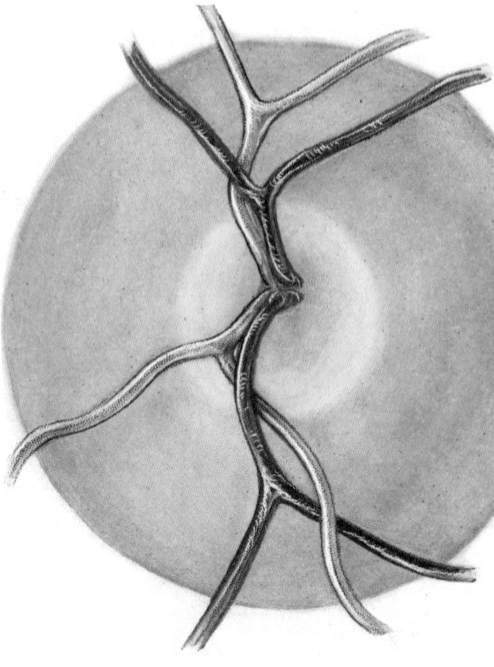

FIGURE 57.3.
The optic disc and vessels in a normal patient. (Reproduced with permission from Sapira JD. The Art and Science of Bedside Diagnosis. *Baltimore: Williams & Wilkins, 1990:182.)*

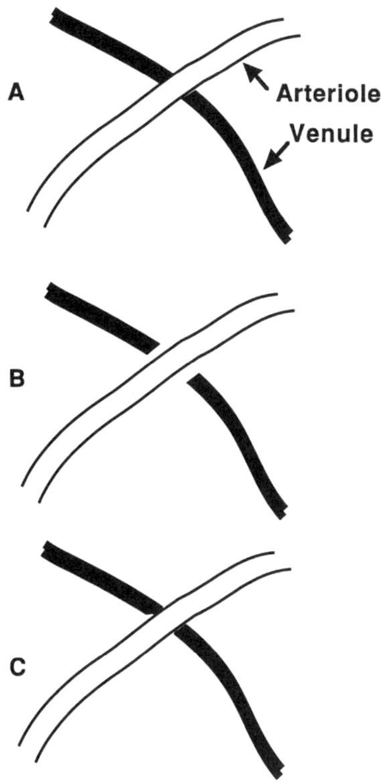

FIGURE 57.4.
*The points at which arteries and veins cross are important to assess. In normal patients (**A**), the crossings show no interaction between the vessels. Arteriovenous "nicking" (**B**) more than two disc diameters from the optic nerve represents a thickening of the arteriolar adventitia. Arteriovenous crossings such as that shown in part **C** do not represent true "nicking" and have little diagnostic significance.*

is asked to look directly into the light; however, this technique produces discomfort for the patient, who will quickly look away.

Selected Abnormal Findings

An excellent discussion of abnormal findings and their differential diagnosis is found in the reference by Sapira listed in the suggested readings.

OPTIC DISC

Enlargement of the optic cup suggests an increase in intraocular pressure (Fig. 57.5). This enlargement must be differentiated from papilledema, which is illustrated in Figure 57.6. Deepening of the optic cup, a change in the cup-to-disc ratio, pallor of the disc, and a change in the axis of the cup to the vertical all suggest glaucoma.

ARTERIES AND VEINS

Narrowing, exaggerated arteriovenous crossings, such as those shown in Figure 57.4; neovascularization; and increased tortuosity of the vessels are abnormal and should warrant further investigation. The significance of changes in arteriovenous crossing has been widely debated and is best explored in the suggested readings supplied at the end of the chapter.

RETINA

Some variation in the color of the retina from patient to patient is normal, but the retina itself should be of uniform color throughout. Patches of white, black, or deep red pigmentation are abnormal. Hemorrhages may occur in patients with hypertension, diabetes, leukemia, or severe anemia. Soft exudates or "cotton-wool" spots are flat and white, with indistinct margins. These may be found in many of the same processes noted

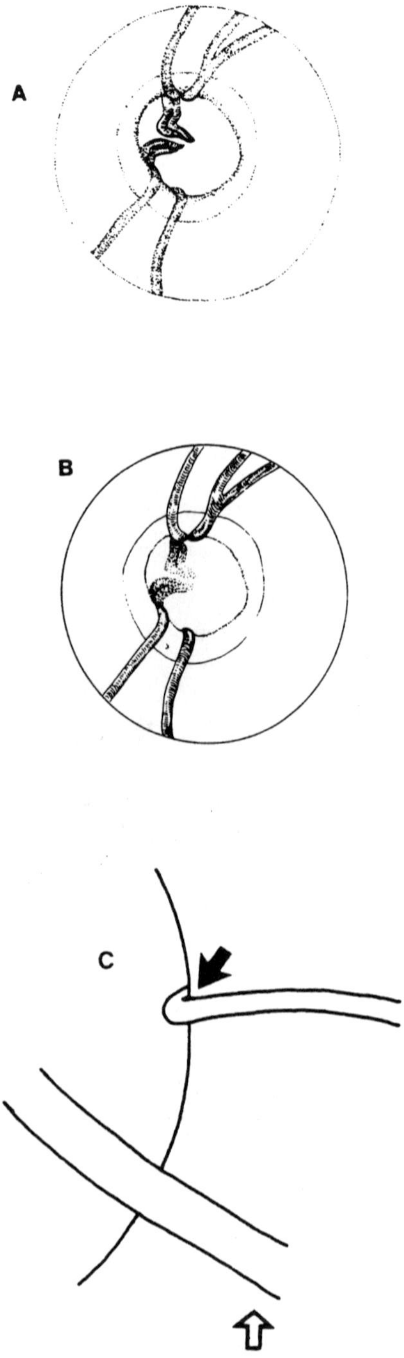

FIGURE 57.5.
A and B *show a disc whose cup is deep. In part* ***A,*** *one can focus on the vessel emerging from the deep cup but cannot as clearly see the vessels as they exit the disc. In part* **B,** *one sees the vessel going under the lip of the disc and the distal vessel emerging, but one cannot see the proximal vessel clearly. In part* **C,** *a normal vessel exits the disc at the bottom (hollow arrow) and a "false-positive" cilioretinal artery exits the disc in a manner faintly suggestive of a true glaucomatous vessel (solid arrow). This cilioretinal artery is always smaller than the normal artery. Furthermore, although the cilioretinal artery exits the disc by coming over the edge like a glaucomatous vessel, the more proximal portion of the artery cannot be identified, as would be the case with a true glaucomatous vessel (compare with* **B***). (Reproduced with permission from Sapira JD.* The Art and Science of Bedside Diagnosis. *Baltimore: Williams & Wilkins, 1990:181.)*

above and are also common in patients with the acquired immunodeficiency syndrome. Hard exudates are more yellowish and have a smoother surface. These are more mature versions of the soft exudates noted above and may be a step on the path to healing.

Special Notes

The greatest risk in using a mydriatic agent is not the precipitation of acute glaucoma but transmitting an ocular infection by way of contamination of the tip of the eye-

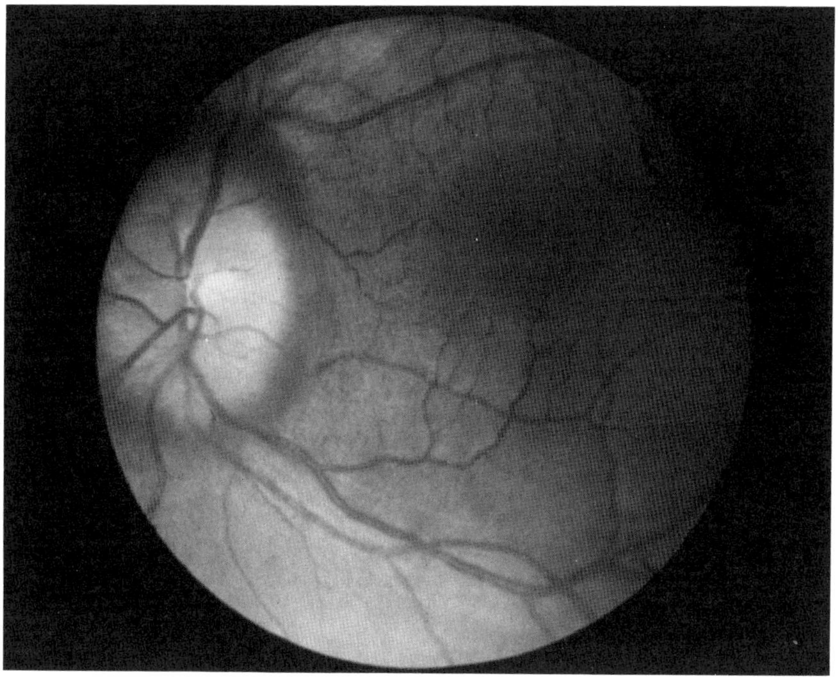

FIGURE 57.6.
Blurring and loss of a distinct disc margin are two of the first signs of papilledema. Normally, there can be slightly less distinction to the temporal margin of a disc without papilledema as compared with its nasal margin. However, no normal disc would have this much blurring, especially at the superior and inferior margins. (Reproduced with permission from Sapira JD. The Art and Science of Bedside Diagnosis. *Baltimore: Williams & Wilkins, 1990:179.)*

dropper. The effects of tropicamide may be reversed through the use of pilocarpine ophthalmic solution.

By approaching the eye from the temporal side, direct illumination of the macula is delayed and with it the discomfort that such stimulation may cause.

Contact lenses worn by either the patient or the examiner may be left in place during the ophthalmoscopic examination. Persons who wear glasses should remove them and use the corrective lens in the ophthalmoscope itself to supply the needed refraction. Patients with severe astigmatism may have to be examined with their glasses in place or referred to a more experienced examiner.

Care should be used when examining the macula because no patient can tolerate direct illumination of the macula for more than a second or two.

Suggested Readings

Potts AM. Diagnostic eye instruments for the general physician. *J Florida Med Assoc* 1994;81:234.

Sapira JD. *The Art and Science of Bedside Diagnosis*. Baltimore: Williams & Wilkins, 1990:155.

Snead MP, Rubinstein MP, Jacobs PM. The optics of fundus examination. *Surv Ophthalmol* 1992;6:439.

Willms JL, Schneiderman H, Algranati PS. *Physical Diagnosis: Bedside Evaluation of Diagnosis and Function*. Baltimore: Williams & Wilkins, 1994:119.

Chapter 58

TONOMETRY

Glaucoma (intraocular hypertension) insidiously leads to irreversible blindness if left untreated. In the United Sates, an estimated 1.5 million patients have some degree of vision loss secondary to glaucoma. Glaucoma is not diagnosed by changes in visual acuity or visual field testing by confrontation techniques. Visual field cuts occur late in the process and progress from nasal arcuate to the temporal fields, sparing central vision until the end. Because of the location of these early field losses, they are not detected by the usual office screening methods. Glaucoma may only be detected by measuring intraocular pressure through tonometry.

Glaucoma exists in three forms: 1) wide-angle or open-angle glaucoma, in which the depth of the anterior chamber is normal; 2) normal-angle or acute-angle glaucoma (rare), in which the anterior chamber is shallow; and 3) the infrequent "miscellaneous" glaucomas, such as "normal pressure" glaucoma, in which pressures are labile. Risk factors for the development of glaucoma are shown in Table 58.1.

Equipment

- Schiötz tonometer, weights (5.5, 7.5, 10.0, and 15.0 g), with conversion chart or similar tonometry device
- Topical ophthalmic anesthetic agent (proparacaine 0.5% or benoxinate 0.4%)

Training/Credentialing

No special credentialing needed; office procedure only.

Coding

92100 (Tonometry services are not typically coded as a separate procedure. Instead, it is performed as a part of a complete evaluation. This code may be used when serial measurements are taken as a part of clinical management.)

Technique

As with most ophthalmologic examinations, the patient's visual acuity should be checked at the onset of the process by using a Snellen wall chart, pocket screening

TABLE 58.1. Risk Factors for the Development of Glaucoma

Age older than 40 years
Black race
Use of corticosteroids
Diabetes mellitus
Family history of glaucoma
Use of mydriatic agents
Use of phenothiazines
Use of sympathomimetic agents

chart, or magazine print held at arm's length. A funduscopic examination is also appropriate at this juncture (see Chapter 57, Funduscopic Examination).

As a part of the screening process for glaucoma, the depth of the anterior chamber of the eye should be evaluated. This can help to identify patients at risk and define the type of glaucoma present (Fig. 58.1). This evaluation is critical if mydriatic agents may be used; these agents can precipitate acute pressure changes in narrow-angle glaucoma. The anterior chamber may be assessed using a pen light shown across the pupil in a tangential manner from the temporal side toward the limbus (Fig. 58.2). The light should follow a path perpendicular to the axis of vision. The light should just barely illuminate the entire iris. If the lens is displaced anteriorly, the central iris forms a nipple-like protrusion.

Tonometric measurements begin with the instillation of one to two drops of local anesthetic in each eye. While the anesthetic agent takes effect, the tonometer should be assembled according to the manufacturer's instructions. If a Schiötz tonometer is used, the lowest weight (5.5 g) should be installed first. The tonometer should be checked for accuracy by using the test block supplied with the instrument.

With the patient supine and keeping a fixed gaze, the nondominant hand is rested lightly on the patient's cheek or forehead and the lids retracted. Care must be used not to exert pressure on the globe itself (Fig. 58.3). The tonometer is grasped by the side arms using the thumb and forefinger and gently rested against the center of the cornea (over the limbus). To obtain valid readings, the tonometer must be vertical and perpendicular to the surface.

The center plunger of the tonometer is elevated by contact with the cornea. The scale reading on the tonometer indicating the degree of this displacement should be noted. The value reflects intraocular pressure, but the actual pressure is measured by translation from the table supplied with the device. For the pressure measurement to be accurate, the scale reading must fall between 4 and 8. If the reading is less than 4, the next higher weight should be added to the tonometer and the measurement repeated. This should continue, with progressively heavier weights, until a reading of 4 to 8 is obtained. The final pressure (in mm Hg) is obtained from the conversion table supplied with the kit.

The tonometer should be carefully cleaned after each use and dissembled at the end of each day.

Selected Abnormal Findings

An intraocular pressure greater than 20 mm Hg should prompt a referral to an ophthalmologist.

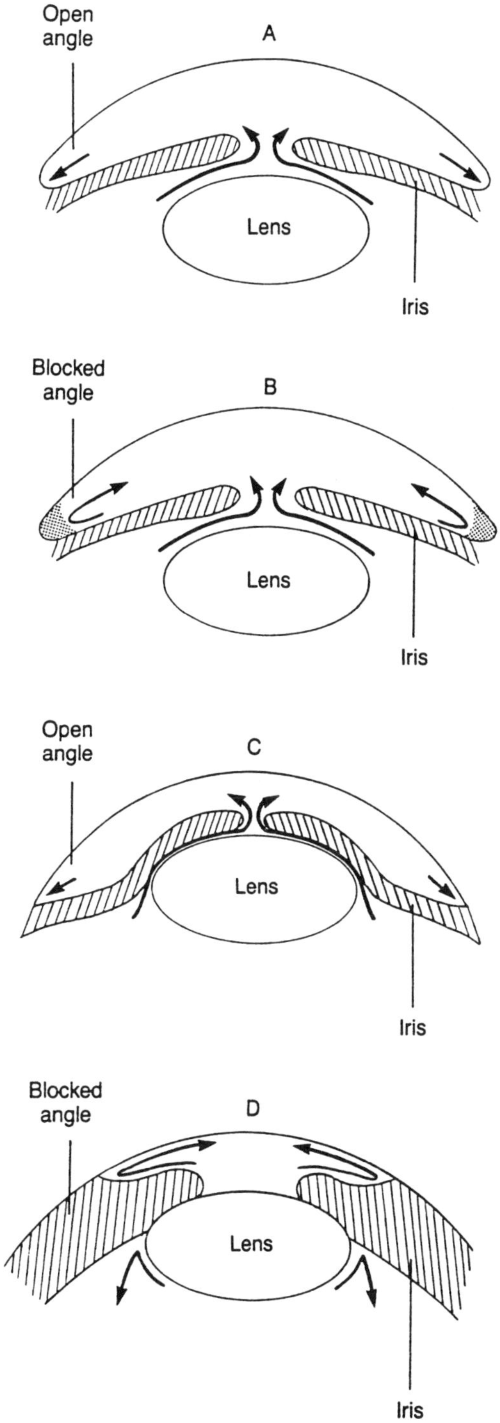

FIGURE 58.1.
A. *A normal eye, showing the flow of the aqueous into the anterior chamber and then the regressing through the canal of Schlemm in the angle.* ***B.*** *The common wide-angle or open-angle glaucoma showing the block at the egress from the anterior chamber. Because there is no anterior displacement of the lens, the anterior chamber depth is normal with this kind of glaucoma.* ***C.*** *Anterior displacement of the lens in senescence or in someone with a propensity to acute-angle glaucoma.* ***D.*** *Anterior displacement of the lens in a patient developing an attack of acute-angle glaucoma after pupillary dilation. As the iris dilates, it occludes both the entrance of the fluid to the anterior chamber and thus its egress. Because the fluid continues to form, the pressure can only increase. Compare to part* ***C****. (Reproduced with permission from Sapira JD, Orient JM.* The Art and Science of Bedside Diagnosis. *Baltimore: Williams & Wilkins, 1990:167.)*

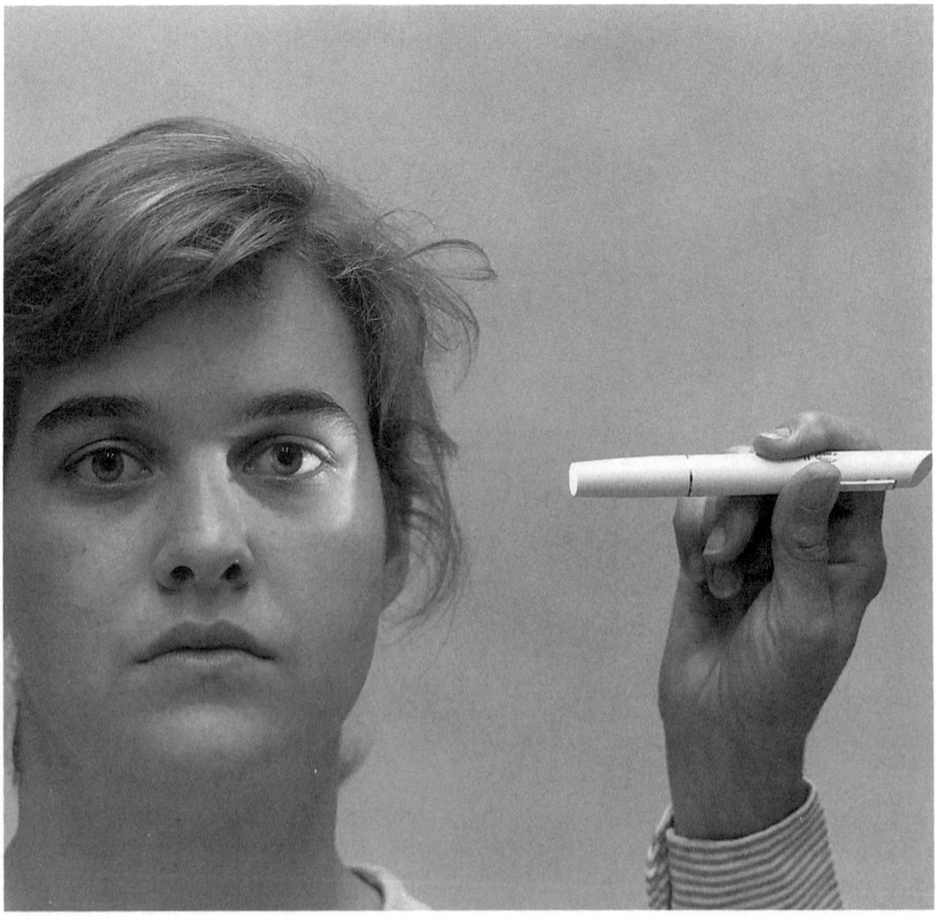

FIGURE 58.2.
"Nipple" test to determine depth of anterior chamber. (Reproduce with permission from Willms JL, Schneiderman H, Algranati PS. Physical Diagnosis: Bedside Evaluation of Diagnosis and Function. *Baltimore: Williams & Wilkins, 1994:119.)*

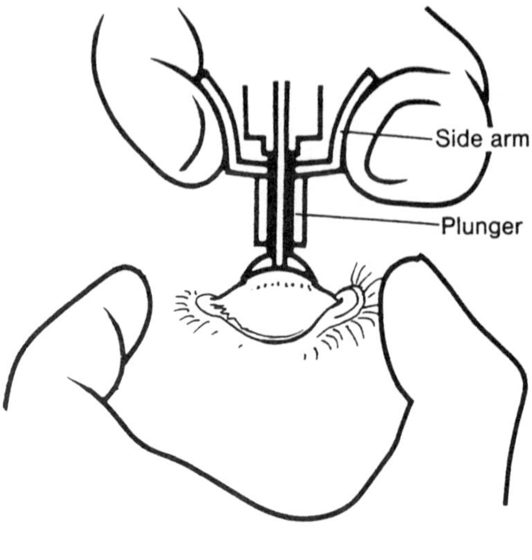

FIGURE 58.3.
Use of a tonometer. Before the tonometer is placed over the cornea, adequate anesthesia of the cornea must be obtained by topical solutions. The plunger of the tonometer will be elevated, indicating the intraocular pressure. (Reproduced with permission from Simon RB, Brenner BE. Emergency Procedures and Techniques. *3rd ed. Baltimore: Williams & Wilkins, 1994:256.)*

Special Notes

Intraocular pressure readings may be falsely elevated if pressure is inadvertently applied to the globe during testing or if the cornea is scarred or inflamed. Trauma to the cornea is rare, but care should still be exercised not to drag the device across the surface of the cornea. The patient should be instructed to contact the physician or seek care if there is any pain, blurring of vision, or exudate.

Suggested Readings

Baum J, Chaturvedi N, Netland PA, et al. Assessment of intraocular pressure by palpation. *Am J Ophthalmol* 1995;119:650.

Bengtsson B. Changes with age in Schiötz and Goldmann readings. *Acta Ophthalmol* 1992;70:350.

Christoffersen T, Fors T, Ringberg U, et al. Tonometry in the general practice setting (I): Tono-Pen compared to Goldmann applanation tonometry. *Acta Ophthalmol* 1993;71:103.

Kooner KS, Cooksey JC, Barron JB, et al. Tonometry comparison: Goldmann versus Tono-Pen. *Ann Ophthalmol* 1992;24:29.

Maldonado MJ, Rodriguez-Galietero A, Cano-Parra J, et al. Goldmann applanation tonometry using sterile disposable silicone tonometer shields. *Ophthalmologica* 1996;103:815.

Midelfart A, Wigers A. Clinical comparison of the ProTon and Tono-Pen tonometers with the Goldmann applanation tonometer. *Br J Ophthalmol* 1994;78:895.

Moreno-Montanes J, Gomez-Demmel E, Lajara-Blesa J, et al. Comparative study of three non-contact tonometers and the Goldmann tonometer. *Ophthalmologica* 1994;208:115.

Moseley MJ, Thompson JR, Deutsch J, et al. Comparison of the Keeler Pulsair 2000 non-contact tonometer with Goldmann applanation. *Eye* 7(Pt 1):127.

Palmberg R, Gutierrez YS, Miller D, et al. Potential bacterial contamination of eyedrops used for tonometry. *Am J Ophthalmol* 1994;117:578.

Ralston ME, Choplin NT, Hollenbach KA, et al. Glaucoma screening in primary care: the role of noncontact tonometry. *J Fam Pract* 1992;34:73.

Sapira JD. *The Art and Science of Bedside Diagnosis*. Baltimore: Williams & Wilkins, 1990:155.

Threlkeld AB, Froggatt JW 3d, Schein OD, et al. Efficacy of a disinfectant wipe method for the removal of adenovirus 8 from tonometer tips. *Ophthalmologica* 1993;100:1841.

Vernon SA. Intra-eye pressure range and pulse profiles in normals with the Pulsair non-contact tonometer. *Eye* 1993;7(Pt 1):134.

Whitacre MM, Stein R. Sources of error with use of Goldmann-type tonometers. *Surv Ophthalmol* 1993;38:1.

Whitacre MM, Stein RA, Hassanein K. The effect of corneal thickness on applanation tonometry. *Am J Ophthalmol* 1993;115:592.

Willms JL, Schneiderman H, Algranati PS. *Physical Diagnosis: Bedside Evaluation of Diagnosis and Function*. Baltimore: Williams & Wilkins, 1994:119.

Wilson MR, Baker RS, Mohammadi P, et al. Reproducibility of postural changes in intraocular pressure with the Tono-Pen and Pulsair tonometers. *Am J Ophthalmol* 1993;116:479.

Chapter 59

VISUAL ACUITY SCREENING

Although many people associate visual acuity screening with school-age children, the importance of periodic screening, especially in the elderly, must not be overlooked. This test is easily administered by the physician or ancillary staff yet can identify a problem that the patient may not have yet recognized. Correcting refractory error may improve the quality of life or decrease the chance of injury. The latter is especially important for the primary care of older women. The ability to provide visual acuity screening is easily acquired and should be made a standard office procedure for most offices.

Equipment

- Snellen, illiterate E ("tumbling E"), or other eye chart
- A well-lit unimpeded hall or other unobstructed 20-foot path over which vision may be tested. (Reverse versions of popular screening charts are available for use with a mirror when a full 20-foot distance is not possible.)
- Standard, near-vision chart for adults (e.g., Rosenbaum Pocket Visual Screener)
- Pinhole cards for persons with severely impaired vision
- Ishihara or Hardy-Rand-Rittler pseudoisochromatic plates for color-vision testing (optional)

Training/Credentialing

No special credentialing needed; office diagnostic procedure only.

Coding

No specific code for visual acuity testing is used. The inclusion of visual acuity testing may justify or support a higher acuity for the other services rendered.

Technique

Visual acuity may be screened using a 20-foot (6-m) distance or a near-vision pocket card. For the standard technique, the patient is placed with an unobstructed view of the test chart located 20 feet distant. The patient is asked to alternatively cover one and then the other of her eyes. With one eye covered, the patient is asked to read the smallest line she can. If the patient can read one line smaller, she should be encouraged to do so. The line at which at least 50% of letters are correctly identified should be noted. This procedure is repeated using the alternate eye; the line should be read in the direction opposite to that just used for the first eye.

For patients who are young, illiterate, or unable to make out specific letters, the illiterate or tumbling E chart may be substituted (Fig. 59.1). This chart consists of symmetrically formed box-like letter "E"s in one of four rotations. The patient is asked to cover one eye as with the Snellen chart and to indicate the direction of the legs of the letter: up, down, right, or left. As with the Snellen chart, the smallest line at which at least 50% of correct responses are obtained should be noted.

When a 20-foot corridor or standard eye chart is not available, pocket screening cards may be used. These are generally held at a distance of one foot and the patient asked to read the smallest line possible. Notations on the card provide an indication of the equivalent distant vision.

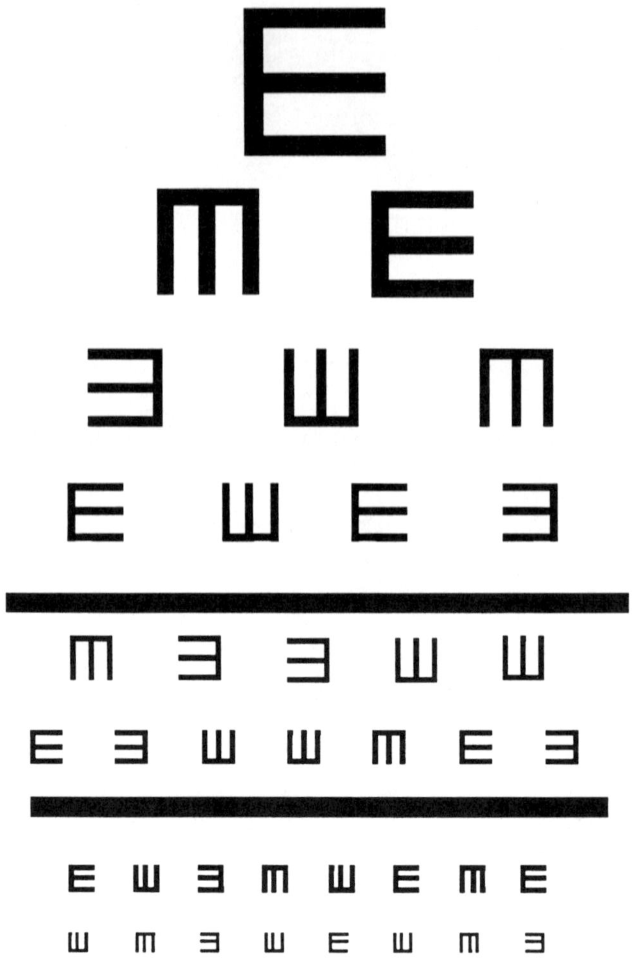

FIGURE 59.1.
The illiterate E or "tumbling E" chart may be used for screening any patient but is specifically designed for screening young or illiterate patients.

Color vision may be tested using charts such as the Ishihara or Hardy-Rand-Rittler pseudoisochromatic sets. These must be viewed with good, white-light illumination and any corrective lenses normally used for near vision. Any figures incorrectly identified should be noted; and these are then compared to the specific instruction set provided to render an interpretation of color vision defect, if any.

Normal Findings

Vision is recorded as the distance from the test chart divided by the distance at which the smallest line correctly read would be visible with normal vision. Therefore, a patient with normal vision will be able to see the line labeled as 20 feet at a distance of 20 feet, resulting in "20/20" vision. If she is able to only read the line labeled as 40 feet at this same distance, her vision would be "20/40," and so forth.

Selected Abnormal Findings

If the patient is unable to read any lines correctly (with corrective lens or a pinhole) she should be advanced toward the chart until the top line may be read. Vision is recorded as the distance in feet over the normal viewing distance for the line. In the case of the largest letter viewed from 10 feet, this would be 10/200 vision.

Special Notes

Significant refractive errors may be corrected by asking the patient to use her corrective lenses or by performing the testing with the patient looking through a pinhole. The use of a pinhole will rectify refractive error but will not correct other difficulties in the visual axis. If a pinhole is used, it must be held close to the eye.

Some authors suggest recording the number of letters incorrectly read as a part of the recording format. In this system, a patient missing two letters on the 20-foot line while reading from a distance of 20 feet would be identified as having "20/20 - 2" vision.

Suggested Readings

Acheson JF, Sanders MD. Vision. *J Neurol Neurosurg Psych* 1995;59:4.

Allen JW, Bose B. An audit of preschool vision screening. *Arch Dis Childhood* 1992;67:1292.

Anonymous. Vision screening in children. U.S. Public Health Service. *Am Fam Phys* 1994;50:587.

Hatch SW. Clinicolegal aspects of practice guidelines for pediatric eye and vision examination. *J Am Optometric Assoc* 1995;66:501.

Limburg H, Vaidyanathan K, Dalal HP. Cost-effective screening of schoolchildren for refractive errors. *World Health Forum* 1995;16:173.

McElearney NL, Waddy RS, Rawll CC. Pre-employment colour vision testing. *OccupMed* 1992;42:19.

Roman F. Eyesight and the public services. *Br J Ophthalmol* 1994;78:794.

Sapira JD. *The Art and Science of Bedside Diagnosis*. Williams & Wilkins, 1990:155.

Willms JL, Schneiderman H, Algranati PS. *Physical Diagnosis: Bedside Evaluation of Diagnosis and Function*. Baltimore: Williams & Wilkins, 1994:128.

Chapter 60

VISUAL FIELDS

Although the assessment of visual fields would seem at first glance to be remote from anything gynecologic, the ability to detect visual field loss is important in the evaluation of pituitary adenomas, stroke, and eye disease (such as glaucoma), which are not infrequently a part of our care. Confrontational testing of visual field is quick and simple. Although it lacks the specificity of more sophisticated methods, it compensates for this in the lack of equipment and specialized training needed.

Equipment

No special equipment is required.

Training/Credentialing

No special credentialing needed; office diagnostic procedure only.

Coding

The testing of visual fields by confrontational methods cannot be billed as a separate item. It is considered a part of an office examination.

Technique

To use the confrontational method of visual field testing, the patient and the examiner must be face to face, at the same level, and roughly 1 m apart. The patient is asked to cover one eye. The examiner covers his or her mirror side and the patient is asked to look directly into the examiner's uncovered eye. It must be remembered that the eye covered is the opposite in side from that of the patient; examiner's left should be used for the patient's right and the right eye for the patient's left.

The examiner begins with his or her arm outstretched toward the lateral (temporal) side, with the hand equidistant between the parties. A moving finger, a pen held in the hand, a colored card, or other hand-held object is used as the object of reference. The patient is asked to report when she can begin to see this object as it is gradually advanced toward the axis of vision. The inward movement must be smooth and remain in a plane equidistant between the patient and examiner and perpendicular to the axis of vision (Fig. 60.1). The point at which the patient first reports the object is visible de-

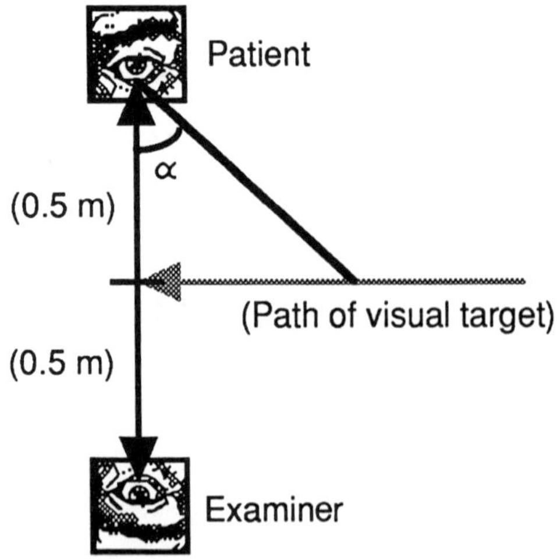

FIGURE 60.1.
By using the confrontational method, the visual field is measured by determining the angle (α) at which the patient can detect a visual target held equidistant between the examiner and the patient.

fines the boundary of the periphery being tested. This procedure is repeated in the superior, inferior, and medial (nasal) fields.

As an alternative method, both eyes remain uncovered and the patient is asked to look at the examiner's nose. Both of the examiner's arms are extended, with the hands placed at the periphery of the examiner's own visual fields. The fingers of one or the other hand are then wiggled and the patient is asked if she saw anything move and, if so, on which side. This technique is repeated for the superior and inferior fields. The finger motions should be varied in pattern from right to left or both so that the patient receives no clue from repetition. This method is faster but provides less specific information.

The findings of confrontational field testing are expressed in the form of degrees relative to the axis of vision. These should be reported separately for each quadrant of each eye. Findings should be recorded in the patient's records.

Normal Findings

Normal peripheral fields should be approximately 90° temporally, 50° nasally, 50° superiorly, and 70° inferiorly. Fields should be symmetric from one side to the other. The examiner's own fields may be used as a control.

Selected Abnormal Findings

The intent of visual field screening is to estimate the integrity of peripheral vision, the optic nerve, the optic chiasm, calcarine radiation, and the occipital lobe function. Because the test only detects major disruptions in this system, it must be viewed as a screening method only. Any abnormalities detected must be further evaluated by referral or more sophisticated mapping. There are no normal variants in visual fields as tested by this method.

Special Notes

The value of confrontational visual field testing is limited by the cooperativeness of the patient and her ability to understand what is being asked of her. The time spent in carefully instructing the patient about her role in this test is vital to obtaining results that have merit or reliability.

As an alternative to moving fingers or other objects as targets for peripheral vision testing, the examiner may choose to hold up a different number of fingers on each hand and ask the patient for the number visible. This variant is more sensitive to retinal function because motion may be detectable while the ability to clearly see and count objects may be lost. If a patient reports having a central scotomata, she may be able to trace the limits of vision using a piece of graph paper.

Suggested Readings

Acheson JF, Sanders MD. Vision. *J Neurol Neurosurg Psych* 1995;59:4.

Adams AJ. Impact of new and emerging instrumentation in optometry. *Optom Vis Sci* 1993;70:272.

Asman P. Computer-assisted interpretation of visual fields in glaucoma. *Acta Ophthalmol Suppl* 1992;206:1.

Ball K, Owsley C. The useful field of view test: a new technique for evaluating age-related declines in visual function. *J Am Optomet Assoc* 1993;64:71.

Cohen JM. An overview of enhancement techniques for peripheral field loss. *J Am Optomet Assoc* 1993;64:60.

Fingeret M. Clinical alternative for reducing the time needed to perform automated threshold perimetry. *J Am Optomet Assoc* 1995;66:699.

Frisen L. High-pass resolution perimetry. A clinical review. *Doc Ophthalmol* 1993; 83:1.

Johnson CA. Role of automation in new instrumentation. *Optom Vis Sci* 1993;70:288.

Johnson CA. The Glenn A. Fry Award Lecture. Early losses of visual function in glaucoma. *Optomet Vis Sci* 1995;72:359.

Levy A, Lightman SL. Diagnosis and management of pituitary tumours. *BMJ* 1994; 308:1087.

Lueck CJ. Investigation of visual loss: neuro-ophthalmology from a neurologist's perspective. *J Neurol Neurosurg Psych* 1996;60:275.

Sandberg MA, Weigel-DiFranco C, Rosner B, et al. The relationship between visual field size and electroretinogram amplitude in retinitis pigmentosa. *Invest Ophthalmol Vis Sci* 1996;37:1693.

Sapira JD. *The Art and Science of Bedside Diagnosis.* Williams & Wilkins, 1990:155.

Stewart WC, Hunt HH. Threshold variation in automated perimetry. *Surv Ophthalmol* 1993;37:353.

Willms JL, Schneiderman H, Algranati PS. *Physical Diagnosis: Bedside Evaluation of Diagnosis and Function.* Baltimore: Williams & Wilkins, 1994:129.

Section VIII

ORTHOPEDIC PROCEDURES AND EVALUATIONS

Chapter 61

ANKLE SPLINTING AND TAPING

Whether it is for an injury sustained in or around the office or as a coach of a children's sports team, gynecologists may be asked to evaluate and stabilize an ankle injury. The first step in the management of ankle sprains or fractures is immobilization. This is especially important in the case of an unstable fracture.

The purpose for emergency splint of any orthopedic injury is threefold: prevent further soft tissue injury; relieve pain; and, in the case of long-bone fracture; reduce the risk for fat embolism. When long-bone trauma is present, the assistance of paramedical personnel for treatment and transportation may be required. When more minor injuries involving the wrist or ankle occur, the gynecologist may be able to render the care required.

Equipment

- Stockinette
- Cotton padding (roll type)
- Elastic roller bandage (2-inch or 3-inch preferred)
- Inflatable splint (Air cast)
- Orthotic brace (Swedo/AOA, ankle ligament protector) (optional)

Training/Credentialing

No special credentialing needed; office procedure only.

Coding

29515	Application of short leg splint (calf to foot)
29540	Strapping; ankle
29550	Strapping; toes

29580	Strapping; Unna boot
99070	Splinting supplies

Technique

Before any attempt is made to stabilize the ankle joint after an injury, the integrity of nerves, vessels, and the skin must be evaluated (see Chapter 63, Ankle Examinations). Elevation of the extremity reduces swelling, promotes drainage, makes examination easier, and improves patient comfort. The application of ice and compression (elastic bandage) also helps this process.

The degree of immobilization and protection needed for any injury depends on the character of the injury itself (Table 61.1). Acute injuries are often treated with casting and cast-splinting, whereas chronic injuries, milder injuries, prophylaxis, and rehabilitation require simple splinting or taping. As a primary care provider, most gynecologists are likely to restrict their involvement to simple splinting and taping as a part of initial first aid care.

TAPING

With the ankle in a position of 90° flexion, pressure pads of cotton or thin felt are applied over the dorsum of the foot, the Achilles tendon region, and other potential pressure points. If possible, the skin of these areas should be shaved and prepared with a light spray of benzoin to further protect the skin. The pressure pads should be held in place using a thin elastic underwrap. Tape (1.5-inch to 2-inch) should be placed in a combination stirrup and transverse anchoring pattern. The emphasis of the pattern used should be to resist inversion of the joint while allowing plantar and dorsiflexion and some degree of eversion.

SPLINTING

Splinting covers both the applications of restrictive devices for short-term immobilization and orthotic devices for longer-term use. These methods are best suited for controlling ligament instability.

One of the most popular varieties of splints available are the inflatable types. These are made of a double-walled construction with a zipper fastening that allows place-

TABLE 61.1. Indications for Ankle Immobilization by Type

Taping
- Prophylaxis (e.g., protection during athletic participation)

Simple splinting
- Long-term stabilization
- Prophylactic support (requiring more protection than offered by taping)
- Rehabilitation
- Stable distal interosseous ligament sprain
- Stable lateral sprain

Rigid splinting (plaster)
- Moderate ankle sprain with inability to bear weight
- Severe ankle sprain before surgical intervention
- Unstable ankle fractures before surgery

Casting
- Fracture of calcaneus, talus, navicular, cuboid, cuneiform, or metatarsal bones
- Lateral malleolar fracture
- Severe lateral ankle sprains
- Stable ankle fracture

ment of the device. These splints are inexpensive and take up little room when deflated, making them ideal for an office first aid kit or coach's sideline bag. These splints are only useful for sprains or fractures of the ankle and should not be used if the leg may be fractured. Care must also be used in the inflation of these splints so that perfusion is not compromised. These splints must not be applied over clothing because wrinkles in the cloth may lead to pressure damage or blisters. The correct placement of an air splint is shown in Figure 61.1.

A pillow splint is a simple alternative to an air splint for emergency use (Fig. 61.2). This splint is fashioned by wrapping an ordinary pillow tightly around the lower leg and foot and securing it in place with safety pins. Towels may be used with wooden splints or other flat rigid material to form a makeshift support (Fig. 61.3).

A common type of splint used to stabilize ankle sprains and fractures is the posterior splint. Posterior splints allow ice packs to be applied while maintaining adequate immobilization. This type of splint uses plaster strips applied over a stockinette and cotton base. A commercially available rigid plastic or metal brace may also be used and is more convenient than plaster to have on hand. The splint must extend from the ball of the foot to just below the knee (Fig. 61.4). The supporting plaster or brace should be applied along the back of the ankle, and an additional lateral brace should be used. The bracing material is secured with an outer layer of stockinette and an elastic wrap. When properly applied, free movement of the knee is allowed while the ankle joint is fully supported.

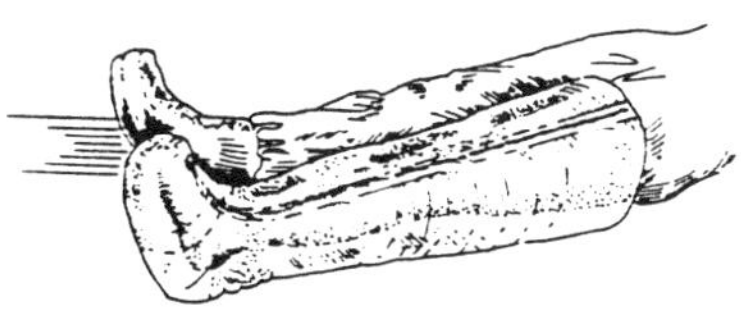

FIGURE 61.1.
An inflatable splint is shown applied over the leg and thigh in a patient with a fractured ankle. (Reproduced with permission from Simon RR, Brenner BE. Emergency Procedures and Techniques. *Baltimore: Williams & Wilkins, 1994:218.)*

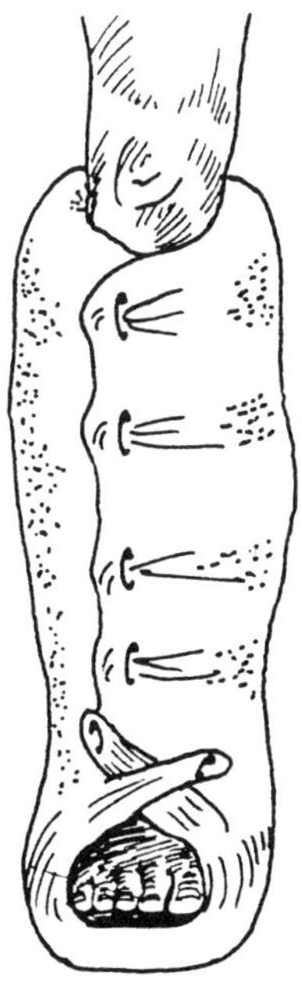

FIGURE 61.2.
A pillow splint may be easily fashioned from an ordinary pillow and safety pins. (Reproduced with permission from Simon RR, Brenner BE. Emergency Procedures and Techniques. *Baltimore: Williams & Wilkins, 1994:218.)*

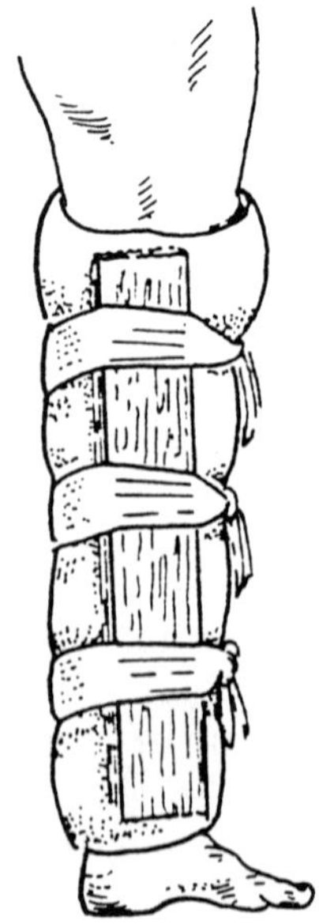

FIGURE 61.3.
A splint fashioned from towels and wooden splints. Towels are wrapped to protect the involved extremity, and wooden slabs are applied to both sides of the extremity; the entire device is secured with rags or pieces of towel. (Reproduced with permission from Simon RR, Brenner BE. Emergency Procedures and Techniques. *Baltimore: Williams & Wilkins, 1994:219.)*

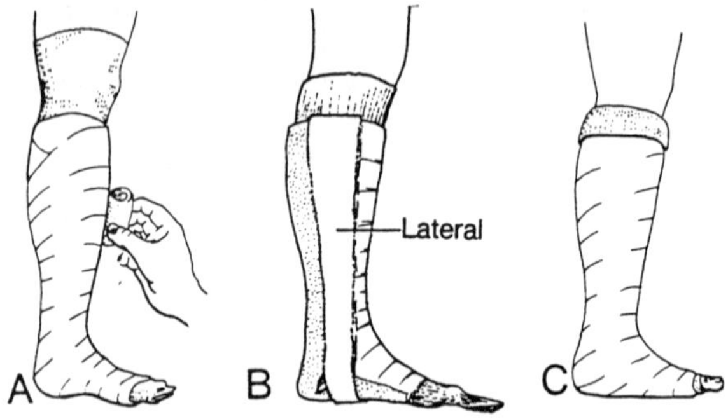

FIGURE 61.4.
The application of a posterior splint to the ankle. The posterior splint extends from the ball of the foot at the metatarsal heads to the posterior aspect of the knee just below the flexor crease. To add stability, a U-shaped lateral splint extends around the medial and lateral sides of the ankle. Commercial posterior splints are currently available. (Reproduced with permission from Simon RR, Brenner BE. Emergency Procedures and Techniques. *Baltimore: Williams & Wilkins, 1994:234.)*

Special Notes

For young or potentially uncooperative patients, an overly large and bulky dressing may reduce the chance that the patient will tamper with or remove the bandaging. The bulk and complexity of the dressing also provide additional immobilization. When applied for the stabilization of an acute injury, a splint should not be removed until x-ray evaluation has been performed.

If an open fracture is to be splinted, the skin puncture site should be dressed with a sterile gauze or other dressing before the application of the splint. When the ankle is wrapped with an elastic bandage, each turn should overlap the previous one by roughly one half the width of the material being used (e.g., 1 inch for a 2-inch bandage).

Suggested Readings

Cox JS. Surgical and nonsurgical treatment of acute ankle sprains. *Clin Orthop Related Res* 1985;198:118.

Homes DS, Kautman JJ. Plaster splints: techniques and indications. *Am Fam Phys* 1984;30:215.

Hume EL, McKeag DB. Soft-tissue ankle injuries: the need for compulsive assessment and therapy. *Emerg Med Rept* 1984;5:45.

Karlsson J, Sward L, Andreasson GO. The effect of taping on ankle stability. Practical implications. *Sports Med* 1993;16:210.

Simon RR, Brenner BE. *Emergency Procedures and Techniques*. Baltimore: Williams & Wilkins, 1994:198.

Smith RW, Reischl SF. Treatment of ankle sprains in young athletes. *Am J Sports Med* 1986;14:465.

Yamamoto T, Kigawa A, Xu T. Effectiveness of functional ankle taping for judo athletes: a comparison between judo bandaging and taping. *Br J Sports Med* 1993;27:110.

Chapter 62

WRIST SPLINTING AND TAPING

During a fall, the natural protective action is to extend the arms in an effort to break the fall. This places the hands, wrists, and forearms at risk for sprains or fractures. Whether as initial support until definitive treatment is possible or as actual treatment, splinting of the wrist is a commonly indicated procedure that should be familiar to all physicians.

Equipment

- Stockinette
- Cotton padding (roll type)
- Elastic roller bandage (2-inch or 3-inch preferred)
- Inflatable splint (air cast)
- Orthotic brace (optional)

Training/Credentialing

No special credentialing needed; office procedure only.

Coding

29125	Application of short-arm splint (forearm to hand); static
29126	dynamic
29130	Application of finger splint; static
29131	dynamic
29260	Strapping; elbow or wrist
29280	Strapping; hand or finger
99070	Splinting supplies

Technique

As noted in Chapter 61 (Ankle Splinting and Taping), the integrity of nerves, vessels, and the skin must be evaluated before any attempt is made to stabilize the wrist after an injury. Elevation of the arm reduces swelling, promotes drainage, makes examination easier, and improves patient comfort. The application of ice and compression (elastic bandage) are also helpful.

Wrist sprains and forearm fractures are stabilized using splinting techniques. For acute injuries in which a fracture is likely, an air splint provides rapid immobilization

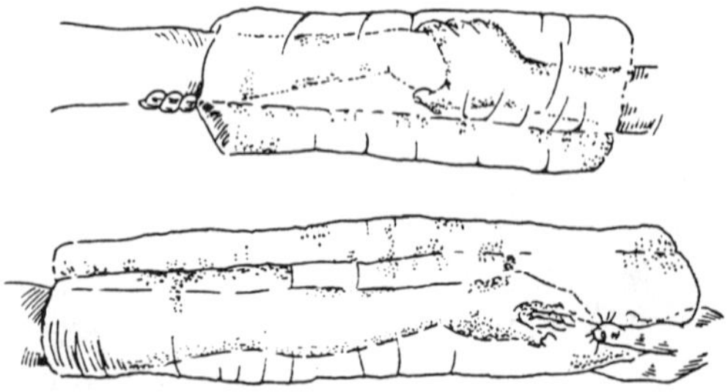

FIGURE 62.1.
The deflated splint is applied by applying traction to the injured extremity and then feeding the splint from over the physician's forearm and hand onto the injured extremity. While traction is maintained, the splint is inflated. (Reproduced with permission from Simon RR, Brenner BE. Emergency Procedures and Techniques. *Baltimore: Williams & Wilkins, 1994:218.)*

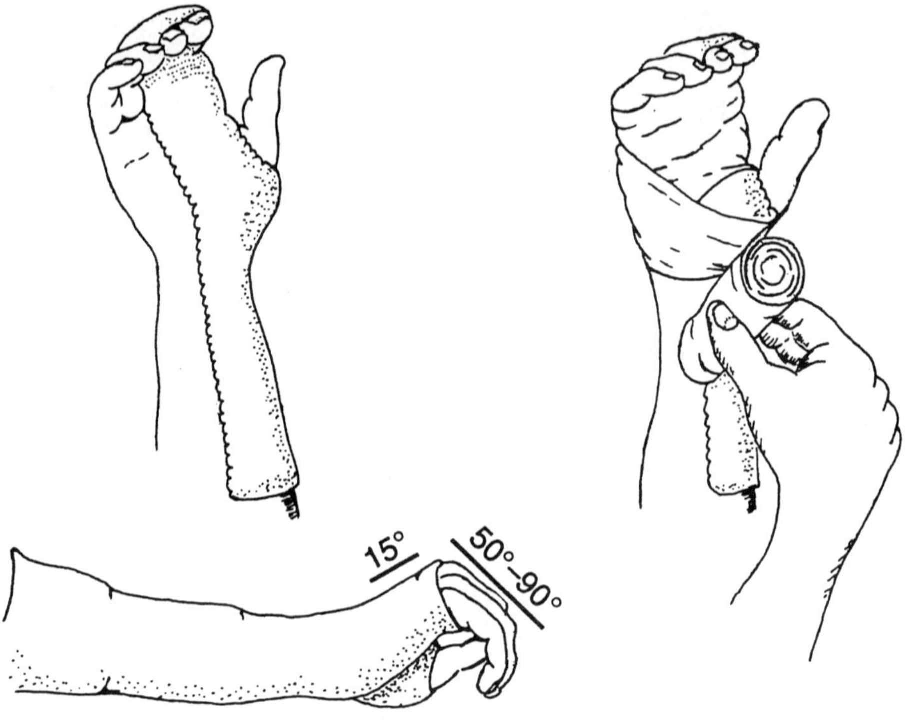

FIGURE 62.2.
Wrist splints may be made using commercially available splints or may be fabricated using strips of casting plaster. The rigid portion of the splint is secured to the arm and hand with elastic bandage wrappings. Note that the wrist is splinted at 15° of extension with the metacarpophalangeal joints at 50–90° of flexion. (Reproduced with permission from Simon RR, Brenner BE. Emergency Procedures and Techniques. *Baltimore: Williams & Wilkins, 1994:226.)*

in an easily stored and applied form. To apply this type of splint, the deflated splint is placed over the examiner's own forearm and the injured limb is grasped (Fig. 62.1). While gentile traction is applied, the splint is fed over the injured arm and inflated. Care must be used when inflating the splint so that perfusion is not compromised. Air splints must not be applied over clothing because wrinkles in the cloth may lead to pressure damage or blisters.

Rigid splints are commercially available or may be made from strips of plaster. These may be secured to the arm and hand using elastic bandage wrappings, as shown in Figure 62.2. When splints of this type are applied to the lateral or medial aspect of the hand (gutter splint), they can be very useful for immobilizing phalangeal fractures. A similar type of splint may be made using rigid material over the anterior and posterior aspects of the arm and hand, as shown in Figure 62.3. This type of support is well suited to wrist sprains and the initial stabilization of fractures of the distal forearm. A slightly more elaborate form of this splint is the sugar tong splint shown in Figure 62.4.

For many minor wrist or hand injuries, the tasks of immobilization and wound protection may be combined in the form of the universal hand dressing (Fig. 62.5). The universal hand dressing may also be used for treating lacerations, burns, and tendinitis. The position in which the universal hand dressing immobilizes the hand provides

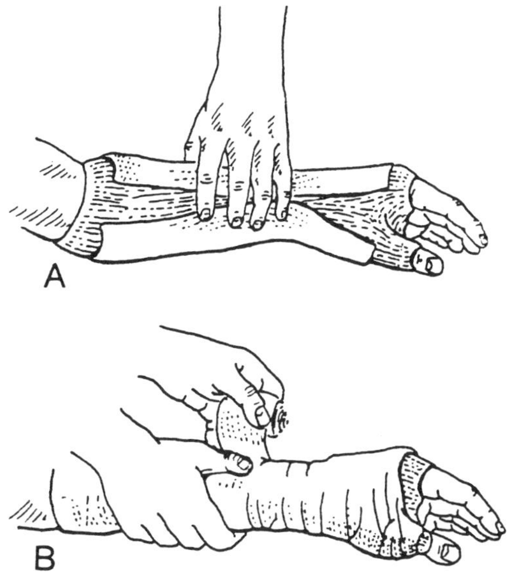

FIGURE 62.3.
An anterior–posterior splint of the forearm. The splint can be extended to make a long-arm anterior–posterior splint by extending the slabs to above the elbow. ***A.*** *Stockinette is applied over the forearm. After this, an anterior and a posterior plaster slab are applied.* ***B.*** *The anterior and posterior slabs are held in position with an Ace wrap. (Reproduced with permission from Simon RR, Brenner BE.* Emergency Procedures and Techniques. *Baltimore: Williams & Wilkins, 1994:232.)*

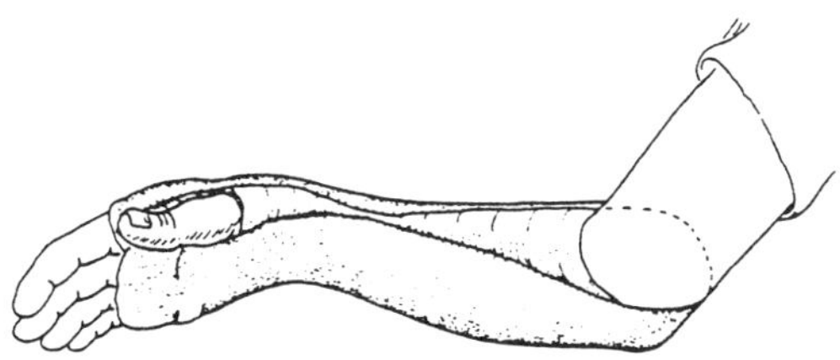

FIGURE 62.4.
The sugar tong splint is best suited to situations in which it is desirable to maintain the forearm in some degree of supination or pronation. This type of splint may also be used for the initial stabilization of fractures of the distal humerus. (Reproduced with permission from Simon RR, Brenner BE. Emergency Procedures and Techniques. *Baltimore: Williams & Wilkins, 1994:232.)*

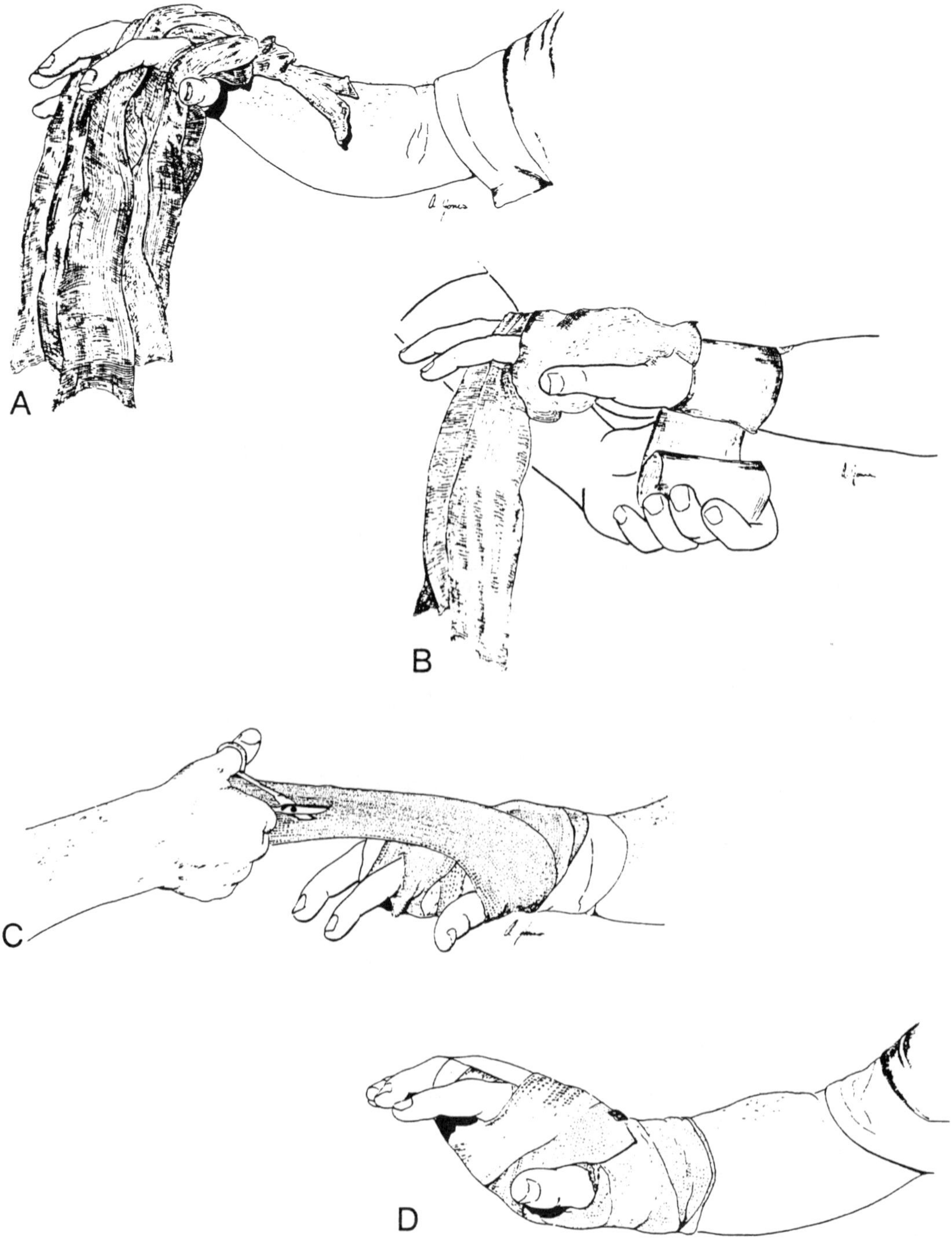

FIGURE 62.5.

Universal hand dressing. ***A.*** *Gauze fluffs are inserted between the fingers.* ***B.*** *A Kerlex gauze roll is then used to wrap between the fingers.* ***C.*** *An elastic bandage is then applied over the gauze. Note that the elastic bandage is placed over the fingers with a hole cut into the bandage for the fingers to pass through.* ***D.*** *When the elastic wrap is being applied, the wrist should be propped at 15° of extension, which allows the metacarpophalangeal joint and interphalangeal joints to be placed in the position noted in the diagram and allows for relaxation of the hand and maximum drainage. The dressing can be extended to the distal interphalangeal joints whenever this is necessary. (Reproduced with permission from Simon RR, Brenner BE.* Emergency Procedures and Techniques. *Baltimore: Williams & Wilkins, 1994:230.)*

optimal lymphatic drainage and is a functionally resting position for all of the joints. The position of the hand should be similar to that shown in Figure 62.2 (15° of flexion at the wrist, 50° of flexion at the metacarpophalangeal joint, and 20–30° of flexion at the interphalangeal joints). The thumb should be positioned as shown in Figure 62.5*A*. Gauze fluffs may be placed between the fingers, the fingers and thumb, and the palmar surface of the hand and extended to the forearm. A gauze roll is used to hold this material in place, followed by an elastic bandage. Tape may be used to secure the elastic bandage in place, if desired.

It is often desirable to augment wrist or forearm splints with the use of a sling. Three types of sling are commonly used to treat upper extremity injuries: the common sling, the collar and cuff, and the stockinette Velpeau dressing (Fig. 62.6). The common sling is most often used to treat upper extremity injury. This type of sling may be easily made from a triangular bandage or a square scarf. Commercial slings are also acceptable.

Special Notes

When applied for the stabilization of an acute injury, a splint should not be removed until x-ray evaluation has been performed. Most injuries to the hand or wrist are accompanied by much swelling. This swelling produces a significant portion of the pain of injury and can impede the healing process. As a result, it is wise to have the patient keep the arm elevated and to use ice packs (if possible) for the first 24 hours after the injury.

There is a tendency to wrap the wrist with elastic bandages that are too narrow; for most patients, a 2-inch or 3-inch bandage works best. The use of 1-inch wraps results in a lumpy wrapping that may apply uneven pressure and result in discomfort or skin damage.

Finger splints may be used to support strains or sprains but should not be used when there is a fracture.

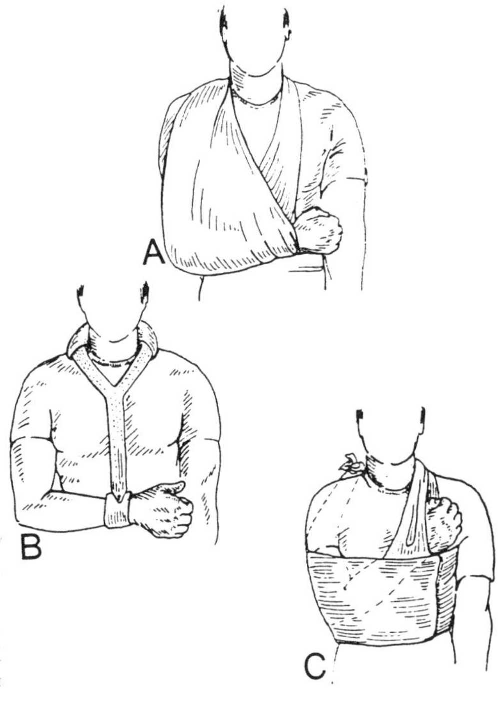

FIGURE 62.6.
***A.** A common sling. **B.** A collar and cuff. **C.** Stockinette Velpeau dressing. (Reproduced with permission from Simon RR, Brenner BE.* Emergency Procedures and Techniques. *Baltimore: Williams & Wilkins, 1994:233.)*

Suggested Readings

Boozer JA, Sanson MS, Soutas-Little RW, et al. Comparison of the biomedical motions and forces involved in high-profile versus low-profile dynamic splinting. *J Hand Ther* 1994;7:171.

Curtin M. Development of a tetraplegic hand assessment and splinting protocol. *Paraplegia* 1994;32:159.

Fricker R, Hintermann B. Skier's thumb. Treatment, prevention and recommendations. *Sports Med* 1995;19:73.

Gill DR, Smith KL, Harvey FJ. Plaster of Paris splintage for the hand: volar or dorsal? *Aust N Z J Surg* 1994;64:547.

Hoeyberghs JL. The use of a polyurethane in hand splinting. *J Hand Ther* 1993;6:319.

Krajnik SR, Bridle MJ. Hand splinting in quadriplegia: current practice. *Am J Occup Ther* 1992;46:149.

Simon RR, Brenner BE. *Emergency Procedures and Techniques.* Baltimore: Williams & Wilkins, 1994:198.

Smoot EC. Long arm splinting of the pediatric upper extremity. *Plast Reconstruct Surg* 1995;95:1328.

Takami M, Fukui K, Saitou S, et al. Application of a shape memory alloy to hand splinting. *Prosth Orthot Intl* 1992;16:57.

Chapter 63

ANKLE EXAMINATIONS

Ankle injuries are common in everyday life; with commonality, comes the probability that the gynecologist will be called on professionally or otherwise to evaluate the ankle. The steps involved in a screening examination are simple and may be easily accomplished in the office without specialized training or equipment.

Equipment

No special equipment is required.

Training/Credentialing

No special credentialing needed; office procedure only.

Coding

The ankle examination cannot be billed as a separate item. It is considered a part of an office examination.

Technique

The evaluation of the ankle consists of inspection, palpation, and special maneuvers. When an injury is involved, a careful history must supplement these modalities.

HISTORY

When the ankle is injured, the nature of the trauma and the force involved should be determined. The extent and type of disability noted immediately after the injury should also be assessed. If the patient was unable to walk immediately after the injury, radiographic evaluation is generally warranted. The use of heat or cold immediately after the injury may alter the presenting symptoms and findings.

INSPECTION

Erythema, edema, ecchymosis, and joint effusions may be noted on simple inspection. Effusion produces a bulging beneath the extensor tendons and a fullness just anterior to the lateral and medial collateral ligaments. When an effusion is present, the foot tends to be held in slight dorsiflexion and inversion. When the joint is viewed from behind, fullness will be seen in the normal fossae behind the malleoli. If there is doubt, comparison to the opposite (normal) side should establish the change.

PALPATION

The joint should be palpated to detect tenderness and swelling that is not apparent on inspection. The area thought to be least tender should be palpated first. Because the lateral ankle is affected in roughly 85% of injuries, the evaluation of the lateral ligaments is of special importance. When forced inversion of the ankle has occurred, there will be tenderness anterior and possibly inferior to the lateral malleolus rather than the malleolus itself. Tenderness over the tendons below and behind the lateral malleolus is typical of chronic stenosing tenosynovitis of the peroneal tendon sheath. If a fracture is possible, touch sensation of the nerves of the foot should be assessed.

SPECIAL MANEUVERS

Special maneuvers are used to evaluate the function of the ankle joint. These include the active and passive range of motion (see Chapter 68, Range of Motion Testing). Because range of motion varies from patient to patient, comparison to the normal side should be made when injury or symptoms are restricted to a single ankle. Active range, passive range, and special provocative tests may be difficult to perform because of pain but should be performed wherever possible. The degree to which pain is present and interferes with motion should be noted and recorded.

Active range of motion should be evaluated, covering dorsiflexion, plantar flexion, inversion, and eversion of the foot (Fig. 63.1). Plantar flexion of the toes and extension of the great toe should also be tested. These same motions may be tested passively by gently moving the joint through the expected range.

Special provocative tests should be included when ankle symptoms are present. The anterior drawer test is performed by stabilizing the lower leg with one hand while

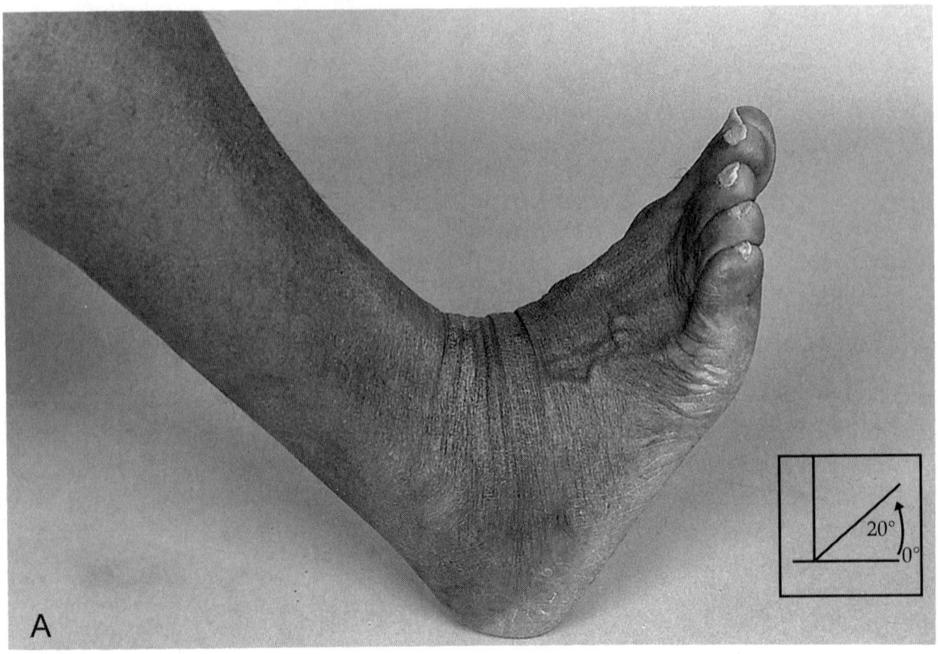

FIGURE 63.1 *(continued)*.
Ankle and foot. ***A.*** *Dorsiflexion of foot. (continued)*

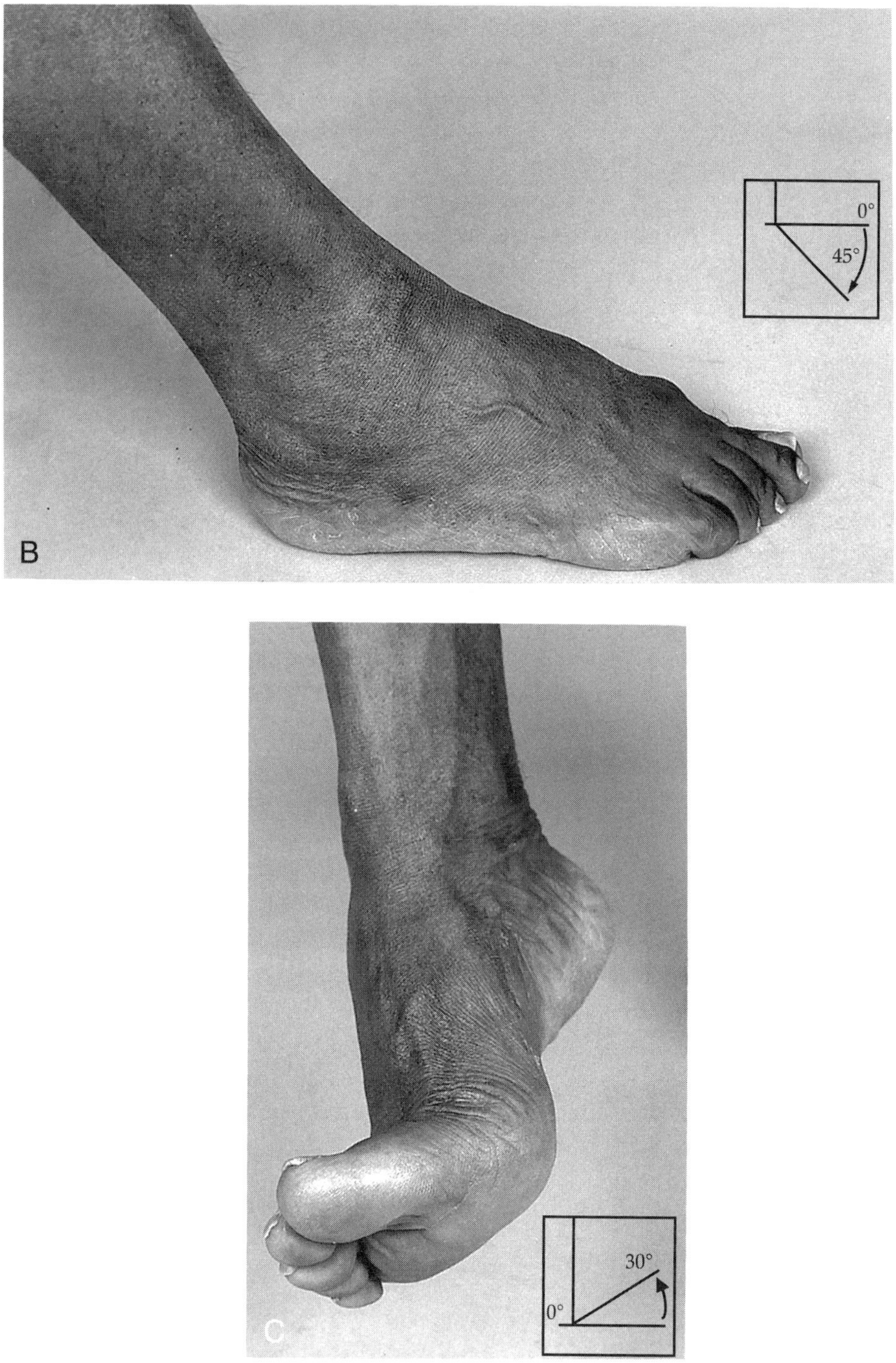

FIGURE 63.1 *(continued).*
B. *Plantar flexion of foot.* ***C.*** *Inversion of foot. (continued)*

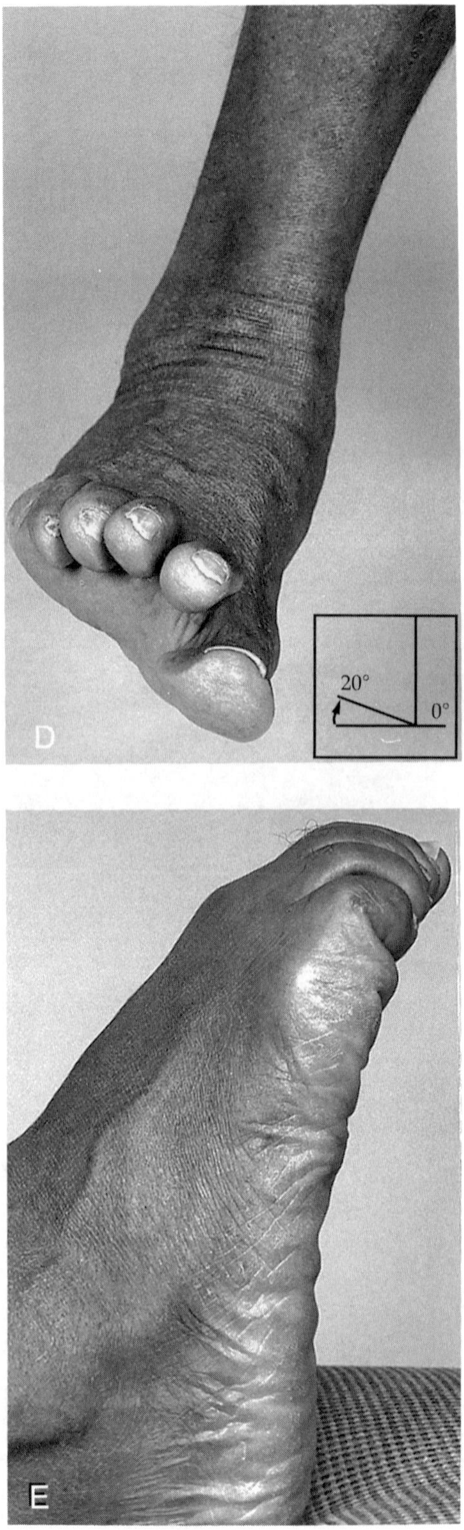

FIGURE 63.1 *(continued).*
D. *Eversion of foot.* ***E.*** *Plantar flexion of toes. (continued)*

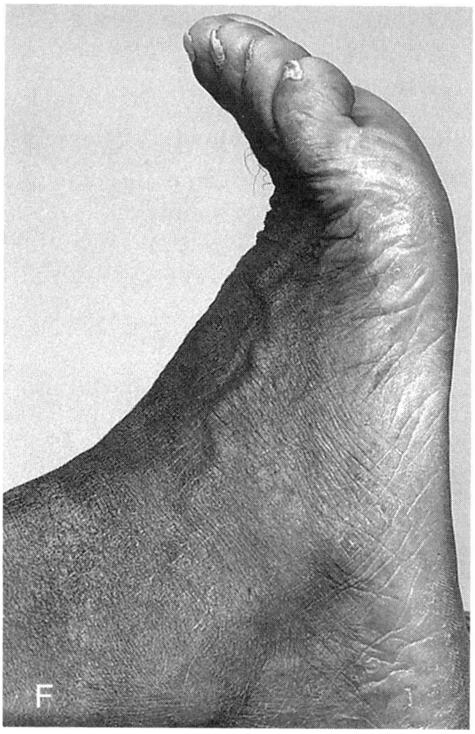

FIGURE 63.1 ***(continued).***
F. *Extension of the great toe (hallux). (Reproduced with permission from Willms JL, Schneiderman H, Algranati PS.* Physical Diagnosis: Bedside Evaluation of Diagnosis and Function. *Baltimore: Williams & Wilkins, 1994:402–403.)*

the heal is grasped by the other hand. Force is applied to the calcaneus to displace the talus forward. Laxity suggests a tear of the anterior talofibular ligament. The talar tilt test is accomplished by again stabilizing the leg and inverting the ankle by drawing the foot medially and upward. Laxity demonstrated by this test suggests a calcaneofibular ligament tear. The last provocative test is the syndesmosis squeeze test. In this test, the proximal fibula is compressed against the tibia by a gentle squeeze over the upper portion of the lower leg. Pain localized distally in the ankle indicates a fibular fracture, interosseus membrane disruption, or damage to the distal tibiofibular syndesmosis.

The integrity of the Achilles tendon may be assessed by having the patient kneel with her foot off the edge of a chair or with the patient supine with her foot off the end of the examining table. The muscles of the calf are compressed and the foot observed. When the Achilles tendon is intact, the foot should plantar flex (Thompson test).

Selected Abnormal Findings

Ecchymosis extending proximally from the ankle to the lower leg suggests the possibility of tibiofibular syndesmotic injury. Radiography should be done under the following conditions: pain in the area of the medial or lateral malleolus or the immediately adjacent area, bone tenderness over the posterior edge or tip of the medial or lateral malleolus, inability to bear weight immediately after the injury or at the time of examination, or pain in the midfoot with bone tenderness over the base of the fifth metatarsal or the navicular bone.

Enlargement, laxity, excessive passive range of motion, or crepitation on passive movement of the ankle joint (Charcot's joint) may be seen in patients with diabetic peripheral neuropathy. Proprioception and general touch sensation may be diminished in these patients.

When an obvious gap between the tip of the malleolus and the talus is seen during ankle inversion, an avulsion of the lateral malleolar ligament should be suspected.

It may be difficult to distinguish between dependent edema and the edema of ankle arthritis. Comparison with the opposite side, the presence of pitting, pain with passive movement, or the presence of edema elsewhere (e.g., presacral edema) may help to make the differentiation.

Special Notes

The ankle should always be examined while uncovered, necessitating the removal of socks or stockings.

Suggested Readings

Ferkel RD, Fasulo GJ. Arthroscopic treatment of ankle injuries. *Orthoped Clin North Am* 1994;25:17.

Haglund-Akerlind Y, Eriksson E. Range of motion, muscle torque and training habits in runners with and without Achilles tendon problems. *Knee Surg Sports Traumatol Arthrosc* 1993;1:195.

Hopkinson WJ, St. Pierre P, Ryan JB, et al. Syndesmosis sprains of the ankle. *Foot Ankle* 1990;10:325.

Kaikkonen A, Kannus P, Jarvinen M. A performance test protocol and scoring scale for the evaluation of ankle injuries. *Am J Sports Med* 1994;22:462.

Liu SH, Jason WJ. Lateral ankle sprains and instability problems. *Clin Sports Med* 1994;13:793.

Michelson JD, Magid D, Ney DR, et al. Examination of the pathologic anatomy of ankle fractures. *J Trauma* 1992;32:65.

Oloff LM, Sullivan BT, Heard GS, et al. Magnetic resonance imaging of traumatized ligaments of the ankle. *J Am Podiatr Med Assoc* 1992;82:25.

Rubin A, Sallis R. Evaluation and diagnosis of ankle injuries. *Am Fam Physic* 1996;54:1609.

Sapira JD. *The Art and Science of Bedside Diagnosis*. Williams & Wilkins, 1990:429.

Steill IG, Greenberg GH, McKnight RD, et al. A study to develop clinical decision rules for the use of radiography in acute ankle injuries. *Ann Emerg Med* 1992;21:384.

Thermann H, Hoffmann R, Zwipp H, et al. The use of ultrasonography in the foot and ankle. *Foot Ankle* 1992;13:386.

Willms JL, Schneiderman H, Algranati PS. *Physical Diagnosis: Bedside Evaluation of Diagnosis and Function*. Baltimore: Williams & Wilkins, 1994:400.

Chapter 64

KNEE EXAMINATIONS

Of all major joints, the knee is the most vulnerable to trauma. Unlike other joints, knee joint function has no normal variants; this potentially eases the process of appraisal for the infrequent evaluator.

Equipment

No special equipment is required.

Training/Credentialing

No special credentialing needed; office procedure only.

Coding

The knee examination cannot be billed as a separate item. It is considered a part of an office examination.

Technique

As with the examination of the ankle joint discussed in Chapter 63 (Ankle Examinations), the assessment of the knee may be divided into separate phases: inspection, palpation, and function tests. For most evaluations of the knee, the patient should rest comfortably in the supine position with the legs well supported. For tests of flexion, the patient may be examined while sitting on the edge of the examination table with the legs freely dangling. Many specialized test of knee function are available, some of which are beyond the scope of the primary care setting. A brief summary of these tests, arranged by focus, is shown in Table 64.1.

INSPECTION

Swelling, discoloration, or misalignment of the knee should be evaluated by inspection. Inspection should be done with the knee fully extended and the quadriceps muscle fully relaxed unless these positions are contraindicated. The patient should be asked to point to the area of symptoms. Pain occurring one-fourth of the way posterior from the anterior edge of the medial side of the knee, just above the end of the tibia, suggests the possibility of damage to the medial meniscus. Pain midway from front to

TABLE 64.1. Tests of Knee Function[a]

Knee joint effusion
Fluctuation test
Patella ballottement test
Stroke test
Ligamentous instability
Abduction stress test
Adduction stress test
Apley's distraction test
Drawer sign
Ghormely's test
Lachman's test
Quadriceps active test
Slocum's test
Meniscus instability
Apley's compression test
Bounce home test
General Varus test
McMurray's test
Modified Helfet's test
Retreating meniscus test
Steinman's tenderness displacement test
Patella tests
Dreyer's test
Patella apprehension test
Patella grinding test

[a]A full discussion of tests not reviewed here may be found in the references by Cipriano and Sapira contained in the list of suggested readings.

back over the medial (tibial) collateral ligament suggests damage to this ligament. Pain in either of these locations points to the need for specialized tests.

Recognizing deformity of the knee is the simplest way to detect effusion, but this technique lacks sensitivity. Obliteration of the normal indentations medial and lateral to the patella indicates effusion but is unreliable in obese patients. For these patients, ballottement of the knee during the palpation phase is required.

PALPATION

Palpation of the knee and surrounding tissues should reveal the presence of heat, swelling, or tenderness. The presence of any of these in an asymmetric distribution about one knee, or on one side and not the other, suggests the presence of an abnormality. When the presence of an effusion is sought, ballottement, the bulge test, or Mann's test should be used.

Ballottement (Tap Test)

Ballottement is performed by pressing the suprapatellar pouch with one hand and with the other pushing sharply posteriorly into the trochlear grove (the track on the front of the femur in which the patella sits) and then release (Fig. 64.1). A click may be heard as the patella taps the femur. When effusion is present, the fluid wave rebounds from the edges of the joint cavity and the patella pops back against the examining fingers.

The Bulge Test (Stroke Test)

This test can detect effusions of as little as 4 mL. To perform the test, squeeze the suprapatellar pouch and milk the fluid out of it and out of the medial part of the cavity by pressing just medial to the patella, producing a small concavity. Immediately stroke or briskly tap the lateral aspect, causing a fullness to bulge outward on the medial side (Fig. 64.2). This bulge should appear promptly and should not be the result of simple tissue displacement.

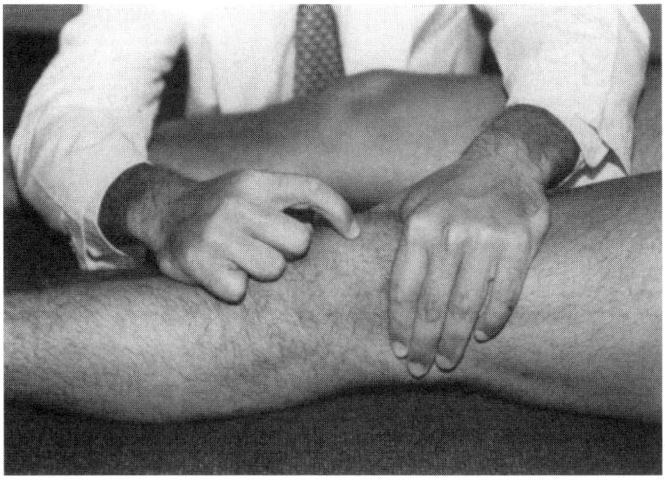

FIGURE 64.1.
An alternate method of performing ballottement: with one hand encircle and place downward pressure above the upper side of the patella; with the other hand, push the patella against the femur with the finger. If fluid is present, the patella will elevate when pressure is applied. When the patella is pushed down, it will strike the femur with a palpable tap. (Reproduced with permission from Cipriano JJ. Photographic Manual of Regional Orthopaedics and Neurological Testing. *2nd ed. Baltimore: Williams & Wilkins, 1991:174.)*

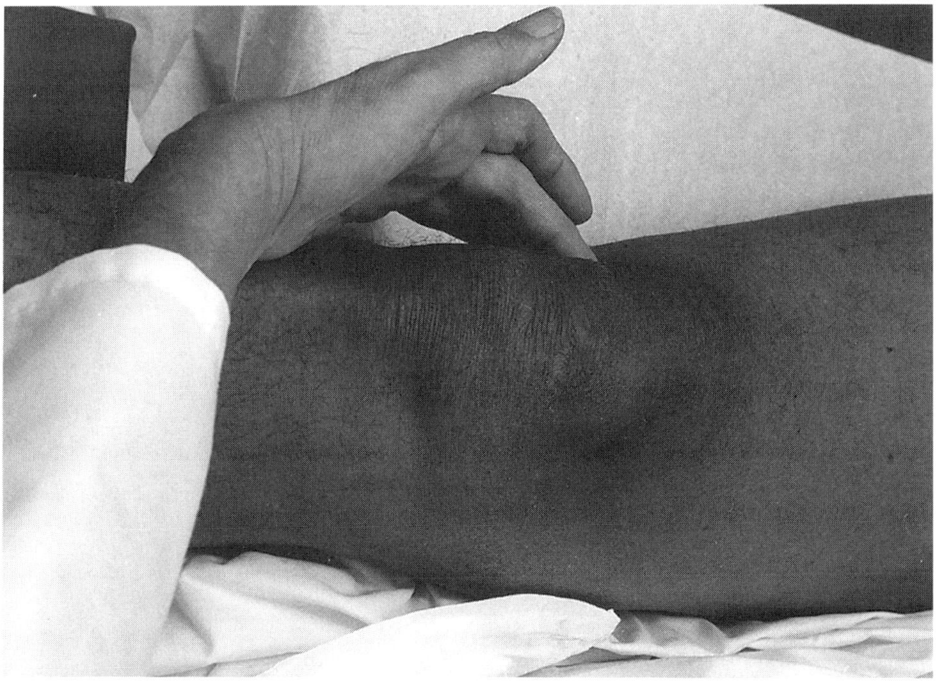

FIGURE 64.2.
Technique of "pushing" small knee effusion from lateral aspect to produce a bulge on the medial side of the knee. (Reproduced with permission from Willms JL, Schneiderman H, Algranati PS. Physical Diagnosis: Bedside Evaluation of Diagnosis and Function. *Baltimore: Williams & Wilkins, 1994:434.)*

Mann's Test

This test is the most sensitive for detecting small effusions. The Mann test relies on the observation of the hollows on either side of the patellar ligament. When the knee is extended, a hollow may be seen or felt just below the patella. As the knee is flexed, these hollows will fill in. In the abnormal knee, the filling takes place at a lower angle of flexion. If the filling is not under undue pressure when it is first noted, a finger on either side of the ligament may be used to rock the intra-articular fluid back and forth.

FUNCTION TESTS

Muscle strength and range of motion testing (see Chapters 67 and 68) should be performed if they have not already been done and are not contraindicated by concerns of fracture or pain. Stance and gait (see Chapter 54, Screening Tests for Gait) should also be reviewed. Function or provocative tests are used to assess the integrity of the cruciate ligaments and the menisci of the knee joint.

Test of Ligaments

The simplest test of ligamentous function is the drawer test. The cruciate ligaments tether the tibia to the femoral condyles. When these ligaments are intact, movement of the tibia on the femur is limited. To perform the drawer test, the patient may be examined with the legs dangling from the end of the examination table or with the leg flexed and the foot resting on the bed (Fig. 64.3). The fingers are wrapped around the knee, resting in the popliteal fossa with the thumbs on the medial and lateral sides of the knee joint. The tibia is drawn forward to test the function of the anterior cruciate ligament (Fig. 64.4). If the ligament is intact, little

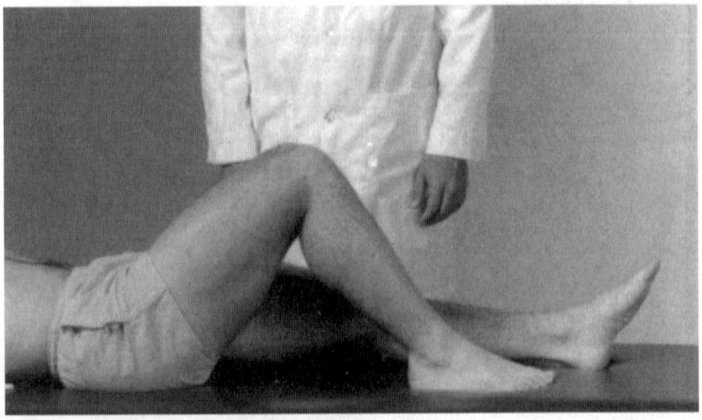

FIGURE 64.3. *The function of the cruciate ligaments may be assessed in the supine position by having the patient draw the knee upward with the foot resting on the table. (Reproduced with permission from Cipriano JJ.* Photographic Manual of Regional Orthopaedics and Neurological Testing. *2nd ed. Baltimore: Williams & Wilkins, 1991:165.)*

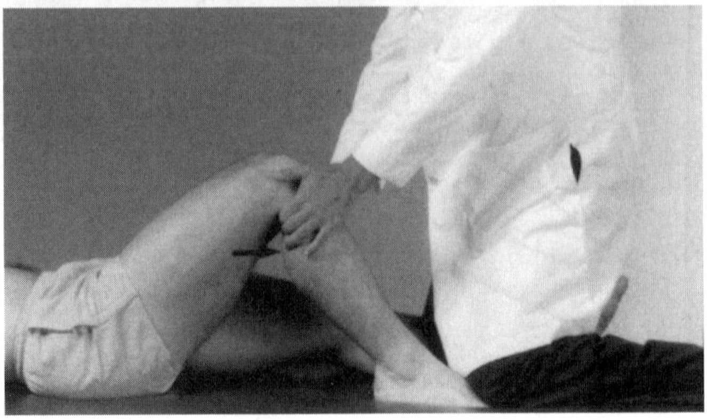

FIGURE 64.4. *The function of the anterior cruciate ligaments is tested when the leg is pulled forward. (Reproduced with permission from Cipriano JJ.* Photographic Manual of Regional Orthopaedics and Neurological Testing. *2nd ed. Baltimore: Williams & Wilkins, 1991:165.)*

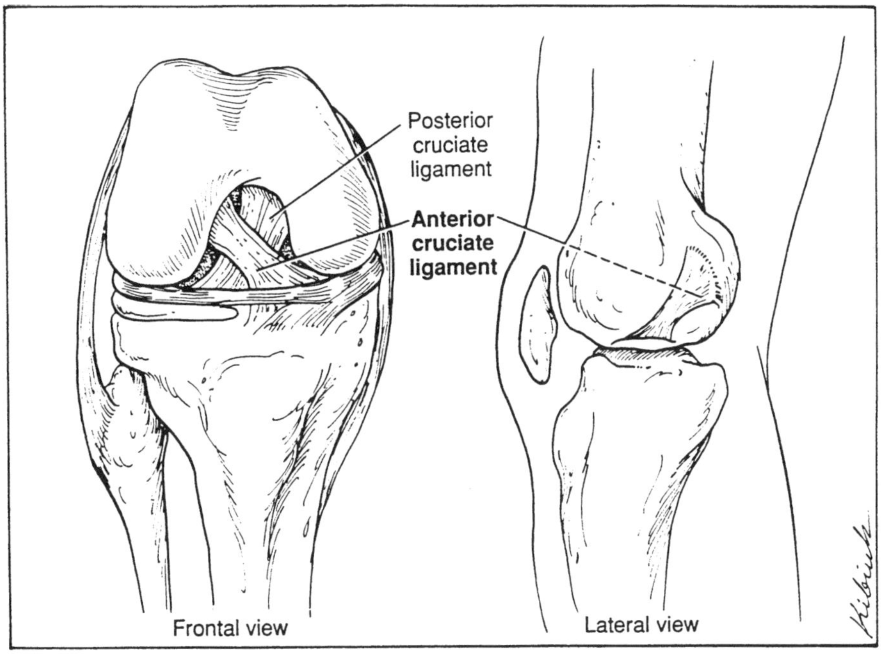

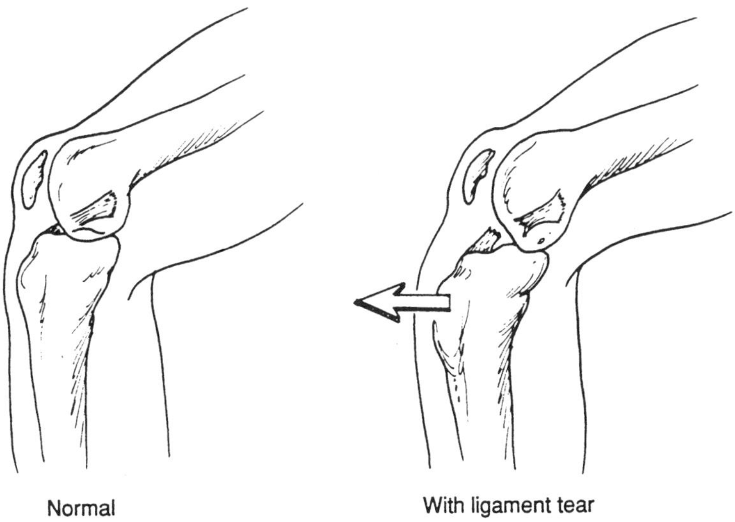

FIGURE 64.5.
When the anterior cruciate ligament has been disrupted, it cannot resist forward displacement. (Reproduced with permission from Cipriano JJ. Photographic Manual of Regional Orthopaedics and Neurological Testing. *2nd ed. Baltimore: Williams & Wilkins, 1991:166.)*

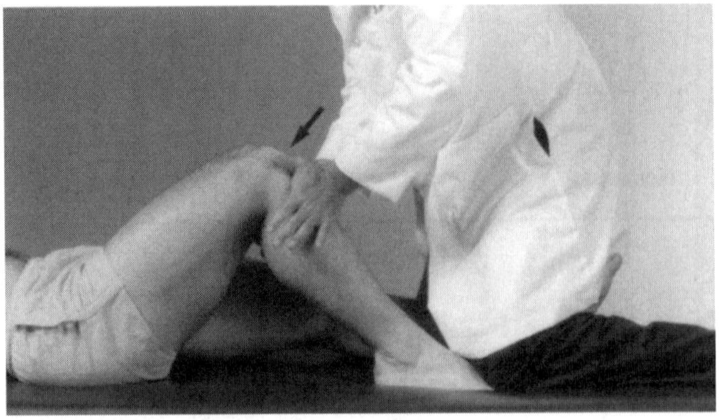

FIGURE 64.6. *The function of the posterior cruciate ligaments is tested when the leg is pushed backward. (Reproduced with permission from Cipriano JJ.* Photographic Manual of Regional Orthopaedics and Neurological Testing. *2nd ed. Baltimore: Williams & Wilkins, 1991:165.)*

movement is detected; if the ligament has been ruptured, the tibia is felt to move forward in a drawer-like manner (Fig. 64. 5). In a similar way, the tibia should be pushed back under the femur (Fig. 64.6). The normal knee resists movement, whereas a knee with a torn posterior cruciate ligament moves backward (Fig. 64.7). Under normal conditions, little movement should be detected, but a comparison to the opposite side is always advisable.

Tests of Menisci

The condition of the menisci may be checked using relatively simple office tests. The simplest test, the McMurray test, provides information about the posterior horns of both the medial and lateral menisci. In this test the foot is maximally externally rotated as the knee is flexed and extended (Fig. 64.8). The test is repeated with the foot maximally internally rotated (Fig. 64.9). If pain is experienced or a click is felt, these tests indicate medial or lateral meniscus damage, respectively. Some patients with abnormally lax cartilaginous attachments may have a false-positive test result. A click in these persons should not be accompanied by pain. Other tests for the presence of damage to the menisci may be performed but are more involved. These are well covered in the suggested readings included with this chapter.

Creaking in the knee joint can suggest arthritis or chondromalacia. This is tested with three maneuvers: 1) move the patella passively in a cephalad-caudad dimension several times, 2) swing the patella left and right, and 3) wiggle the femur and tibia and then flex the knee. If the creaking is found in only the last maneuver, arthritis of the knee is most likely. If creaking is found with only the first two maneuvers, chondromalacia of the patella is suspected. Creaking with all three procedures suggests chondromalacia of the femur.

Selected Abnormal Findings

Many disorders of the knee lead to the build-up of excess fluid that may be easily detected by the nonorthopedist. Detection of this fluid indicates disease or trauma but is seldom specific as the cause.

Tenderness in the area of the medial collateral ligament may be caused by problems with that ligament or with the medial meniscus. Maximal tenderness over the femoral end suggests a tear of the ligament, whereas maximal tenderness directly over the joint line in front of the ligament is more consistent with a bucket-handle tear of the medial meniscus. Tenderness of these types must be evaluated with the knee flexed because the patient may not exhibit tenderness to palpation while the knee is extended.

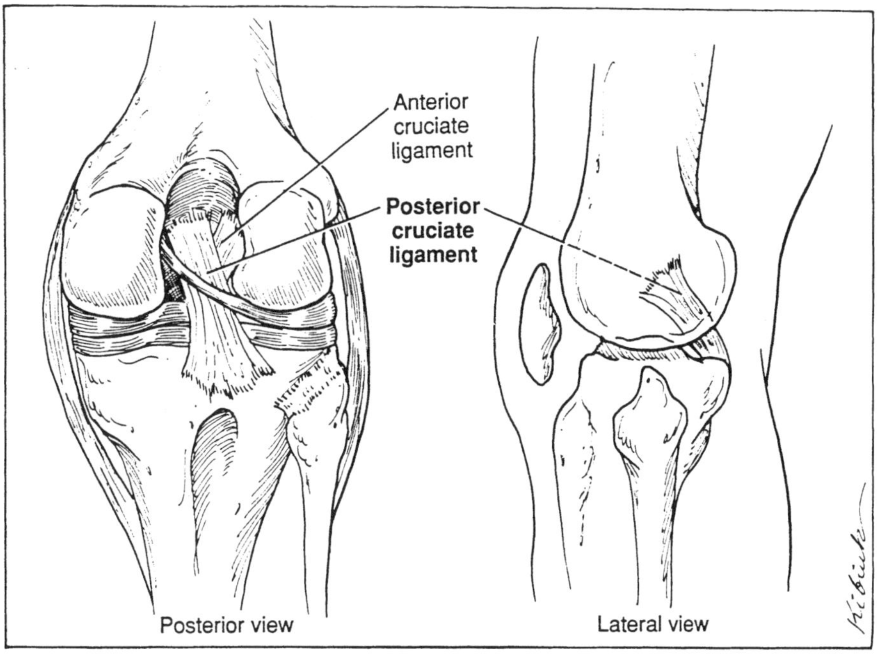

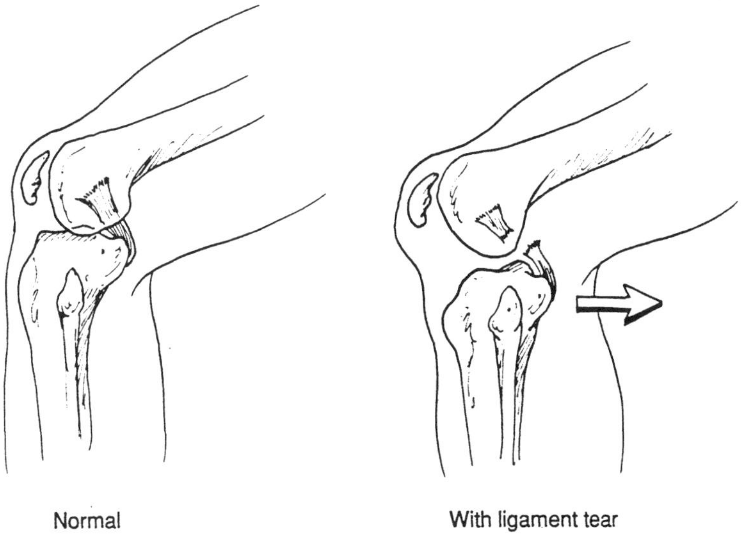

FIGURE 64.7.

When the posterior cruciate ligament has been disrupted, it cannot resist backward displacement. (Reproduced with permission from Cipriano JJ. Photographic Manual of Regional Orthopaedics and Neurological Testing. *2nd ed. Baltimore: Williams & Wilkins, 1991:167.)*

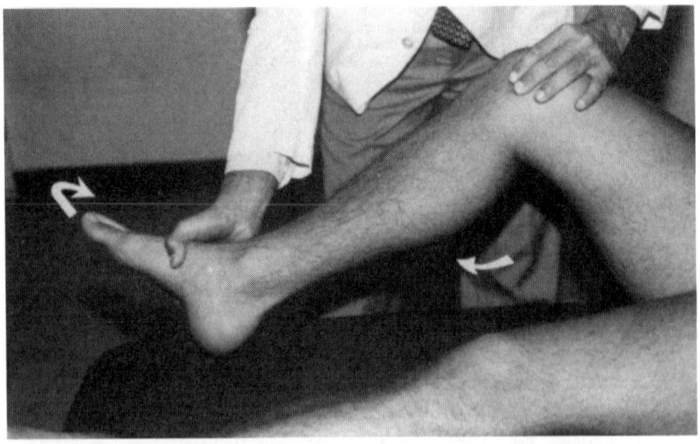

FIGURE 64.8.
If the medial meniscus has been torn, pain or a click will be felt as the knee is flexed and extended with the foot externally rotated. (Reproduced with permission from Cipriano JJ. Photographic Manual of Regional Orthopaedics and Neurological Testing. *2nd ed. Baltimore: Williams & Wilkins, 1991:160.)*

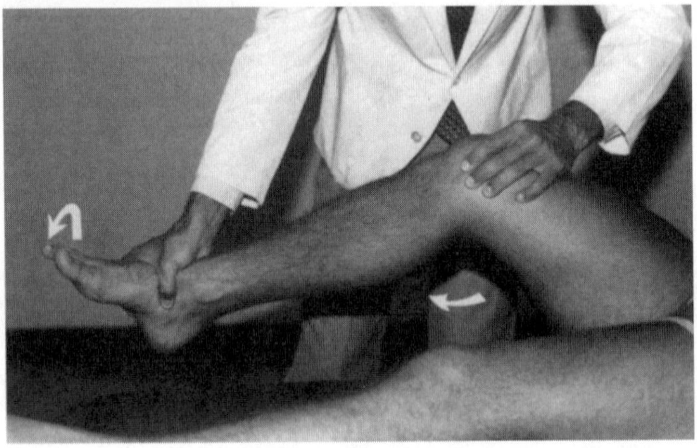

FIGURE 64.9.
If the lateral meniscus has been torn, pain or a click will be felt as the knee is flexed and extended with the foot internally rotated. (Reproduced with permission from Cipriano JJ. Photographic Manual of Regional Orthopaedics and Neurological Testing. *2nd ed. Baltimore: Williams & Wilkins, 1991:160.)*

A fractured patella may be detected by running a fingernail along the anterior surface, moving from cephalad to caudad. The nail will get stuck in the groove made by the fracture.

Suggested Readings

Cipriano JJ. *Photographic Manual of Regional Orthopaedic and Neurological Tests.* 2nd ed. Baltimore: Williams & Wilkins, 1991:155.

Sapira JD. *The Art and Science of Bedside Diagnosis.* Williams & Wilkins, 1990:426.

Willms JL, Schneiderman H, Algranati PS. *Physical Diagnosis: Bedside Evaluation of Diagnosis and Function.* Baltimore: Williams & Wilkins, 1994:433.

Chapter 65

SHOULDER EXAMINATIONS

The shoulder is a complex yet incomplete ball-and-socket joint, articulating with the scapula at the glenoid fossa. Because of its almost constant use, the shoulder is exposed to stress and trauma that may present in many forms, including referred chest or breast pain. The ability to perform screening assessments of shoulder function in the primary care setting allows early diagnosis and referral when a problem exists or reassurance when findings are normal.

Equipment

No special equipment is required.

Training/Credentialing

No special credentialing needed; office diagnostic procedure only.

Coding

Shoulder examination cannot be billed as a separate item. It is considered a part of an office examination.

Technique

Many specialized tests of shoulder function are available, some of which are beyond the scope of the primary care setting. A brief summary of these tests, arranged by focus, is shown in Table 65.1.

Examination of the shoulders should begin with inspection of both joints from the front and back. No clothing should interfere with the examination. Symmetry from one side to the other, contour, and relative height should be noted. Unusual loss of rounding in the frontal plane or an increased prominence of the greater tuberosity of the humerus is abnormal. Enlargement, as if by shoulder pads, is abnormal and should be assessed for texture.

Screening for normal range of motion may be accomplished by having the patient

TABLE 65.1. Tests of Shoulder Function[a]

Bursitis or tenosynovitis
- Drawbarn's test
- Speed's test
- Subacromial push-button test
- Yergason's test

Dislocation
- Anterior apprehension test
- Calloway's sign
- Dugas test
- Posterior apprehension test

Range of motion (See Chapter 68, Range of Motion Testing)

Tendinitis
- Apley scratch test
- Neer and Welsh impingement sign
- Supraspinatus tendinitis test

Tendon instability or torn rotator cuff
- Abbott-Saunders test
- Biceps tendon stability
- Drop arm
- Ludington's test
- Transverse humeral ligament test
- Yergason's test

[a]A full discussion of tests not reviewed here may be found in the references by Cipriano and Sapira contained in the list of suggested readings.

TABLE 65.2. Apley Scratch Test

Have the patient do the following:
- Reach behind the head and scratch the superomedial angle of the opposite scapula (tests abduction and external rotation)
- Reach in front of chest to rest the hand on the opposite shoulder (tests internal rotation and adduction)
- Reach behind the back to touch the inferior angle of the opposite scapula (tests internal rotation and adduction)

stand with her arms at her side with elbows extended. She is then asked to swing her arms upward (in the frontal plane) to touch her palms above her head. This may then be repeated, moving through the sagittal plane to test flexion. Internal rotation may be tested by having the patient reach the back of her hand as high as possible toward her shoulder blade. These maneuvers should be repeated by the examiner, with the joint moved passively through the same range. As an alternative, the Apley scratch test may be used to screen for limitations of motion, asymmetry, and discomfort (Table 65.2). These maneuvers test both external rotation (Fig. 65.1) and internal rotation (Fig. 65.2).

On the basis of the results of these simple screening tests, more specific provocative tests may be indicated. The most common problems that a gynecologist may be called on to diagnose are dislocations, bursitis or tendinitis, and rotator cuff injury (tendon instability).

TESTS FOR DISLOCATION

Acute dislocation of the shoulder may be diagnosed by a suggestive history and the Dugas test: patients with a shoulder dislocation are unable to touch the opposite shoulder with the elbow against the chest wall (Fig. 65.3).

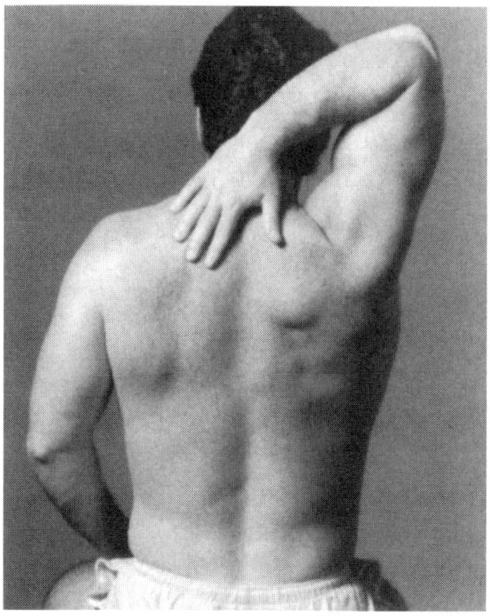

FIGURE 65.1.
Patients with impaired abduction or external rotation are unable to "scratch" the superomedial angle of the opposite scapula. (Reproduced with permission from Cipriano JJ. Photographic Manual of Regional Orthopaedics and Neurological Testing. *2nd ed. Baltimore: Williams & Wilkins, 1991:102.)*

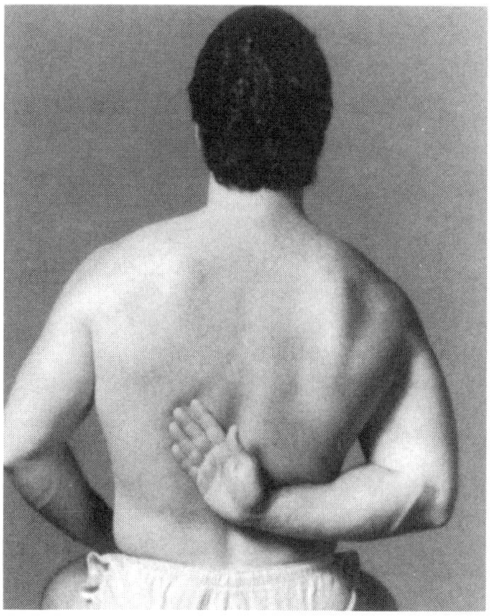

FIGURE 65.2.
Patients with impaired abduction or internal rotation are unable to "scratch" the inferior angle of the opposite scapula. (Reproduced with permission from Cipriano JJ. Photographic Manual of Regional Orthopaedics and Neurological Testing. *2nd ed. Baltimore: Williams & Wilkins, 1991:109.)*

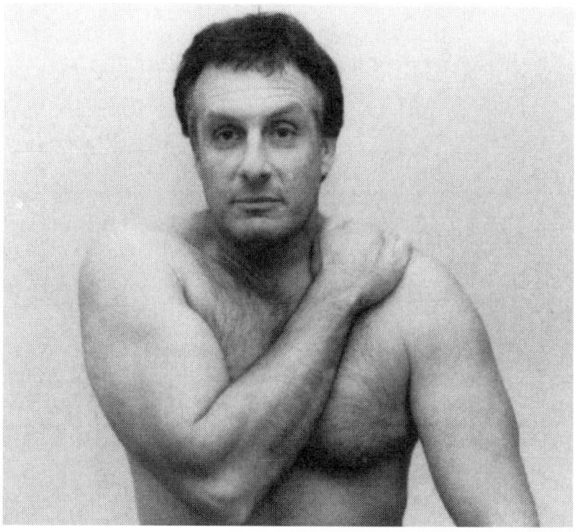

FIGURE 65.3.
Patients with a dislocated shoulder are unable to touch the opposite shoulder while the elbow is held against the chest wall. (Reproduced with permission from Cipriano JJ. Photographic Manual of Regional Orthopaedics and Neurological Testing. *2nd ed. Baltimore: Williams & Wilkins, 1991:114.)*

TESTS FOR BURSITIS OR TENDINITIS

Bursitis is an inflammation in the subacromial bursa located just above the head of the humerus (Fig. 65.4). Inflammation in this bursa causes pain in the shoulder on abduction. When bursitis is present, pressure applied to the subacromial area produces localized pain (Push-button sign, Fig. 65.5). This tenderness decreases if the arm is passively elevated, a position that interposes the deltoid muscle between the bursa and the point of finger pressure (Drawbarn's sign, Fig. 65.6).

Bicipital tenosynovitis produces direct tenderness over the biceps tendon in its groove. This may be demonstrated by flipping the tendon back and forth above its junction with the muscle belly. Speed's test may also be used to identify tenderness in the bicipital groove. In this test, the patient is asked to raise flex the shoulder (elevate it anteriorly) against resistance while the elbow is extended and the forearm is supinated (Fig. 65.7).

Yergason's test is based on the remote production of pain in the bicipital groove or insertion. Pain is produced when the patient is asked to rotate the palm upward against resistance, starting from a resting position with the palm on the anterior thigh.

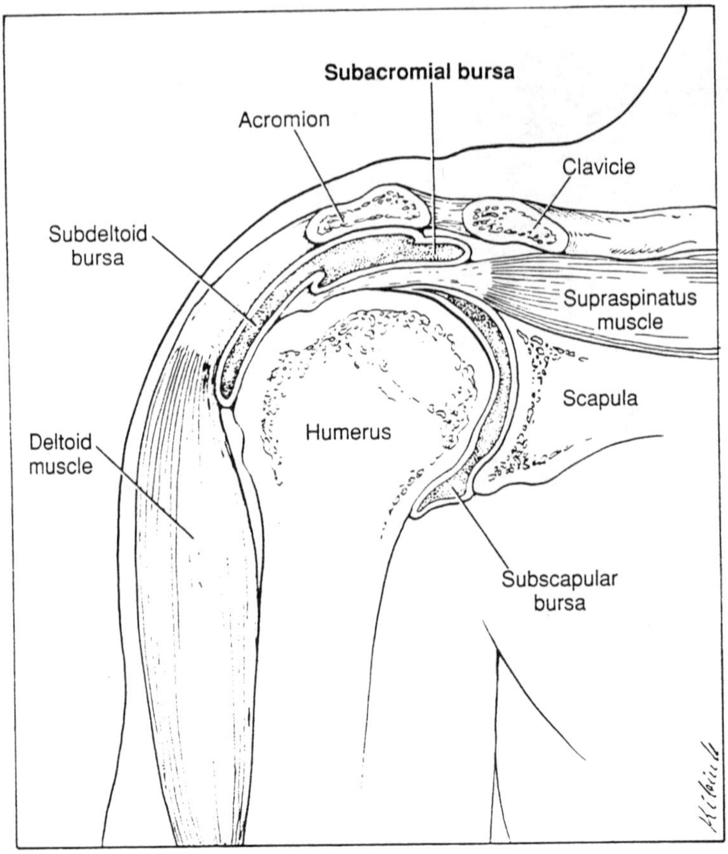

FIGURE 65.4.
The subacromial bursa is located above the head of the humerus and is contiguous with the subdeltoid bursa. (Reproduced with permission from Cipriano JJ. Photographic Manual of Regional Orthopaedics and Neurological Testing. *2nd ed. Baltimore: Williams & Wilkins, 1991:111.)*

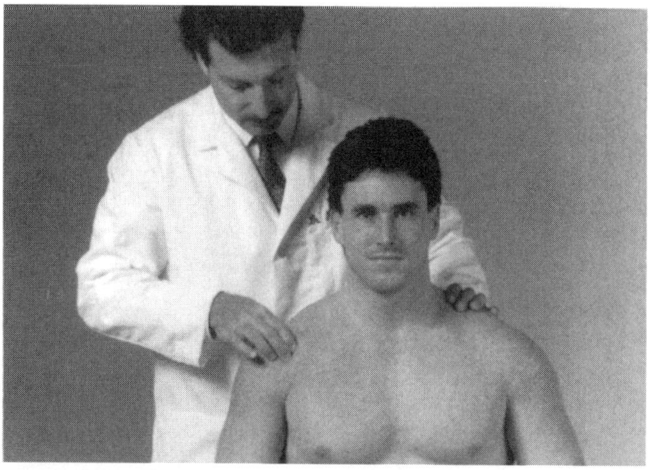

FIGURE 65.5.
Palpation directly over the subacromial bursa elicits localized pain when bursitis is present. (Reproduced with permission from Cipriano JJ. Photographic Manual of Regional Orthopaedics and Neurological Testing. *2nd ed. Baltimore: Williams & Wilkins, 1991:111.)*

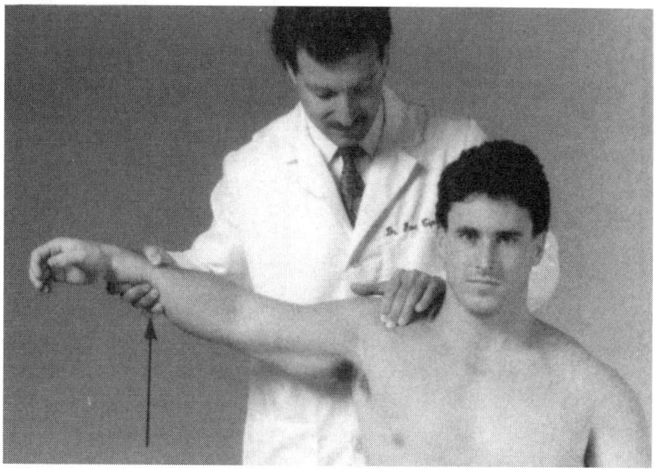

FIGURE 65.6.
When the arm of patients with subacromial bursitis is passively raised, palpation directly over the subacromial bursa becomes less tender. (Reproduced with permission from Cipriano JJ. Photographic Manual of Regional Orthopaedics and Neurological Testing. *2nd ed. Baltimore: Williams & Wilkins, 1991:112.)*

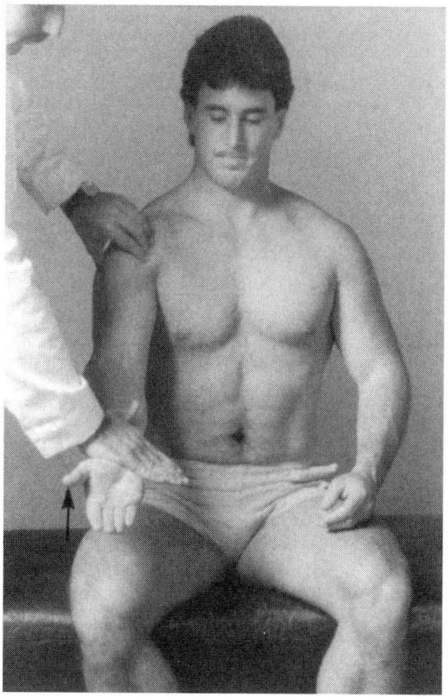

FIGURE 65.7.
Speed's test produces pain or tenderness in the bicipital groove when tendinitis is present. (Reproduced with permission from Cipriano JJ. Photographic Manual of Regional Orthopaedics and Neurological Testing. *2nd ed. Baltimore: Williams & Wilkins, 1991:110.)*

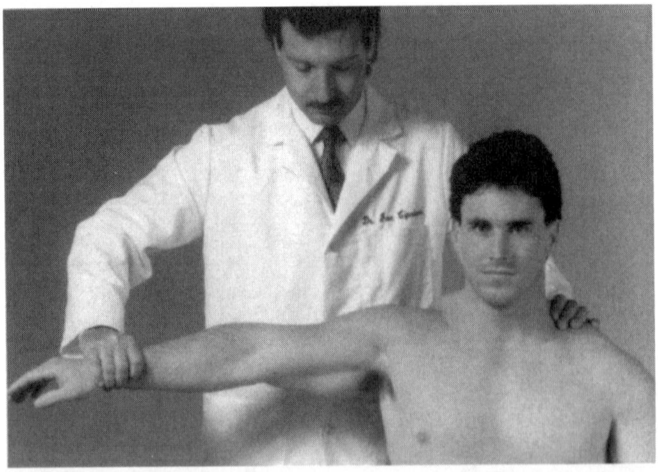

FIGURE 65.8.
Patients with rotator cuff injuries are unable to hold the arm in the horizontal position when resistance is applied. (Reproduced with permission from Cipriano JJ. Photographic Manual of Regional Orthopaedics and Neurological Testing. *2nd ed. Baltimore: Williams & Wilkins, 1991:116.)*

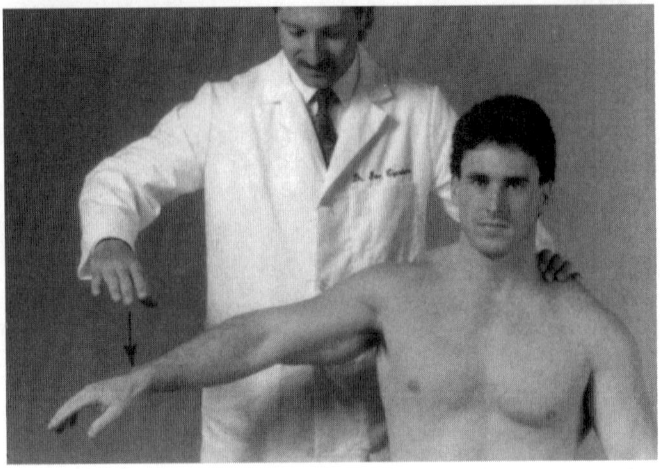

FIGURE 65.9.
Rotator cuff injuries cause inability to gently lower the raised arm from the horizontal plane. (Reproduced with permission from Cipriano JJ. Photographic Manual of Regional Orthopaedics and Neurological Testing. *2nd ed. Baltimore: Williams & Wilkins, 1991:116.)*

TESTS FOR ROTATOR CUFF INJURY (TENDON INSTABILITY)

The drop-arm test is one of the simplest tests for the detection of rotator cuff injury. Rotator cuff injuries impair the ability of the patient to actively abduct the arm. In this test, the patient's arm is passively raised to the horizontal and the patient is asked to maintain her arm in this position while resistance is applied. The patient is then asked to raise her arm over her head, then lower it to the horizontal. Lastly, the patient is asked to lower her arm from the horizontal back to the resting position at her side. Patients with rotator cuff damage are unable to maintain the arm in the horizontal position against resistance (Fig. 65.8), or the arm suddenly falls to the patient's side as it is lowered (Fig. 65.9). More subtle but equally telling is the inability to lower the arm fully to the side in a fluid motion. Some asymmetry is occasionally seen between the dominant and nondominant side, but it should be minimal and should never constitute a "drop."

Suggested Readings

American Association of Orthopedic Surgery. *Method of Measuring and Recording.* Chicago: American Association of Orthopedic Surgery, 1965.

Boublik M, Hawkins RJ. Clinical examination of the shoulder complex. *J Orthop Sports Phys Ther* 1993;18:379.
Cipriano JJ. *Photographic Manual of Regional Orthopaedic and Neurological Tests.* 2nd ed. Baltimore: Williams & Wilkins, 1991:102.
Neviaser JS. Musculoskeletal disorders of the shoulder region causing cervicobrachial pain: differential diagnosis and treatment. *Surg Clin North Am* 1963;43:1703.
Post M, Silver R, Singh M. Rotator cuff tear: diagnosis and treatment. *Clin Orthop Relat Res* 1983;173:78.
Sapira JD. *The Art and Science of Bedside Diagnosis*. Williams & Wilkins, 1990:418.
Willms JL, Schneiderman H, Algranati PS. *Physical Diagnosis: Bedside Evaluation of Diagnosis and Function*. Baltimore: Williams & Wilkins, 1994:406.
Yocum LA. Assessing the shoulder: history, physical examination, differential diagnosis, special tests used. *Clin Sports Med* 1983;2:281.

Chapter 66

BACK EXAMINATIONS

One of the greatest prices humans pay for a bipedal stance is back pain. Back problems can manifest in many ways, including chronic pelvic pain. As a result, facility with screening test of back function is not inappropriate in the gynecologic setting.

Equipment

No special equipment is required.

Training/Credentialing

No special credentialing needed; office diagnostic procedure only.

Coding

Back examination cannot be billed as a separate item. It is considered a part of an office examination.

Technique

The examination of the back begins with inspection of the uncovered back. The normal forward concave (kyphotic) curves of the thoracic and sacral regions should be apparent. The normal lumbar lordosis should also be evident. Exaggerations of these curves (as with the kyphosis of osteoporosis) are abnormal.

Scoliosis (lateral curvature) may be detected by such findings as a high shoulder, a prominent hip, or a projecting shoulder blade. Subtle changes may be detected by asking the patient to lean forward from the hips while examining the patient from behind. Asymmetry of the scapulae or the erector spini muscles masses suggest scoliosis.

After inspection, the back should be palpated. Spasms in the paravertebral muscles are readily detected by palpation, especially if the spasm is unilateral. Point tenderness can be elicited by palpation or gentle percussion over the spinous processes. Tenderness of the spinous processes is a cardinal sign of fracture; thus, if fracture is a possibility, the spinous processes should be evaluated before any attempt is made to move the patient.

The range of motion of the back may be measured by having the patient bend forward and then measuring the distance from the floor of the tip of the middle finger.

The patient should stand without shoes, with the heels at the width of the shoulders, and bend forward as if to touch the toes, but without flexing the hips. Most normal patients will be able to bring the fingertips to about 4 cm from the floor. Because a specific joint is not tested, this test is highly subjective and the standard deviation in normal values is wide (± 6.9 cm). This test may be invalidated by tight hamstrings or tall stature; thus, an abnormal result of this test alone is insufficient to establish a diagnosis. A superior test is the Schober or modified Schober test.

The Schober and modified Schober tests are based on measuring the increase in distance between two marks placed on the spine and measured before and during forward bending. In the original Schober test, a line is drawn between the posterior iliac spines and a mark is placed at this level over the spine. A second mark is placed 10 cm above the first, also in the midline. In the modified Schober test, the top of the sacrum is estimated by drawing a line between the dimples of Venus. Marks are placed over the spine at 10 cm above and 5 cm below this line. In both tests, the patient is asked to bend forward maximally and the distance between marks is remeasured. In the Schober test, normal patients should demonstrate an increase of 4–6 cm. In the modified Schober test, the increase should be between 4.3 and 10.3 cm. Only 2% of normal patients have increases of less than 5 cm in the modified test.

Straight-leg raising tests are used when the sciatic nerve or spinal nerve roots are thought to be involved in the patient's symptoms. The test is performed with the patient supine. The examiner should place his or her hand beneath the lumbar spine to check for a compensatory lordosis. The examiner passively raises the leg (with the knee straight) until pain is experienced or until the leg is raised to 90° at the hip. The test is repeated on the other side. The angle at which pain is experienced should be noted because it suggests the source of the pain (Fig. 66.1). Flexing the hip places the sciatic nerve roots on tension over the intervertebral disc. This generally begins at 35–70° of flexion and is maximal at 70–90°. Involuntarily flexed knee during the straight-leg raising test (buckling sign) suggests sciatic nerve pain. Pain on the side opposite of the raised leg (crossed straight-leg raising sign, Fajersztajn's test) is pathognomonic of disc herniation.

The role of the sacroiliac joint may be evaluated by Patrick's test (Fabere test and sign). In this test, the patient is asked to place the lateral malleolus of the tested leg on the opposite knee. The examiner then pushes the flexed knee downward, toward the examination table. Pain in the hip suggests sacroiliitis.

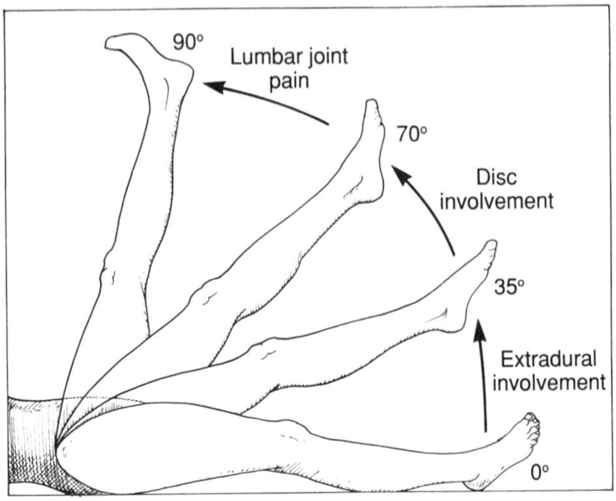

FIGURE 66.1.
The angle at which pain is produced during straight-leg raising can suggest the source of discomfort. (Reproduced with permission from Cipriano JJ. Photographic Manual of Regional Orthopaedics and Neurological Testing. *2nd ed. Baltimore: Williams & Wilkins, 1991:56.)*

Selected Abnormal Findings

Increased lordosis occurs most often as a result of poor posture, pregnancy, and poor footwear (high-heeled shoes). Patients with pain caused by herniated discs or the posterior apophyseal joints report that the pain is located in the back, the buttocks, or the posterior thighs. Pain caused by nerve-root irritation tends to radiate distally to the leg. Pain that is either localized or referred directly to a vertebral body is common in compression fractures and infectious or neoplastic processes.

Pain caused by spinal or nerve compression is increased by any maneuver that increases cerebrospinal fluid pressure. A cough, sneeze, Valsalva maneuver, or gentle head thump causes remote pain that may suggest the area of the lesion.

Irritation of the sciatic nerve root at the level of the intervertebral disc is suggested by an increase in pain when the straight leg is flexed at the hip and the foot is sharply dorsiflexed (Braggard's test, Fig. 66.2).

Special Notes

Mobility of the back, especially flexion, may decrease by as much as 50% between youth and old age.

The straight-leg raising test may be duplicated while the patient is sitting on the end of the examination table with the legs dangling freely. The ankle on the side to be tested is grasped and the knee extended until pain is produced or until the leg is fully extended. Findings in this form of the test should be within 15° of that found with the patient supine.

Because the symptom of chronic back pain is occasionally abused, several tests that differentiate organic and functional disability should be familiar to the examiner. One such test is that noted in the preceding paragraph. In a similar manner, asking the patient to attempt to touch her toes while sitting with straight legs should duplicate the findings made while the patient was standing (Aird's test). In Magnuson's test, the site

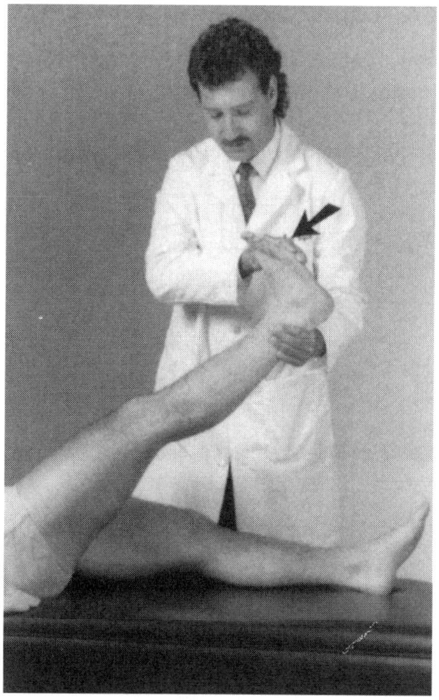

FIGURE 66.2.
Dorsiflexion of the foot with the straight leg flexed to 35° at the hip causes pain that occurs in the back or radiates (Braggard's test). Dull pain in the posterior thigh indicates tight hamstring muscles. (Reproduced with permission from Cipriano JJ. Photographic Manual of Regional Orthopaedics and Neurological Testing. *2nd ed. Baltimore: Williams & Wilkins, 1991:59.)*

of pain indicated by the patient is marked with a small amount of chalk dust. After several other maneuvers or tests, the patient is asked again to indicate the site; the results are then compared. Lastly, both legs may be raised simultaneously. Patients with nerve-root disease are often able to have the legs raised to a higher level than in the single leg version; patients whose disease is not located in the spine report pain at a markedly lower level.

Suggested Readings

American Association of Orthopedic Surgery. *Method of Measuring and Recording.* Chicago: American Association of Orthopedic Surgery, 1965.

Chadwick PR. Examination, assessment and treatment of the lumbar spine. *Physiotherapy* 1984;70:2.

Charnley J. Orthopedic signs in the diagnosis of disc protrusion with special reference to the straight-leg-raising test. *Lancet* 1951;1:156.

Cipriano JJ. *Photographic Manual of Regional Orthopaedic and Neurological Tests.* 2nd ed. Baltimore: Williams & Wilkins, 1991:48.

Cram RH. Sign of sciatic nerve root pressure. *J Bone Joint Surg* 1953;358:192.

Edgar MA, Park WM. Induced pain patterns on passive straight-leg-raising in lower lumbar disc protrusion. *J Bone Joint Surg* 1974;56B:658.

Fahrni WH. Observations on straight-leg-raising with special reference to nerve root adhesions. *Can J Surg* 1966;9:44.

Hudgins WR. The crossed-straight-leg-raising test. *N Engl J Med* 1977;297:1127.

Macnab I. *Backache.* Baltimore: Williams & Wilkins, 1977.

Mayer TG, Tencer AF, Kristoferson S, et al. Use of non-invasive techniques for quantification of spinal range-of-motion in normal subjects and chronic low back dysfunction patients. *Spine* 1984;9:588.

McGregor AH, McCarthy ID, Hughes SP. Motion characteristics of the lumbar spine in the normal population. *Spine* 1995;20:2421.

Merrit JL, McLean TJ, Erickson RP, et al. Measurement of trunk flexibility in normal subjects: reproducibility of three clinical methods. *Mayo Clin Proc* 1986;61:192.

Moll JMH, Wright V. Normal range of spinal mobility. *Ann Rheum Dis* 1971;30:381.

Sapira JD. *The Art and Science of Bedside Diagnosis.* Baltimore: Williams & Wilkins, 1990:421.

Urban LM. The straight-leg-raising test: a review. *J Orthop Sports Phys Ther* 1981;2:117.

Chapter 67

MUSCLE STRENGTH TESTING

The evaluation of the strength and integrity of various muscle groups may provide specific clues to local and systemic disease. In the primary care setting, a familiarity with muscle strength screening is reasonable and may help avoid unnecessary consultation or referral.

Equipment

No special equipment is required.

Training/Credentialing

No special credentialing needed; office diagnostic procedure only.

Coding

95831	Muscle testing, manual (separate procedure); extremity (excluding hand) or trunk, with report
95832	hand (with or without comparison with normal side)
95833	total evaluation of body, excluding hands
95834	total evaluation of body, including hands

Technique

The strength and integrity of muscles are evaluated by their function in moving joints and providing resistance to external force supplied by the examiner and gravity. The effectiveness of the muscle may be graded in several ways (Table 67.1), but all reflect overall ability of the muscle to provide force. To be accurate, any test must isolate the action of the muscle of interest apart from the action of other adjacent muscles. This is accomplished by placing the joint served by the muscle in a defined position and evaluating forces in a specific direction. Some of these positions and directions are outlined for commonly tested muscles in Table 67.2. For most tests, the examiner pro-

TABLE 67.1. Scale Used to Rate Muscle Strength[a]

CHARACTER OF MUSCLE STRENGTH	RESPONSE	GRADE	PERCENTAGE
Against resistance and gravity	Normal	5	100%
Against gravity and some resistance	Good	4	75%
Against gravity only	Fair	3	50%
Motion with gravity eliminated	Poor	2	25%
Muscle contraction without joint motion	Trace	1	10%
No evidence of contraction	None	0	0%

[a]Muscle strength may be rated using several scales.

TABLE 67.2. Testing Motor Function

MUSCLES TESTED	MANEUVER
Sternocleidomastoids Profundi colli	*Neck flexion.* Have supine patient raise head from the bed. Place your hand on her forehead and instruct her to push against it.
Longissimus capitis and cervicis Trapezius	*Neck extension.* Place patient prone, with head extending beyond the top of the table. Place your hand on her occiput and ask her to push against it.
Rectus abdominus	*Trunk flexion.* Have patient lie on a firm surface with knees flexed. Hold her knees and have her do a sit-up.
Iliopsoas	*Flexion of hip.*[a] Have the seated patient lift her thigh from the table and resist your effort to push it down.
Gluteus maximus "Hamstrings" (semi-membranosus, semitendinosus, biceps femoris)	*Extension of hip.* Have patient lie prone. With her knee extended, have her extend the thigh (i.e., lift it up from the table) and resist your effort to push it down.
Gluteus medius and minimus	*Abduction of hip.*[a] Have patient lie on her side, raise the upper leg to about 45°, and resist your effort to push it down.
Adductors, gracilis, and pectineus	*Adduction of hip.*[a] Have patient lie on her side with both legs straight. Have her raise both legs off the table and resist your effort to push down on the lower leg.
Obturator, quadratus femoris, pyriformis, gemelli	*External rotation of hip.*[a] Have patient lie supine with one foot resting on the table and the leg to be tested dangling beyond the edge of the table, with the knee at a 90° angle. Have her rotate the leg so that the foot moves medially, until the lower leg makes an angle of about 30° with the vertical. Place your hand above the medial malleolus and have her resist your effort to push the leg down to a vertical position.
Gluteus medius and minimus	*Internal rotation of hip.*[a] Similar to the above, except that patient rotates leg so that the foot moves laterally. Place your hand above the lateral malleolus and have her resist your effort to push the leg toward the vertical.
"Hamstrings"	*Flexion of knee.* Have patient lie prone, flexing the leg at right angles. Place one hand on her thigh and one on the Achilles tendon. Have the patient resist your effort to pull the foot down to the table.
Quadriceps femoris	*Extension of knee.*[a] Have patient lie supine, with her knee extended and at the edge of the table. Place one hand on her thigh and one at the ankle. Have her resist your effort to push the foot toward the floor.
Gastrocnemius, soleus, plantaris (triceps surae)	*Plantar flexion of ankle.*[a] Have the patient stand on the leg to be tested and raise her heel a couple of inches from the floor. (If strength is not a grade 5, repeat against examiner's resistance with patient supine.)

TABLE 67.2 *(continued).* Testing Motor Function

MUSCLES TESTED	MANEUVER
Tibialis anterior	*Dorsiflexion of ankle.*[a] With the patient supine, place your hand on the dorsum of her foot and have her pull the foot up (toward her face) against your resistance.
Tibialis anterior, tibialis posterior	*Inversion (supination) of foot.*[a] Have the patient invert the foot (if she is sitting, the big toe will be farther from the floor). Place your hand under the foot from the lateral side and have the patient resist as you try to pull the foot down into neutral position.
Extensor digitorum longus, peroneus longus and brevis	*Eversion (pronation) of foot.*[a] Have the patient evert the foot and hold that posture as you try to pull the foot back into neutral position.
Flexor hallucis longus and brevis, flexor digitorum longus	*Flexion of toes.*[a] Place one hand under the tips of the patient's toes and the other hand on top of the toes. Push upward on the tips of the toes as the patient pushes down.
Extensor hallucis longus, extensor digitorum longus	*Extension of toes.*[a] Place one hand on the dorsum of the foot and the fingertips of the other on the dorsal side of the toes. Have the patient push her toes against your fingertips as you resist.
Serratus anterior	*Abduction and upward rotation of scapula.* With her arms in front of her, have the patient push hard against some immovable object. Observe the medial borders of the scapulae, which should remain close to the thoracic wall.
Rhomboids	*Adduction and downward rotation of scapulae.* Have the patient brace her shoulders backward against resistance. The muscle bellies can be felt and sometimes seen.
Levator scapulae Trapezius (upper)	*Elevation of the shoulders.*[a] Have the patient shrug her shoulders against resistance.
Deltoid	*Abduction of shoulder.*[a] Have patient maintain abduction against resistance. To test the deltoid muscle, the angle between the arm and the patient's chest must be more than 15° but less than 90°.
Supraspinatus	*Abduction of shoulder.* With her arm at her side, have patient try to abduct the arm against resistance.
Pectoralis major	*Adduction of shoulder.* Have the patient adduct the arm against resistance. (If the arm is above the horizontal, the clavicular part is tested; if the arm is below the horizontal, the sternocostal part of the muscle is tested.)
Latissimus dorsi, teres major	*Extension of shoulder.* Have the patient lie prone with arms at her side and lift the arm off the table as you resist.
Coracobrachialis Anterior deltoid	*Flexion of shoulder.*[a] With patient seated on the examining table, have her lift the upper arm against resistance (with elbow extended), so as to parallel the thighs.
Infraspinatus	*External (lateral) rotation of shoulder.* Have the patient keep her elbow at her side and have her try to carry the flexed forearm backward against resistance. The muscle belly can be felt over the scapula. Alternately, have the patient lie prone, with shoulder abducted to 90° and elbow flexed 90°, with her hand pointed toward her head. Place one hand at her wrist and have her resist your effort to push her forearm toward the floor.
Subscapularis, teres major, latissimus dorsi	*Internal (medial) rotation of shoulder.* Have the patient lie prone as in testing external rotation, except that her hand points toward her feet. Have her resist your effort to push her wrist toward the floor.
Biceps, brachialis	*Flexion of elbow.*[a] Have the patient flex her elbow and resist your attempt to straighten her arm. (Put one hand on the patient's humerus and the other at the wrist.)

TABLE 67.2 *(continued)*. Testing Motor Function

MUSCLES TESTED	MANEUVER
Triceps	*Extention of elbow.*[a] Position the patient's arm so that it is parallel to the ground, to eliminate the effect of gravity on the forearm. Have her extend the forearm against resistance, starting from an angle of about 130°.
Biceps, supinator	*Supination of forearm.* Have the patient extend her arm by her side, with the hand in supination (palm forward), and resist your attempt to pronate the hand.
Pronator teres	*Pronation of forearm.* Have the patient extend her arm by her side, with the hand in pronation, and resist your attempt to supinate the hand.
Flexor carpi radialis	*Flexion of wrist.* (a) Have the patient try to flex the wrist toward the radial side against resistance.
Flexor carpi ulnaris	*Flexion of wrist.* (b) Place the patient's hand, palm upward, on the table with the fingers extended. Have the patient try to abduct the little finger strongly against resistance. If the flexor carpi ulnaris is intact, the tendon can be seen and felt as it fixes the point of origin of abductor digiti minimi, even when the abductor digiti minimi is paralyzed.
Extensor carpi radialis longus	*Extension of wrist.* (a) With the patient's fingers extended, have the patient try to extend the wrist to the radial side against resistance.
Extensor carpi ulnaris	*Extension of wrist.* (b) With the patient's fingers extended, have the patient try to extend the wrist to the ulnar side against resistance.
Abductor pollicis longus	*Abduction of thumb.* (a) With the patient's thumb in the plane of the palm, have the patient try to abduct it at right angles against resistance.
Abductor pollicis brevis	*Abduction of thumb.* (b) Place the patient's thumb so that the nail is in a plane at right angles to the palm, with a fountain pen or similar object between thumb and palm. Have the patient try against resistance to bring the edge of her thumb to a point vertically above its original position, maintaining the nail in the original plane.
Adductor pollicis	*Adduction of thumb.* Have the patient resist your attempt to abduct the thumb. (Alternately, have the patient try against resistance to hold a strip of paper between the thumb and the palm, with the thumb lying along the palmar aspect of the index finger, its nail in a plane at right angles to the palm.)
Flexor pollicis longus and brevis	*Flexion of thumb.* Fix the proximal phalanx of the thumb between your thumb and index finger. Have the patient flex the terminal phalanx and resist your effort to extend it by pulling with your index finger.
Extensor pollicis (a) brevis and (b) longus, respectively	*Extension of thumb.* Have the patient resist attempts to flex the thumb at (a) the metacarpophalanged joint and (b) the intraphalangeal joint.
Opponens pollicis and opponens digiti quinti	*Opposition of thumb and fifth finger.* Have the patient touch her thumb and little finger together, while you try to pull them apart using the thumbs of both hands.
Lumbricales	*Flexion of fingers at metacarpophalangeal joints (MCPs).* Keeping the patient's fingers extended at the proximal and distal interphalangeal joints, have the patient flex at the MCPs, and maintain flexion while you attempt to extend the fingers by exerting pressure with your thumb.
Extensor digitorum communis, extensor indicis proprius, extensor digiti quinti proprius	*Extension of fingers at MCPs (while flexed at the interphalangeal joints).* Fix the metacarpals and have the patient try to keep her fingers extended at the MCPs while you exert pressure on the proximal phalanges.

TABLE 67.2 *(continued)*. Testing Motor Function

MUSCLES TESTED	MANEUVER
Flexor digitorum sublimis	*Flexion of fingers.* Using your index finger, fix the proximal phalanx in extension at the MCP joint and have the patient flex at the PIP joint and resist your attempts to straighten the finger, using your other index finger.
Flexor digitorum profundus	*Flexion of fingers.* Fix the second phalanx in extension, using your index finger, and have the patient flex the distal phalanx and resist attempts to straighten it.
Extensor digitorum communis and interossei	*Extension of fingers.* With the patient's wrist and fingers extended at all joints, have the patient resist attempts to flex the fingers by pressing on the middle phalanges.
First dorsal interosseus and abductor digiti quinti	*Abduction of fingers.* With the patient's fingers in extension, have the patient try to abduct the index finger and then the little finger against resistance.
Palmar interossei	*Adduction of fingers.* With the patient's fingers in extension, and close together, have the patient try to spread the fingers, while you exert resistance.

[a]Indicates items routinely tested.

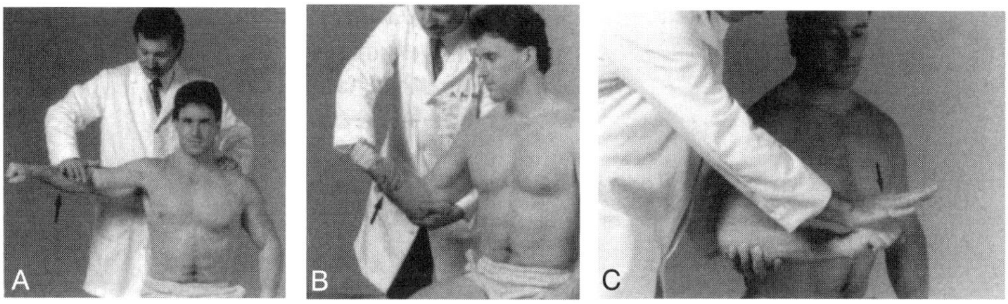

FIGURE 67.1.
*The strength of muscles in the upper extremity may be easily tested while the patient is seated. Shown are methods of testing shoulder abduction (**A**), elbow flexion (**B**), and wrist extension (**C**). (Reproduced with permission from Cipriano JJ.* Photographic Manual of Regional Orthopaedic and Neurological Tests. *2nd ed. Baltimore: Williams & Wilkins, 1991:224, 226.)*

vides resistance while the patient attempts to move the limb or joint (Fig. 67.1). This same principle is used even when smaller muscles, such as the intrinsic muscles of the hands or feet, are evaluated (Fig. 67.2).

When muscle strength is tested, the stability of the joint must be secured (Fig. 67.3). This provides direct feedback about the health of that joint but also provides protection from injury or spurious effects from other muscle groups.

Normal Findings

Although some variation from patient to patient and from one side to the other is acceptable, most muscles should be able to resist the effects of both gravity and the resistance of the examiner. In many tests, the examiner's own strength in providing resistance provides the touchstone for assessment.

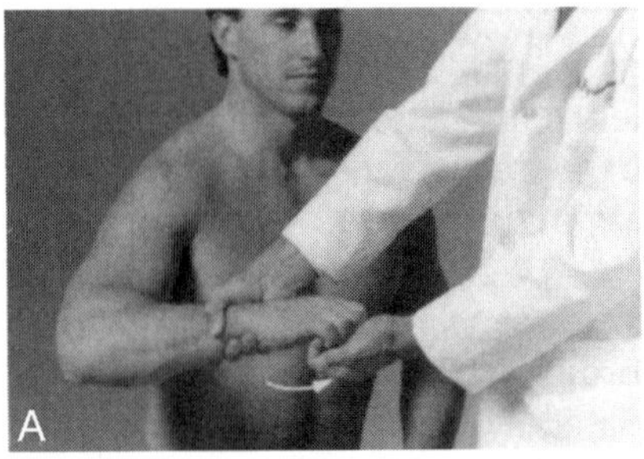

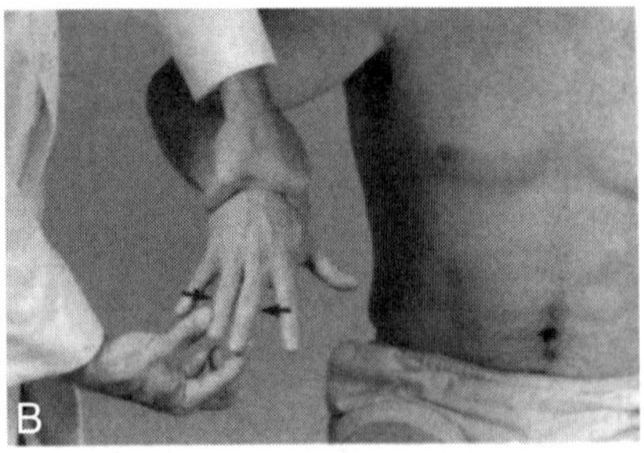

FIGURE 67.2.
*Muscles of the hand are generally evaluated as a unit unless specific deficits are suspected. Shown are flexion (**A**) and abduction of the fingers (**B**). (Reproduced with permission from Cipriano JJ.* Photographic Manual of Regional Orthopaedic and Neurological Tests. *2nd ed. Baltimore: Williams & Wilkins, 1991:230.)*

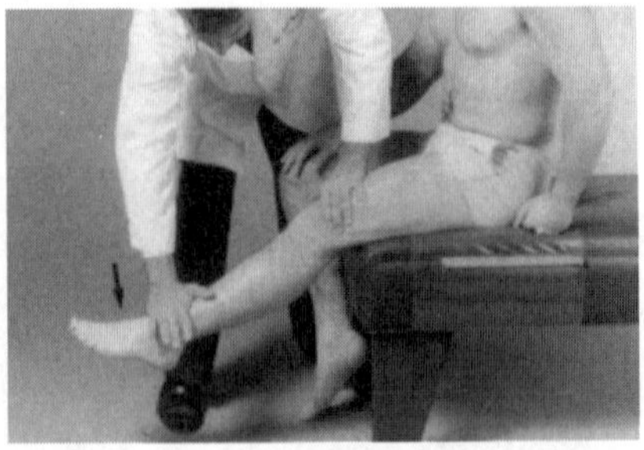

FIGURE 67.3.
When large joints are tested, the joints should be stabilized. Shown is the testing of knee extension. (Reproduced with permission from Cipriano JJ. Photographic Manual of Regional Orthopaedic and Neurological Tests. *2nd ed. Baltimore: Williams & Wilkins, 1991:236.)*

Special Notes

When joint disease or contracture is present, results of muscle testing are inconclusive. If an evaluation of muscle function is required in these circumstances, the assistance of a specialist should be enlisted.

Suggested Readings

Brandsma JW. Manual muscle strength testing and dynamometry for bilateral ulnar neuropraxia in a surgeon. *J Hand Ther* 1995;8:191.

Brandsma JW, Schreuders TA, Birke JA, et al. Manual muscle strength testing: intraobserver and interobserver reliabilities for the intrinsic muscles of the hand. *J Hand Ther* 1995;8:185.

Cipriano JJ. *Photographic Manual of Regional Orthopaedic and Neurological Tests.* 2nd ed. Baltimore: Williams & Wilkins, 1991:221.

Merlini L, Dell'Accio D, Granata C. Reliability of dynamic strength knee muscle testing in children. *J Orthop Sports Phys Ther* 1995;22:73.

Sapira JD. *The Art and Science of Bedside Diagnosis*. Baltimore: Williams & Wilkins, 1990:481.

Vernon HT, Aker P, Aramenko M, et al. Evaluation of neck muscle strength with a modified sphygmomanometer dynamometer: reliability and validity. *J Manip Physiol Ther* 1992;15:343.

Willms JL, Schneiderman H, Algranati PS. *Physical Diagnosis: Bedside Evaluation of Diagnosis and Function.* Baltimore: Williams & Wilkins, 1994:387.

Chapter 68

RANGE OF MOTION TESTING

When patients present with joint symptoms, a careful examination often suggests a diagnosis or indicates the need for consultation. Joints are evaluated for the presence of erythema, swelling, heat, tenderness, crepitus, deformity, misalignment, and function. Range of motion testing is used to assess this last item.

Equipment

- Goniometer or protractor to measure angle of motion

Training/Credentialing

No special credentialing needed; office diagnostic procedure only.

Coding

95851	Range of motion measurements and report (separate procedure); each extremity (excluding hand) or each trunk section (spine)
95852	hand, with or without comparison with normal side

Technique

Joints should be reviewed for their range of function by both active and passive testing. If restricted motion is found, the angle through which the joint can move should be documented. This may be done using a simple protractor or an angle meter (goniometer) specifically designed for the purpose. The joint or joints to be tested should be placed at rest and palpated for erythema, swelling, heat, tenderness, crepitus, or deformity. The presence of significant findings suggests a need for consultation. The tests of motion used varies somewhat by joint as follows. Specific, detailed examination techniques for selected joints are detailed in separate chapters.

SHOULDER

The shoulder is an incomplete ball-and-socket joint, articulating with the scapula at the glenoid fossa. Screening may be accomplished by having the patient stand with her

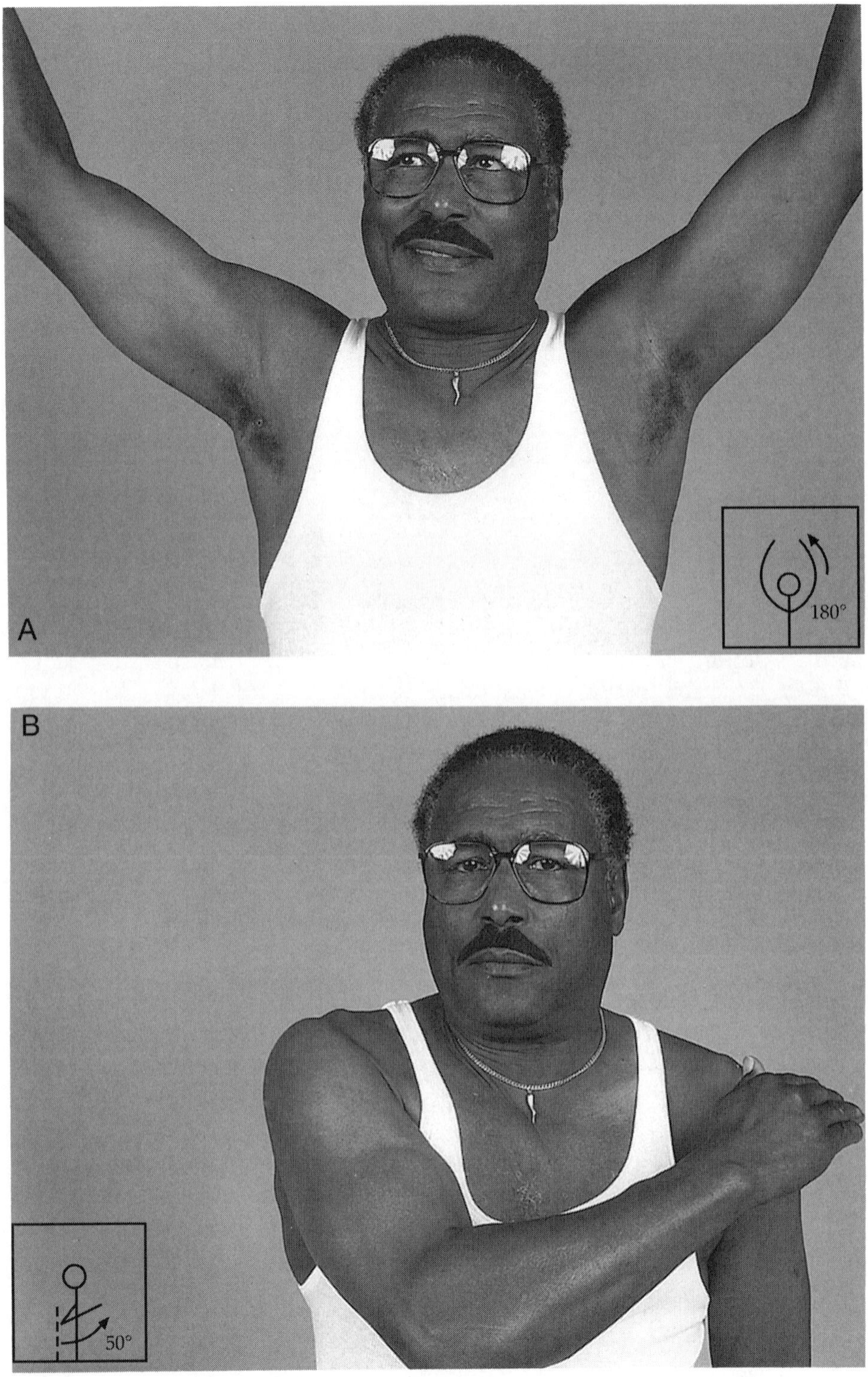

FIGURE 68.1.

*Range of motion of the shoulder is evaluated by having the patient raise her arms upward in the frontal plane (**A**). Adduction is tested by having the patient draw her arm across the chest (**B**). (Reproduced with permission from Willms JL, Schneiderman H, Algranati PS.* Physical Diagnosis: Bedside Evaluation of Diagnosis and Function. *Baltimore: Williams & Wilkins, 1994:406.)*

arms at her side with elbows extended. The patient is then asked to swing the arms upward (in the frontal plane) to touch her palms above her head (Fig. 68.1). This may then be repeated, moving through the sagittal plane to test flexion (Fig. 68.2). Internal rotation may be tested by having the patient reach the back of her hand as high as pos-

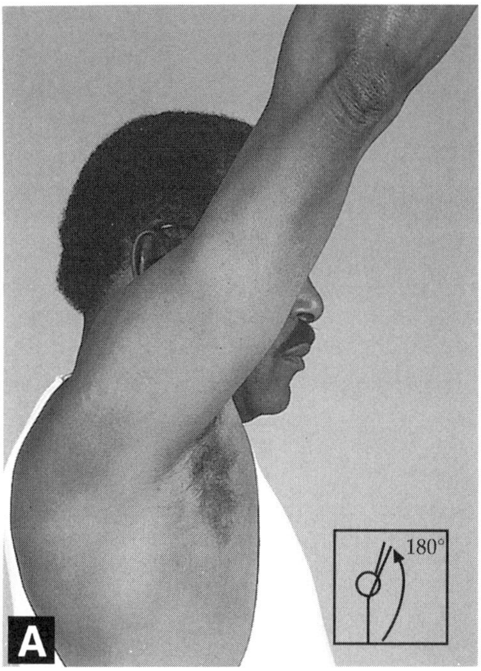

FIGURE 68.2 *(continued).*
*Flexion (**A**) (continued)*

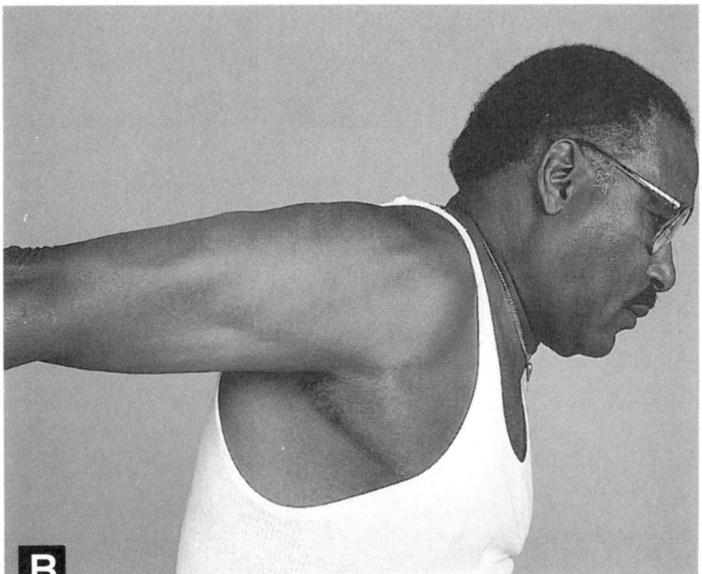

FIGURE 68.2 *(continued).*
*and extension (**B**) of the shoulder are tested in the sagittal plane. (Reproduced with permission from Willms JL, Schneiderman H, Algranati PS.* Physical Diagnosis: Bedside Evaluation of Diagnosis and Function. *Baltimore: Williams & Wilkins, 1994:407.)*

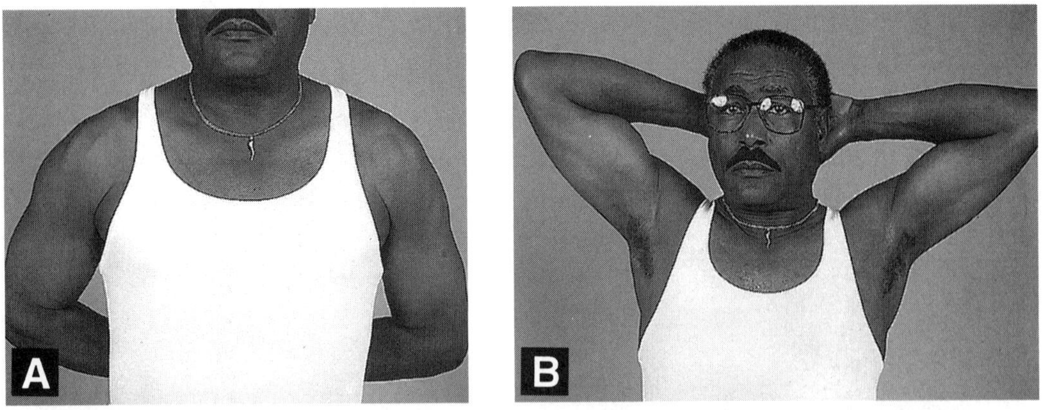

FIGURE 68.3.
*In testing internal rotation of the shoulder, the hands are clasped behind the back (**A**). In testing of external rotation, the hands are clasped behind the head (**B**). (Reproduced with permission from Willms JL, Schneiderman H, Algranati PS.* Physical Diagnosis: Bedside Evaluation of Diagnosis and Function. *Baltimore: Williams & Wilkins, 1994:407.)*

sible toward her shoulder blade (Fig. 68.3). These maneuvers should be repeated by having the examiner move the joint passively through the same range.

ELBOW

The hinge joint of the elbow permits motion in only one plane: flexion and extension (Fig. 68.4). Pronation and supination may be tested with the elbow and hand fully extended (Fig. 68.5). The carrying angle (often abnormal in some genetic syndromes) should only be assessed with the palms outward.

WRIST

Flexion and extension (Fig. 68.6) and ulnar-radial deviation are measured from a zero point measured with the hand in the axis of the forearm. The degree of flexion achieved is generally greater than the degree of extension.

FINGERS (METACARPOPHALANGEAL JOINT)

The metacarpophalangeal joints may be evaluated individually or screened as a unit. Both finger spread and flexion should be assessed (Fig. 68.7).

HIP

Despite the ball-and-socket character of the hip, this joint has less mobility than the shoulder. The ability of the hip to flex is most easily measured with the patient in the supine position (Fig. 68.8). In this position, the ability of the hip joint to rotate (Fig. 68.9) and be abducted (Fig. 68.10) may also be gauged. Hip extension may be better assessed while the patient is standing.

KNEE

The knee is best examined with the patient sitting and the knee comfortably suspended as for reflex testing. The knee of the normal patient should only be capable of extension and flexion, with little side-to-side mobility as befits a complex hinge joint (Fig. 68.11).

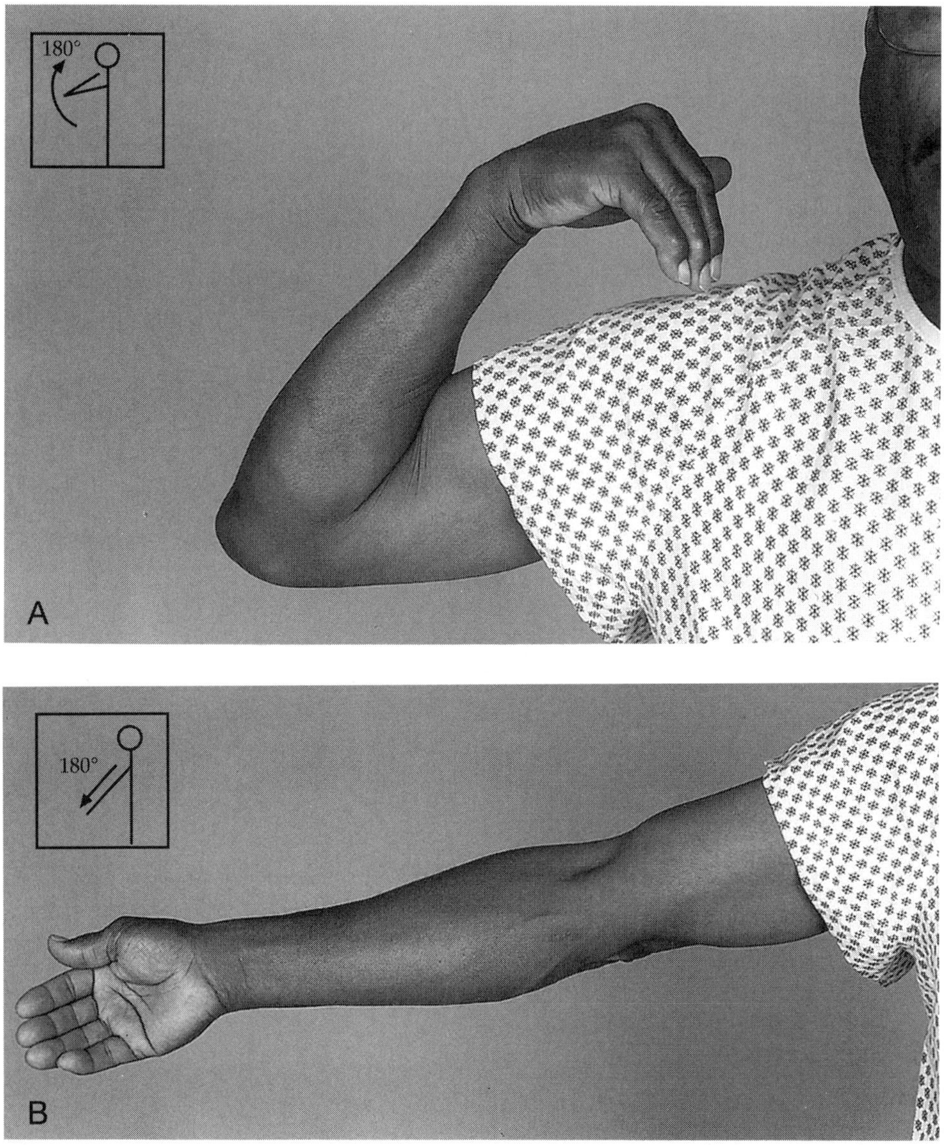

FIGURE 68.4.
*Flexion (**A**) and extension (**B**) of the elbow are easily evaluated. (Reproduced with permission from Willms JL, Schneiderman H, Algranati PS.* Physical Diagnosis: Bedside Evaluation of Diagnosis and Function. *Baltimore: Williams & Wilkins, 1994:408.)*

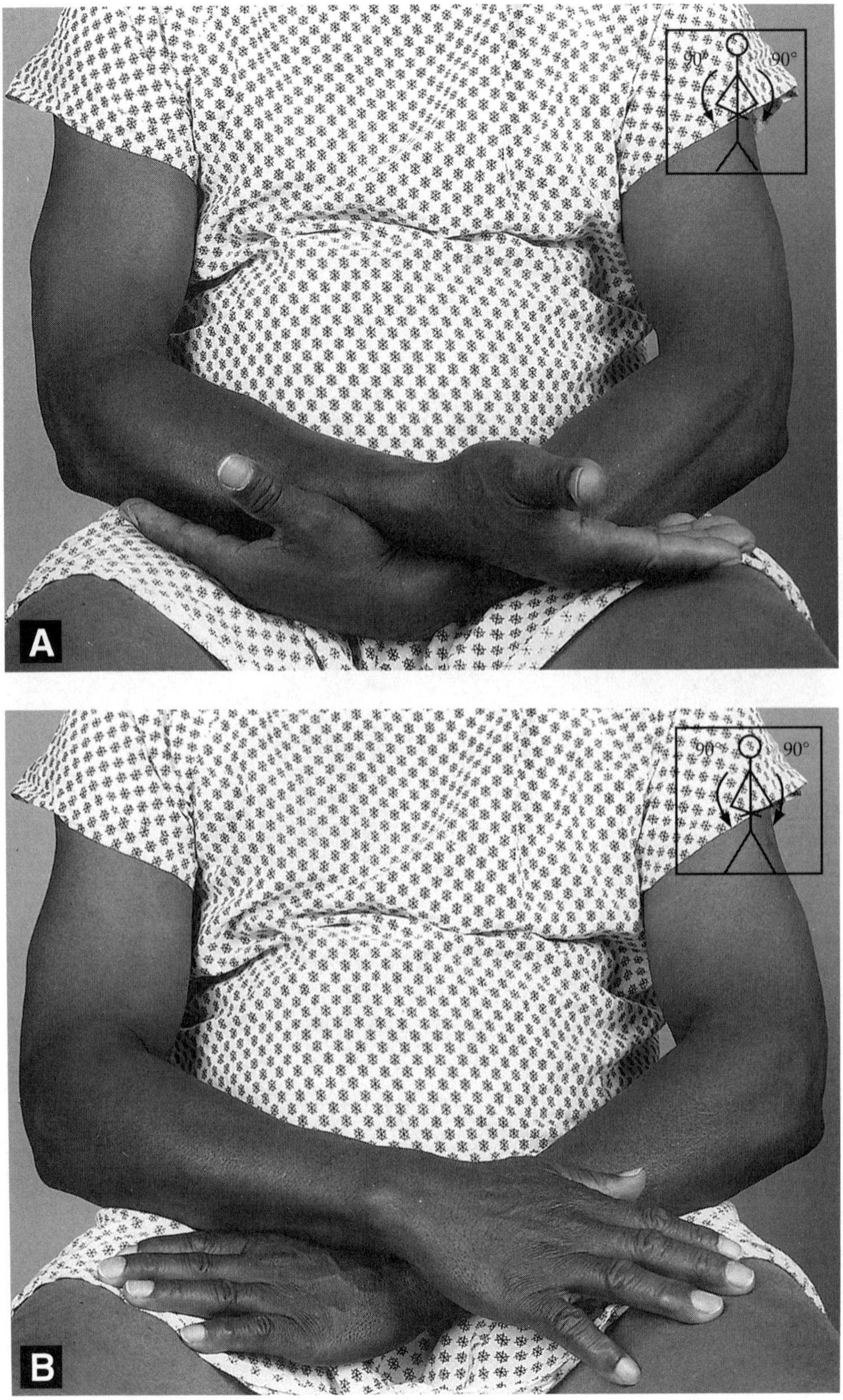

FIGURE 68.5.
*Supination (**A**) and pronation (**B**) are measured by degree of rotation. (Reproduced with permission from Willms JL, Schneiderman H, Algranati PS.* Physical Diagnosis: Bedside Evaluation of Diagnosis and Function. *Baltimore: Williams & Wilkins, 1994:409.)*

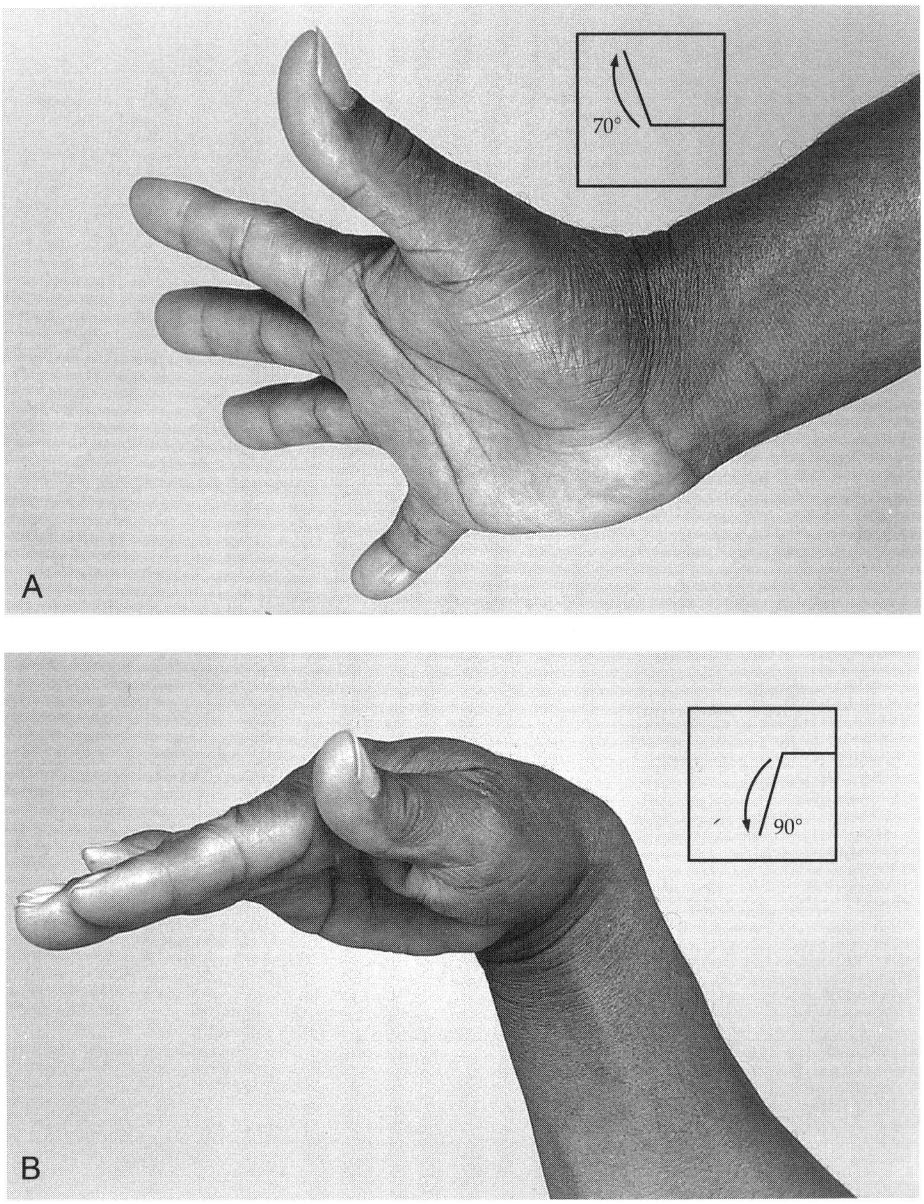

FIGURE 68.6.
*Extension (**A**) and flexion (**B**) of the wrist are measured from the plane of the forearm. (Reproduced with permission from Willms JL, Schneiderman H, Algranati PS.* Physical Diagnosis: Bedside Evaluation of Diagnosis and Function. *Baltimore: Williams & Wilkins, 1994:410.)*

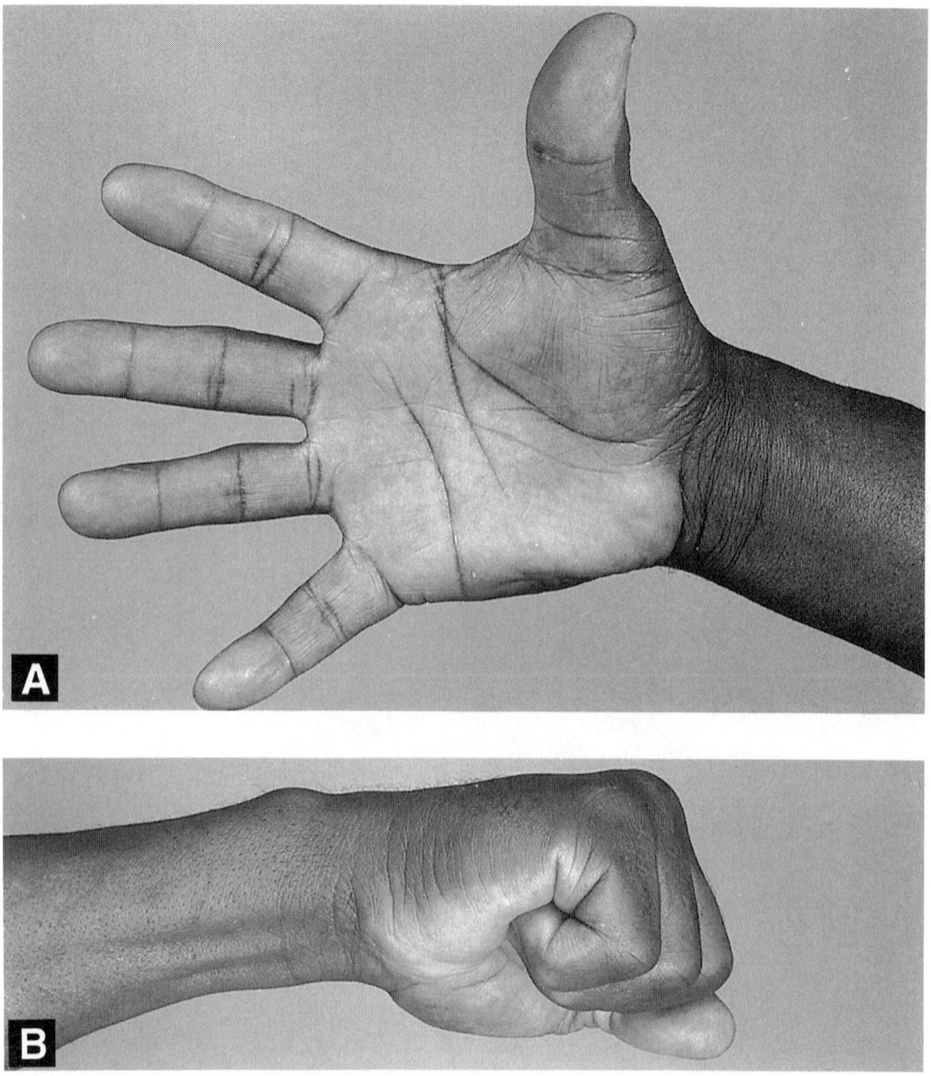

FIGURE 68.7.
*Finger flair (**A**) and flexion (**B**) may be evaluated as a group. Abnormal findings should be confirmed by individual testing. (Reproduced with permission from Willms JL, Schneiderman H, Algranati PS.* Physical Diagnosis: Bedside Evaluation of Diagnosis and Function. *Baltimore: Williams & Wilkins, 1994:411.)*

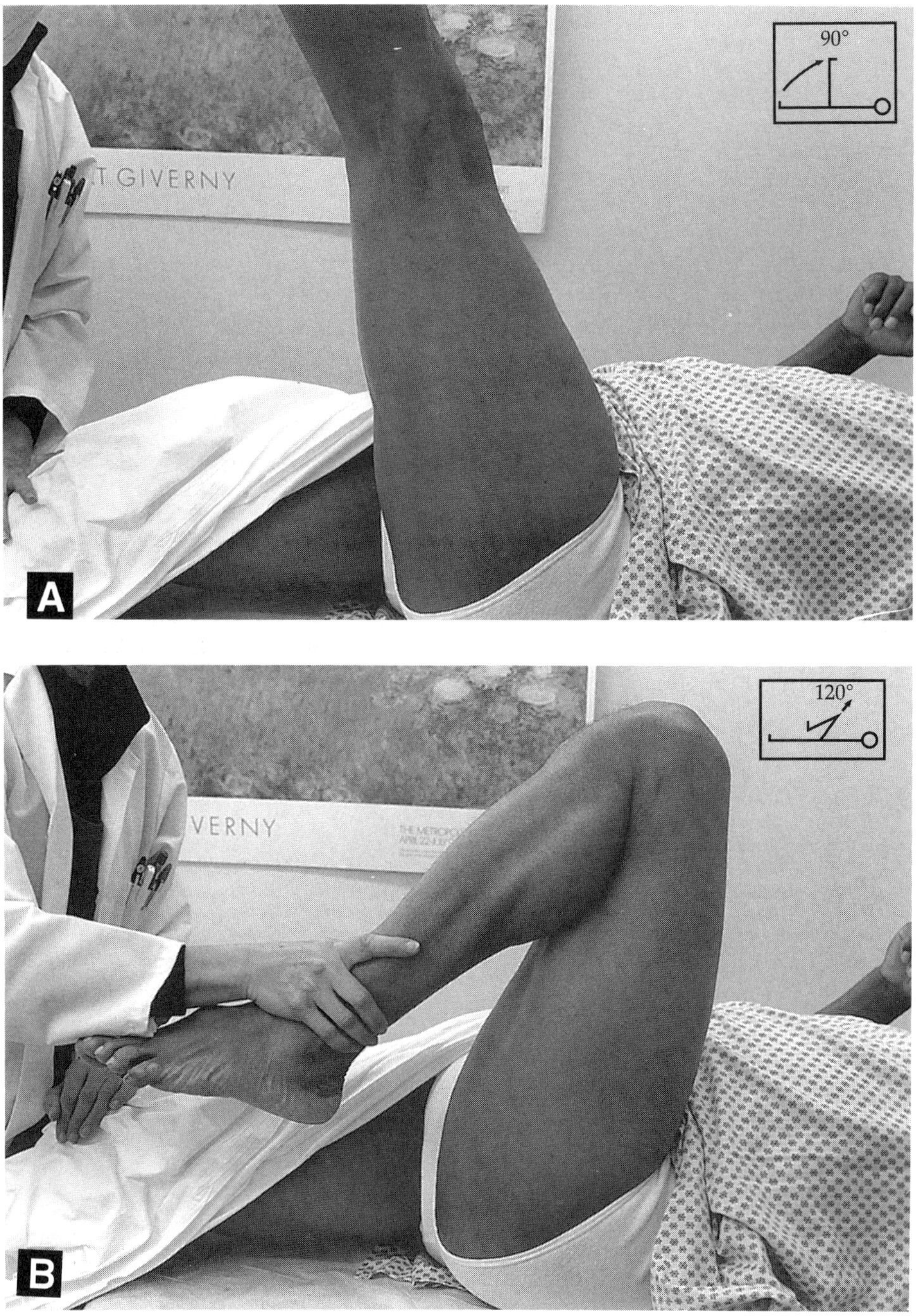

FIGURE 68.8.
*Hip range of motion is tested with the patient supine. Flexion should be tested with the knee both extended (**A**) and flexed (**B**). (Reproduced with permission from Willms JL, Schneiderman H, Algranati PS.* Physical Diagnosis: Bedside Evaluation of Diagnosis and Function. *Baltimore: Williams & Wilkins, 1994:398.)*

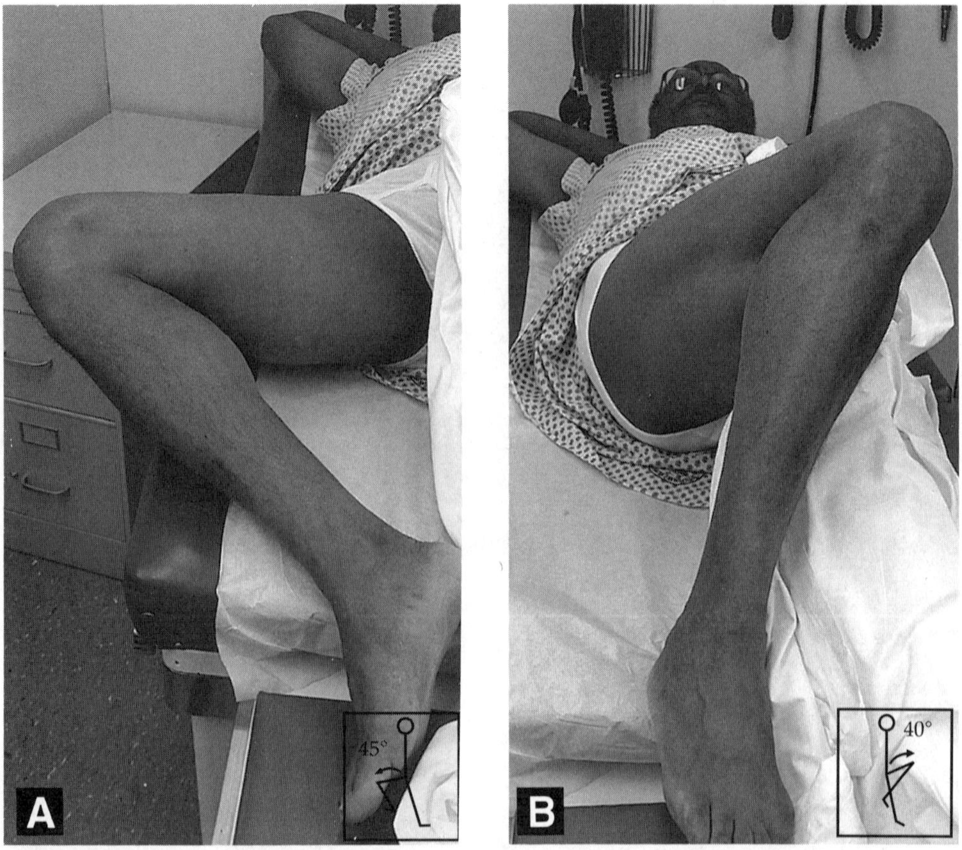

FIGURE 68.9.
*External (**A**) and internal (**B**) rotation range of motion is tested with the patient supine and the knee flexed. (Reproduced with permission from Willms JL, Schneiderman H, Algranati PS.* Physical Diagnosis: Bedside Evaluation of Diagnosis and Function. *Baltimore: Williams & Wilkins, 1994:399.)*

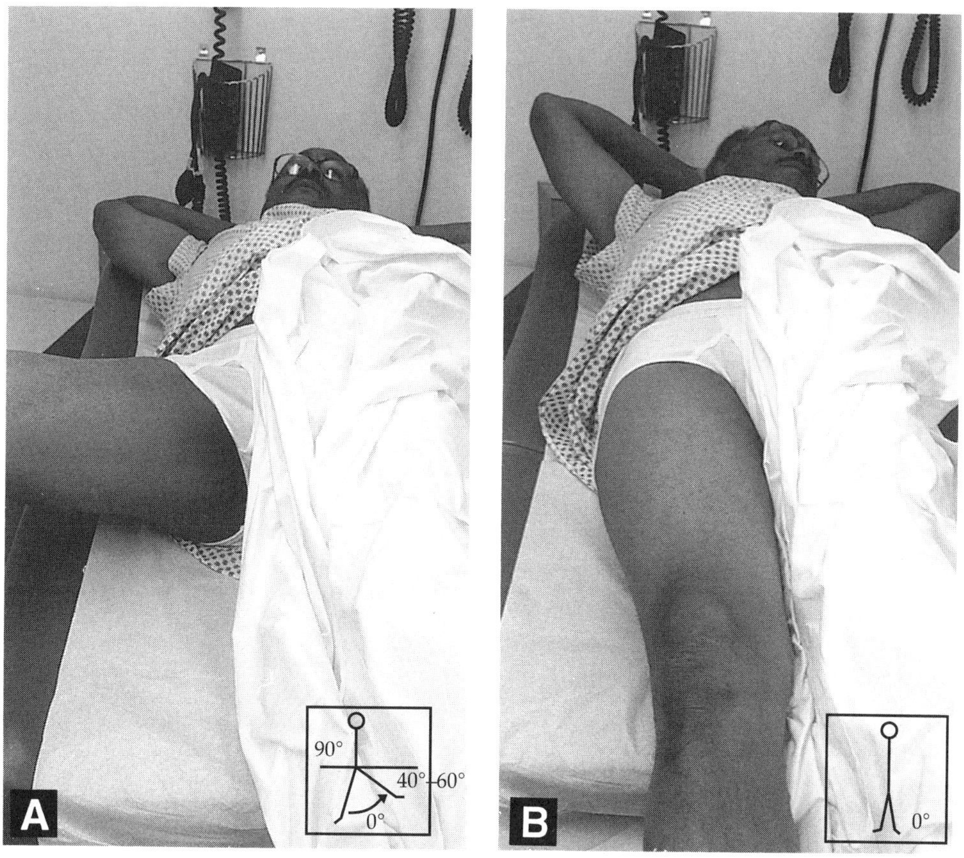

FIGURE 68.10.
A. Abduction. B. Adduction. Note that the adducted hip is in a rest or baseline position. (Reproduced with permission from Willms JL, Schneiderman H, Algranati PS. Physical Diagnosis: Bedside Evaluation of Diagnosis and Function. *Baltimore: Williams & Wilkins, 1994:400.)*

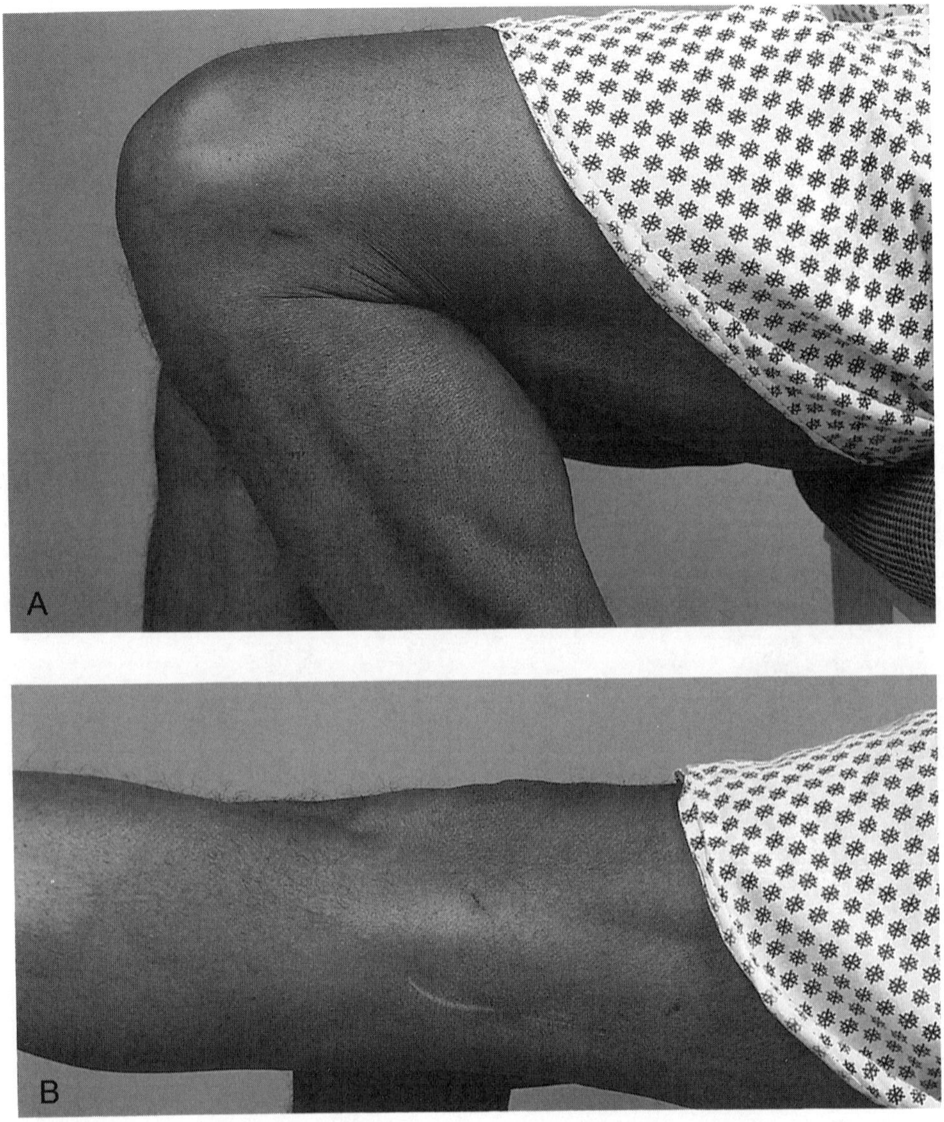

FIGURE 68.11.
Range of motion of the knee with the patient seated. ***A,*** *Flexion.* ***B,*** *Extension. (Reproduced with permission from Willms JL, Schneiderman H, Algranati PS.* Physical Diagnosis: Bedside Evaluation of Diagnosis and Function. *Baltimore: Williams & Wilkins, 1994:401.)*

ANKLE

The ankle joint is actually a complex set of articulations that allow movement in more than one plane. The articulation of the distal tibia and fibula with the talus allow for flexion (Fig. 68.12), whereas the transverse tarsal joint and the subtalar articulation allow rotation (Fig. 68.13). For adequate evaluation of ankle motion, the foot should be examined without either shoes or stockings.

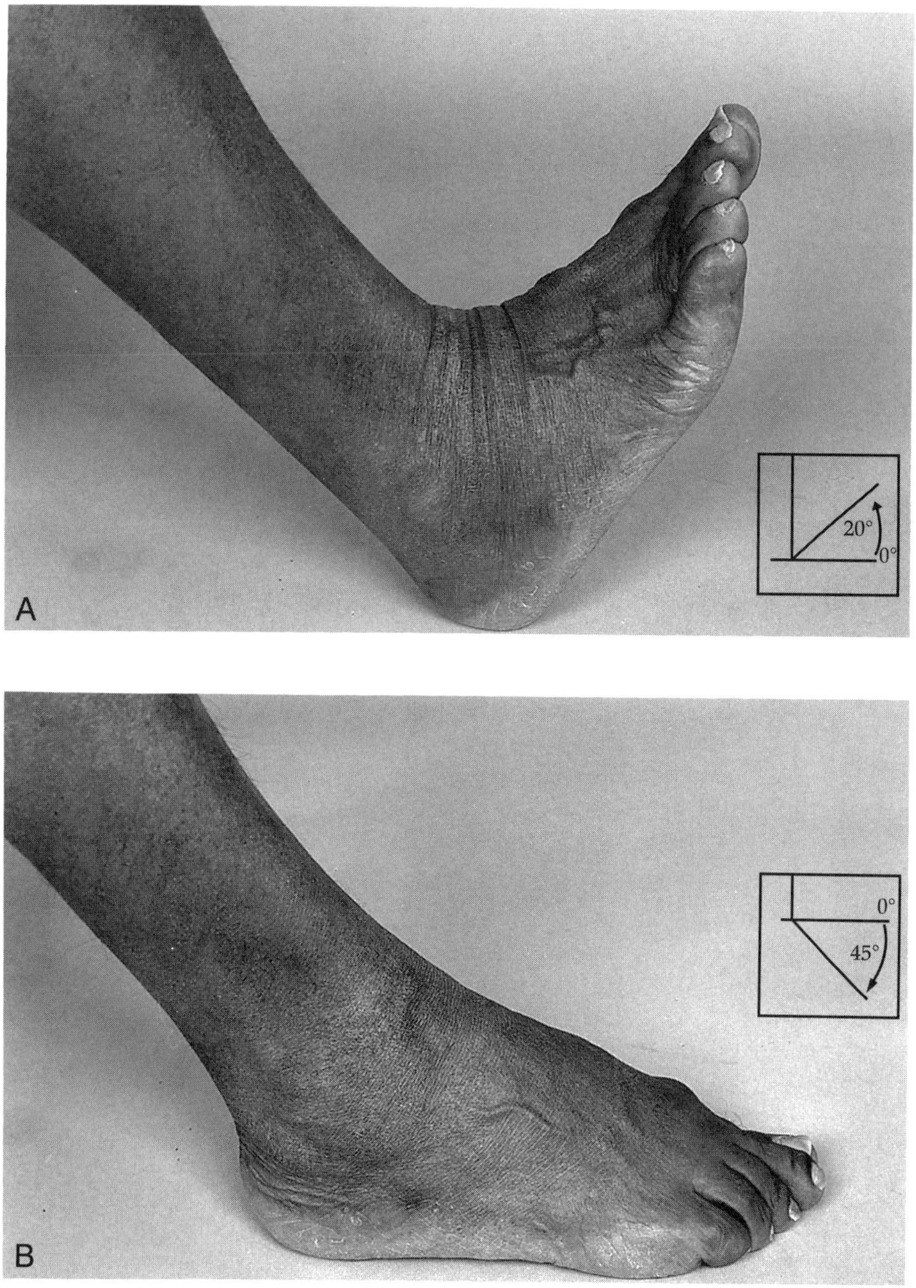

FIGURE 68.12.
*Dorsiflexion (**A**) and plantar flexion (**B**) of the ankle are performed with the foot in the midline. (Reproduced with permission from Willms JL, Schneiderman H, Algranati PS.* Physical Diagnosis: Bedside Evaluation of Diagnosis and Function. *Baltimore: Williams & Wilkins, 1994:402.)*

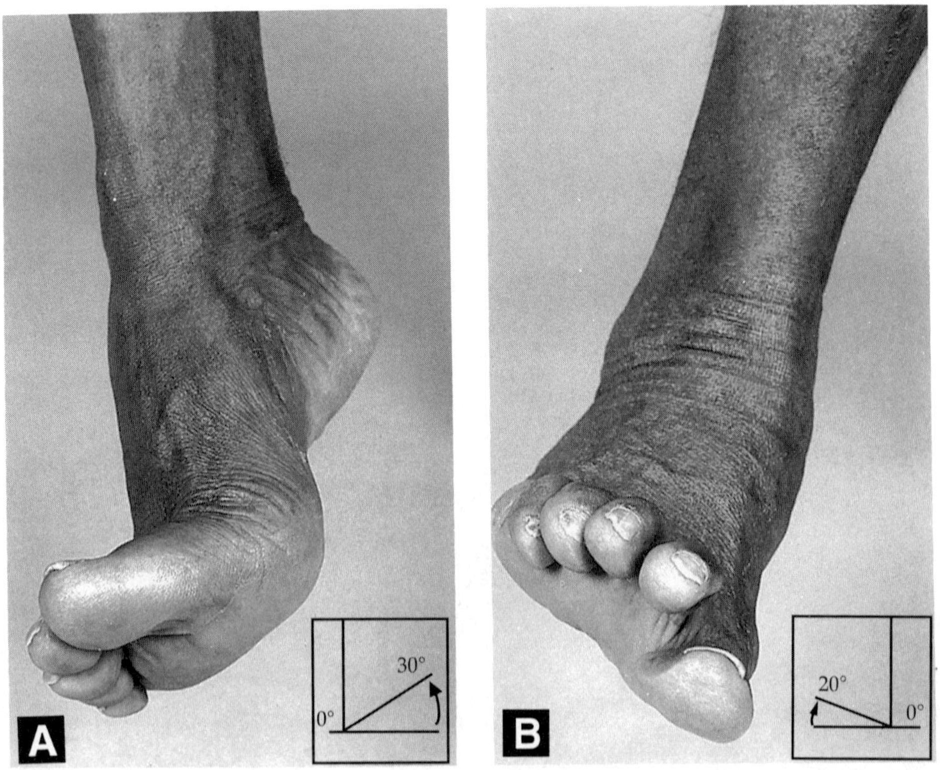

FIGURE 68.13.
*Shown are inversion (**A**) and eversion (**B**) testing of the foot. (Reproduced with permission from Willms JL, Schneiderman H, Algranati PS.* Physical Diagnosis: Bedside Evaluation of Diagnosis and Function. *Baltimore: Williams & Wilkins, 1994:403.)*

CERVICAL SPINE

Cervical spine mobility should be examined with care; if there is any possibility of instability, examination should be avoided. Conditions that suggest this possibility include trauma, rheumatoid arthritis, and ankylosing spondylitis.

SPINE

To test forward flexion of the spine, the patient should stand (without shoes) and bend forward as if to touch her toes, but without flexing the hips. Because a specific joint is not tested, a high degree of subjectivity is inherent in this test.

Normal Findings

Normal ranges of motion for commonly tested joints are shown in Table 68.1. Some variation may be seen from patient to patient and from one side of the body to the other. This variability should generally be in the range of 5 to 10° or less. Pain or resistance to motion should be minimal.

Selected Abnormal Findings

Significant restriction or asymmetry of motion suggests abnormality. Consultation should be based on the severity of the symptoms reported by the patient and the findings at evaluation.

TABLE 68.1. Expected Range of Motion for Selected Joints

JOINT	ACTION	RANGE
Shoulder	Abduction (frontal plane)	0–180°
	Flexion (forward)	0–180°
	Rotation (internal, external while upper arm is parallel to floor)	0–90°
Elbow	Flexion-extension	0–160°
	Pronation	0–90°
	Supination	0–90°
Wrist	Flexion-extension	90–70°
	Deviation (ulnar-radial)	50–20°
Fingers (Metacarpo-phalangeal)	Flexion-extension	90–30°
Hip	Extension	0–15°
	Flexion (with knee flexed)	0–120°
	Flexion (with knee extended)	0–90°
	Abduction	0–40°
	Internal rotation	0–40°
	External rotation	0–45°
Knee	Hyperextension-flexion	−15–130°
Ankle	Plantar flexion-dorsiflexion	−45–20°
	Inversion-eversion	−30–20°
Cervical spine	Flexion	45°
	Extension	60°
	Rotation	60–80°
	Lateral bending	40°
Spine	Extension	0–30°
	Lateral motion	0–50°
	Trunk rotation	90°
	Low thoracic-lumbar rotation	30°

Special Notes

If the patient experiences more pain and resistance to motion performed actively rather than passively, the pain probably reflects extra-articular structures (muscle or tendons). Intra-articular sources of pain create symptoms that are constant regardless of the mechanism of motion.

When hip motion is measured, it is important to keep the pelvis and spine fixed to avoid compensatory mobility in these structures that might be confused with mobility of the hip itself. When mobility of the thoracic and lumbar spine is being evaluated, the examiner should look for rotation that accompanies forward bending. This is a sensitive indicator of scoliosis.

When active joint motion cannot be accomplished but passive range is normal, the joint should be exonerated and muscular or neural function implicated.

Suggested Readings

Andrews JR, Wilk KE, Satterwhite YE, et al. Physical examination of the thrower's elbow. *J Orthop Sports Phys Ther* 1993;17:296.

Boublik M, Hawkins RJ. Clinical examination of the shoulder complex. *J Orthop Sports Phys Ther* 1993;18:379.

Cipriano JJ. *Photographic Manual of Regional Orthopaedic and Neurological Tests.* 2nd ed. Baltimore: Williams & Wilkins, 1991:221.

McGregor AH, McCarthy ID, Hughes SP. Motion characteristics of the lumbar spine in the normal population. *Spine* 1995;20:2421.

Robinson ME, O'Connor PD, Shirley FR, et al. Intrasubject reliability of spinal range of motion and velocity determined by video motion analysis. *Phys Ther* 1993; 73:626.

Sapira JD. *The Art and Science of Bedside Diagnosis*. Baltimore: Williams & Wilkins, 1990:417.

Willms JL, Schneiderman H, Algranati PS. *Physical Diagnosis: Bedside Evaluation of Diagnosis and Function*. Baltimore: Williams & Wilkins, 1994:387.

Chapter 69

TRIGGER POINT INJECTION

Musculoskeletal pain frequently radiates, or is referred to, areas quite distant from the source of the nociceptive signal. On occasion, a "trigger point" may be identified that induces or reproduces the patient's symptoms. Variously called trigger points, spots, zones, or areas, these hypersensitive areas overlie muscles and induce spasm and pain. Trigger points are frequently seen in myofascial pain syndromes and fibromyalgia. Trigger points may be found throughout the body but are most common in the abdominal wall, back, and pelvic floor when pelvic pain is the symptom. When present, trigger points may be treated by injection of steroids or local anesthetics or by "spray-and-stretch" techniques.

Equipment

- Single-agent local anesthetic such as lidocaine (0.5–1% solution, without epinephrine), procaine (1%), chloroprocaine (2%), or bupivacaine (0.125% or 0.25%)
- 22-gauge needle (1-inch to 1.5-inch) or an 18-gauge needle if a multidose vial is used
- 2.5–10 mL syringe
- Skin cleansing solution
- Alcohol wipes
- Sterile gloves (preferred but optional)
- Ice or ethyl chloride spray (optional)
- Skin marking pencil (optional)

Training/Credentialing

No special credentialing needed; office procedure only.

Coding

20550 Injection, tendon sheath, ligament, trigger points or ganglion cyst

Technique

The existence of a trigger point and the point of maximal tenderness must be established before injection therapy can be considered. Most trigger points are located at or near areas of moving or sliding muscle surfaces, but they are not limited to these locations. Gentle palpation over the various muscle groups of the body is done using the flat of the hand or the finger tips. A trigger point is often felt as an extremely taut band of muscle. Compression of this site elicits local tenderness and often reproduces the referred pain. The site of maximal tenderness should be noted and can be marked with a skin marking pencil.

The patient should be made comfortable and warned that the process of injection may briefly increase the referred pain. If this occurs, the increase will pass almost immediately. The skin over the point of maximal tenderness should be disinfected using a skin disinfecting agent or an alcohol wipe. Ice or a spray-type topical anesthetic (e.g., ethyl chloride) may be used to numb the skin before needle insertion. The skin should be held taut and the needle inserted smartly at an acute angle to minimize discomfort. Skin tension should be maintained to minimize bleeding.

A 22-gauge needle is selected for trigger point injection because of the amount of movement within tissue often required to probe for and block a taut muscle bundle. Thinner needles may bend or break under these circumstances. The length of the needle should be sufficient to allow the entire trigger point to be reached without indenting the skin or having the hub at the skin surface. The former unduly distorts landmarks and findings, and the latter prevents the possibility of a lost needle should the needle break or become separated from the hub during the injection maneuvers.

Once the needle has been inserted beneath the skin, the tip should be used as a probe to identify the taut band of muscle responsible for the patient's symptoms. Injection will be less successful if this band is not identified and specifically injected. With the needle at or in the taut muscle band, the syringe is aspirated to ensure against intravascular injection and a small amount (0.5–2 mL) of anesthetic agent is injected. The needle should be withdrawn slightly and then be moved from side to side of this original location, repeating the injection sequence (Fig. 69.1). No more than 10 mL of any anesthetic agent should be used.

The most common complications of trigger point injection are local ecchymoses and a toxic reaction to the anesthetic agent. The latter is best avoided by strictly limiting the total dose given. Infection is rare if the skin is first disinfected and areas of frank infection avoided.

Superficial trigger points may also be treated with a "spray-and-stretch" technique. To use this technique, the trigger point is identified in the same manner as for injection. The area overlying the trigger point is sprayed with a coolant or freezing spray (e.g., ethyl chloride) for several seconds and the muscle is forcibly stretched by passive extension. This may also be augmented by aggressive massage of the affected muscle. This technique is less specific and may be best applied by someone trained in physical therapy or rehabilitative medicine.

Normal Findings

Normal muscle should not be tender on firm compression and does not contain taut bands. Trigger points often respond immediately to therapy, thereby providing direct feedback to confirm the diagnosis. Response to trigger point injection routinely persists longer than the duration of action of the anesthetic agent used. This frequently extends to permanent relief after only one or two injections.

Trigger points may be inactivated by one of several mechanisms: mechanical disrup-

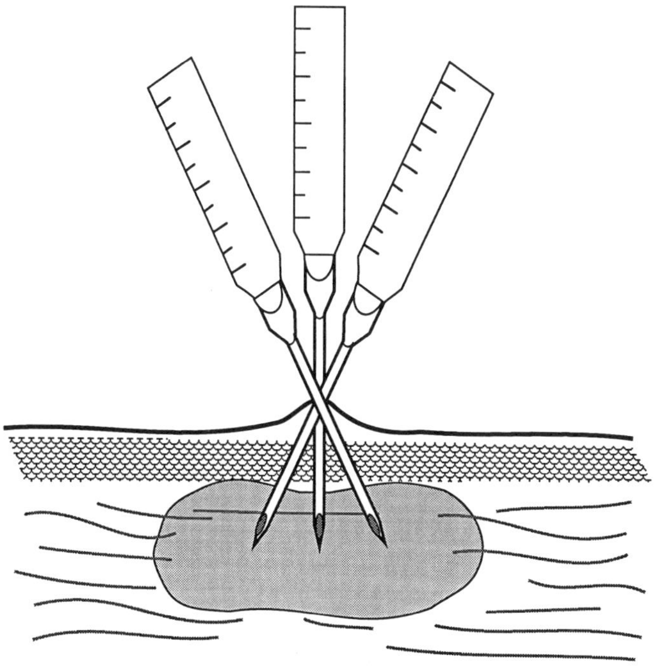

FIGURE 69.1.
A zone of infiltration, including the trigger point and an area immediately surrounding it, should be created by injecting small amounts of anesthetic agent in multiple locations.

tion of abnormal muscle fibers; dilution of nerve-sensitizing substances; depolarization block of nerve fibers by potassium liberated from muscle cells; local vasodilation; interruption of neural feed-back; and focal necrosis. The exact mechanism remains unknown.

Selected Abnormal Findings

Trigger points may occur in skin, ligaments, or periosteum in addition to muscles themselves.

Special Notes

Trigger points may occur to either men or women and at any age but are most common in sedentary middle-age women. The diagnosis of a trigger point is established solely on clinical grounds. No laboratory or imaging studies are available to assist in the diagnosis.

When possible trigger points are evaluated in the lower abdominal wall, care must be taken to separate the origin of the identified tenderness. This is especially true during bimanual pelvic examination. It should be apparent that tenderness is arising from the abdominal wall and not the uterus, adnexa, bladder, or bowel. To aid in this differentiation, ask the patient to lift her head and shoulders off the table or raise her heels with her legs held straight. Pain arising from the abdominal wall will worsen; visceral pain may improve.

Long-term relief may be enhanced through the use of passive stretching, the application of heat or ice, or transcutaneous electrical nerves stimulation (TENS).

Suggested Readings

Adelman A. Abdominal pain in the primary care setting. *J Fam Pract* 1987;25:27.

Bonica JJ. Management of myofascial pain syndromes in general practice. *JAMA* 1957;146:732.

Campbell SM. Regional myofascial pain syndromes. *Rheum Dis Clin North Am* 1989; 15:31.

Carlson CR, Okeson JP, Falace DA, et al. Reduction of pain and EMG activity in the masseter region by trapezius trigger point injection. *Pain* 1993;55:397.

Cheshire WP, Abashian SW, Mann JD. Botulinum toxin in the treatment of myofascial pain syndrome. *Pain* 1994;59:65.

Fine PG. Myofascial trigger point pain in children. *J Pediatrics* 1987;111:547.

Fricton JR. Myofascial pain. *Baillières Clin Rheumatol* 1994;8:857.

Garnett JB. Intercostal neuralgia as a cause of abdominal pain and tenderness. *Surg Gynecol Obstet* 1926;42:625.

Garvey TA, Marks MR, Wiesel SW. A prospective, randomized, double-blind evaluation of trigger-point injection therapy for low-back pain. *Spine* 1989;14:962.

Gerwin RD. Neurobiology of the myofascial trigger point. *Baillières Clin Rheumatol* 1994;8:747.

Graff-Radford SB, Reeves JL, Baker RL, et al. Effects of transcutaneous electrical nerve stimulation on myofascial pain and trigger point sensitivity. *Pain* 1989;37:1.

Hong CZ. Lidocaine injection versus dry needling to myofascial trigger point. The importance of the local twitch response. *Am J Phys Med Rehab* 1994;73:256.

Hopwood MB, Abram SE. Factors associated with failure of trigger point injections. *Clin J Pain* 1994;10:227.

Ingber RS. Iliopsoas myofascial dysfunction: a treatable cause of "failed" low back syndrome. *Arch Phys Med Rehab* 1989;70:382.

Ling FW, Slocumb JC. Use of trigger point injections in chronic pelvic pain. *Obstet Gynecol Clin North Am* 1993;20:809.

Maigne JY, Maigne R. Trigger point of the posterior iliac crest: painful iliolumbar ligament insertion or cutaneous dorsal ramus pain? An anatomic study. *Arch Phys Med Rehab* 1991;72:734.

McClaflin RR. Myofascial pain syndrome. Primary care strategies for early intervention. *Postgrad Med* 1994;96:56.

Njoo KH, Van der Does E. The occurrence and inter-rater reliability of myofascial trigger points in the quadratus lumborum and gluteus medius: a prospective study in non-specific low back pain patients and controls in general practice. *Pain* 1994;58:317.

Padamsee M, Mehta N, White GE. Trigger point injection: a neglected modality in the treatment of TMJ dysfunction. *J Pedodont* 1987;2:72.

Phero JC, Raj PP, McDonald JS. Transcutaneous electrical nerve stimulation and myoneural injection therapy for management of chronic myofascial pain. *Dent Clin North Am* 1987;31:703.

Simons DG. Trigger point origin of musculoskeletal chest pain. *South Med J* 1990; 83:262.

Skootsky SA, Jaeger B, Oye RK. Prevalence of myofascial pain in general internal medicine practice. *West J Med* 1989;151:157.

Slocumb JC. Neurologic factors in chronic pelvic pain: trigger points and the abdominal pelvic pain syndrome. *Am J Obstet Gynecol* 1984;149:536.

Theobald GW. The relief and prevention of referred pain. *J Obstet Gynecol Br Eur* 1949;56:447.

Travell JC, Simons DG. *Myofascial Pain and Dysfunction: The Trigger Point Manual.* Baltimore: Williams & Wilkins, 1983.

Wolfe F, Simons DG, Fricton J, et al. The fibromyalgia and myofascial pain syndromes: a preliminary study of tender points and trigger points in persons with fibromyalgia, myofascial pain syndrome and no disease. *J Rheumatol* 1992;9:944.

Section IX

UROLOGIC PROCEDURES

Chapter 70

CIRCUMCISION (NEWBORN AND INFANT)

Although debate lingers about the advisability of newborn circumcision, many patients continue to request this procedure. It remains the most commonly performed surgical procedure (for males) in the United States; more than 60% of newborn males are circumcised. In many locations, this service is performed by the obstetrician, either in the hospital before the baby is discharged or in the office soon after. Some parents request that the physician assist with, or perform, this procedure as a part of a religious ritual. When this is the case, the medical aspects of the procedure may vary slightly, but the basic principles remain unchanged.

Equipment

- Infant restraint board ("papoose" board)
- Sterile gloves
- Sterile drape (one with a small fenestration or several drapes)
- Skin preparation materials (e.g., povidone–iodine and 70% isopropyl alcohol)
- Sterile gauze pads (2-inch × 2-inch or 4-inch × 4-inch)
- 3 hemostats (small tips, 2 curved, 1 straight)
- Small scissors or scalpel (#10 or #11 blade)
- Flexible blunt probe
- Gomco clamp (1.1–1.45 cm) or Plastibell (1.3–1.6 cm) or Mogen clamp (for clamp methods)
- Sterile safety pin, clip, or skin staple (optional)
- Viscous lidocaine (2–5%) or 1% lidocaine without epinephrine, 1-mL syringe, 27-gauge needle for dorsal penile nerve block
- Petrolatum (Vaseline) gauze
- Silver nitrate stick or Monsel's solution
- Small suture (3-0 or 4-0 absorbable) and needle holder (available)

Training/Credentialing

No special credentialing is needed if performed in the office. If the procedure is performed in a hospital, the institution may require specific credentials; these vary by location.

Coding

54150	Circumcision, using clamp or other device; newborn
54152	except newborn
54160	Circumcision, surgical excision other than clamp, device, or dorsal slit; newborn
54161	except newborn
00920	Anesthesia for procedure on male external genitalia; not otherwise specified

Technique

Before circumcision is considered, the possibility of contraindications should be evaluated (Table 70.1). All circumcision techniques begin with the undiapered newborn restrained on an infant (papoose) board. The penis should be inspected to identify the meatus and its location on the glans. Once the anatomy has been confirmed to be normal, anesthesia by way of topical lidocaine or dorsal block (see below) may be administered, if desired. The skin of the penis and the surrounding areas should be disinfected by any suitable method, and sterile drapes should be placed to provide a surgical field.

The specific technique used varies with the type of instrument chosen. Although there are theoretical differences among the three commonly used methods, the final choice is generally based on the personal preference and experience of the operator.

Both the GOMCO clamp and Plastibell begin in the same way: the tip of a hemostat is used to grasp the edge of the foreskin just dorsal to the 3 and 9 o'clock positions (dorsal is the 12 o'clock position). A hemostat or flexible probe is inserted just under the foreskin and swept laterally to bluntly lyse any adhesions present (Fig. 70.1). Care must be taken to avoid disrupting either the ventral attachment or the coronal reflection. The foreskin is tented away from the glans. A straight hemostat inserted along the dorsal line and clamped to a depth of one-third–one-half of the way to the coronal

TABLE 70.1. Contraindications to Newborn Circumcision

Age older than 6–8 weeks (relative)
Age younger than 12 hours
Ambiguous genitalia
Hypospadias
Illness
Less than 1 hour postprandial
Possibility of blood dyscrasia
Prematurity
Undescended testicles (relative)

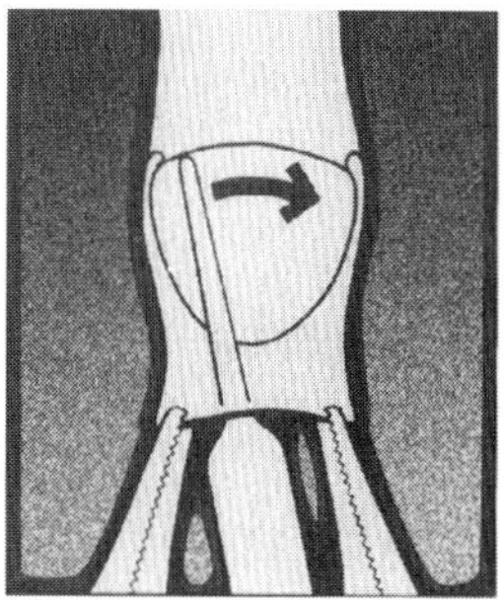

FIGURE 70.1.
After two hemostats are applied to the foreskin, gently separate the adhesions using either the pointed or spatula end of the probe. (Permission to reproduce this material has been granted by the owner, Hollister, Libertyville, IL 60048.)

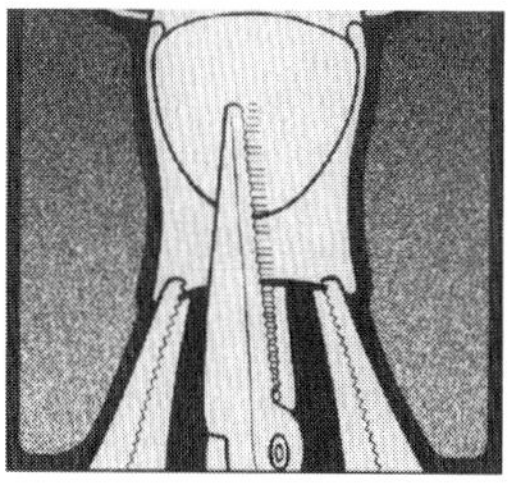

FIGURE 70.2.
Two hemostats should be used to spread the foreskin and another should be used to crush the foreskin where the dorsal slit is to be made. The foreskin should be crushed to a length that is approximately the same as the width of the glans. This can be visualized while the foreskin is being pulled and dissected. (Permission to reproduce this material has been granted by the owner, Hollister, Libertyville, IL 60048.)

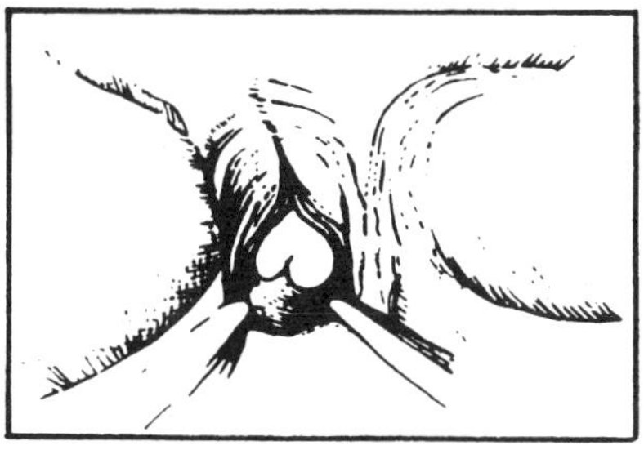

FIGURE 70.3.
The foreskin is incised along the dorsal aspect to a point one-third–one-half of the distance to the coronal reflection. (Used with permission by GOMCO Division of Allied Healthcare Products, St. Louis, MO 63110.)

reflection (Fig. 70.2). The hemostat is allowed to crush the tissue for approximately 1 minute before it is removed; the crushed tissue is then incised by using scissors (Fig. 70.3) . The glans must be avoided during both the clamping and incision process. The foreskin is then retracted, and any further adhesions are removed. The dorsal incision may be extended if needed by repeating the crush and cut process. Depending on the instrument preferred, the procedure may then be complete.

GOMCO CLAMP

The GOMCO clamp consists of a base plate, arm, bell, and thumbscrew (Fig. 70.4) . The bell of the GOMCO clamp is placed under the foreskin, over the glans. This placement may be facilitated by upward traction on the edges of the foreskin grasped by hemostats and by downward pressure on the stem of the bell (Fig. 70.5) . When in a correct position, the bell should rest against the corona.

The bell and foreskin must now be inserted through the opening in the baseplate of the clamp. This may be facilitated by reaching through the opening with a hemostat to help guide the foreskin or by placing a sterile safety pin, clip, or skin staple to hold the edges of the flaps together. These instruments, if used, should hold the distal foreskin in close approximation to the shaft of the bell. When the bell is passed through the baseplate, the foreskin must be brought completely through the opening and evenly drawn up on all sides. The entire length of the dorsal incision must be above the baseplate opening. The stem of the bell is placed into the top of the clamp, and the

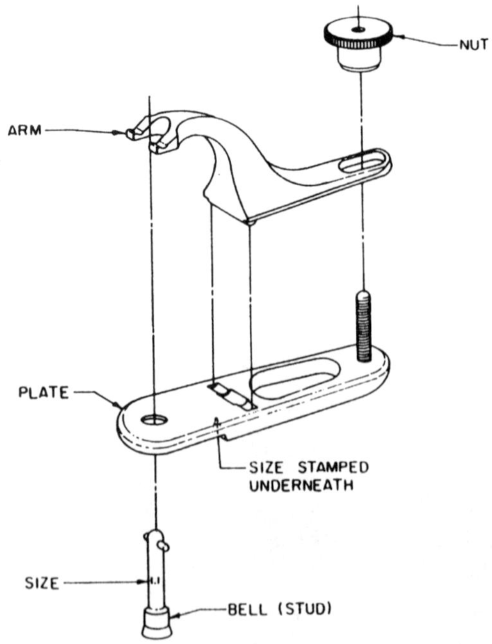

FIGURE 70.4.
The parts of the Gomco circumcision clamp are shown. (Used with permission by GOMCO Division of Allied Health-care Products, St. Louis, MO 63110.)

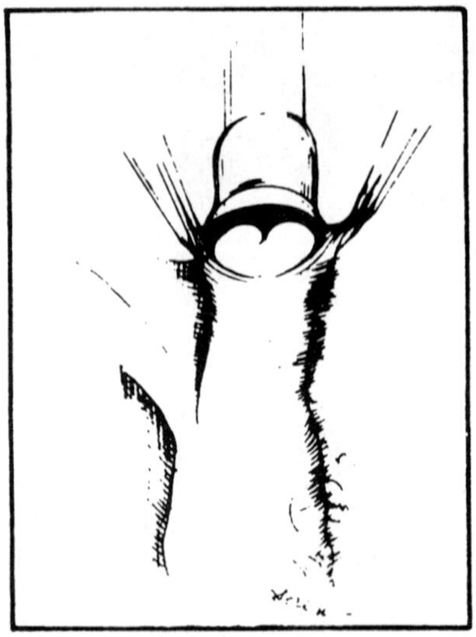

FIGURE 70.5.
The foreskin is drawn up and over the bell of the Gomco clamp using small hemostats for traction. The bell acts to protect the glans of the penis. (Used with permission by GOMCO Division of Allied Healthcare Products, St. Louis, MO 63110.)

thumb screw is gently tightened. The foreskin, bell, and shaft of the penis are again inspected before the final tightening is performed.

A scalpel is used to excise all of the tissue above the baseplate of the clamp (Fig. 70.6). Care must be used to completely incise all layers of tissue and to completely remove any tissue devitalized by the clamp. The GOMCO clamp is loosened and the bell is freed. The foreskin is freed from the bell by gentle traction using a gauze sponge. Hemostasis must be assured and may be assisted by pressure, the application of Monsel's solution, or a fine suture. A petrolatum gauze dressing should be placed and the newborn diapered.

PLASTIBELL

After the foreskin has been dissected free of the glans, the Plastibell string is placed as a loop near the base of the penis. The bell is placed over the glans in much the same way as in the GOMCO technique. The foreskin is pulled upward, ensuring even place-

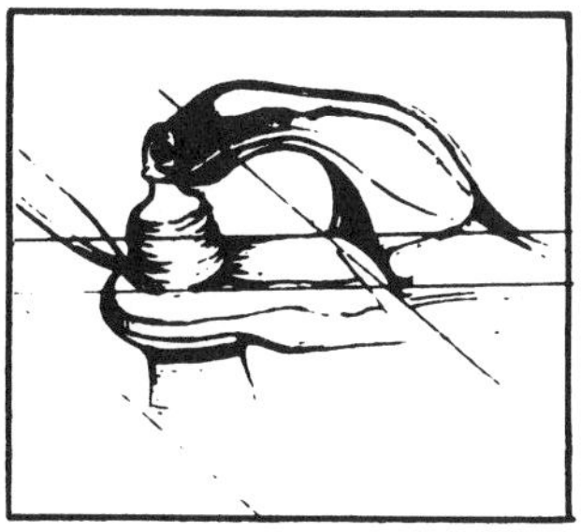

FIGURE 70.6.
When the excess tissue is incised, care must be taken that the scalpel is flush and perpendicular to the bell (parallel to the base plate of the clamp). (Used with permission by GOMCO Division of Allied Healthcare Products, St. Louis, MO 63110.)

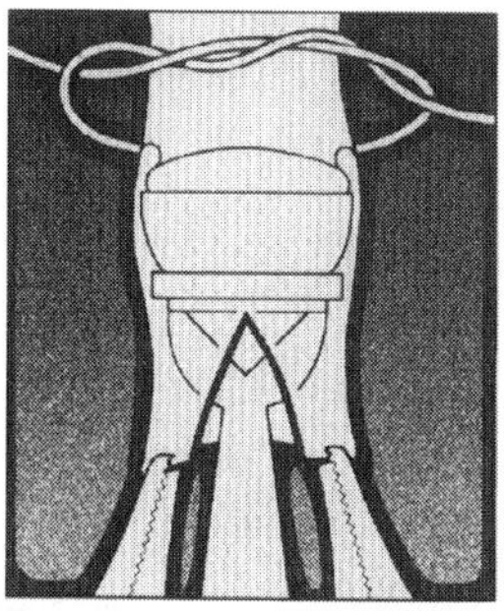

FIGURE 70.7.
The appropriate-sized bell should be placed over the glans so that it prevents undue pressure on ventral vessels. Too small a bell may injure the glans. Too large a bell may eventually slip over the corona and onto the shaft, possibly causing edema and damage to skin and underlying tissue. Apex of dorsal slit should be distal to the bell's groove. The foreskin should be pulled only enough to position the apex of the dorsal slit distal to groove. If excessively pulled, the foreskin may later draw the bell too tightly against or over the glans onto the shaft. Approximately 1.0 cm should separate the sulcus and the groove of the bell where the ligature will be applied. (Permission to reproduce this material has been granted by the owner, Hollister, Libertyville, IL 60048.)

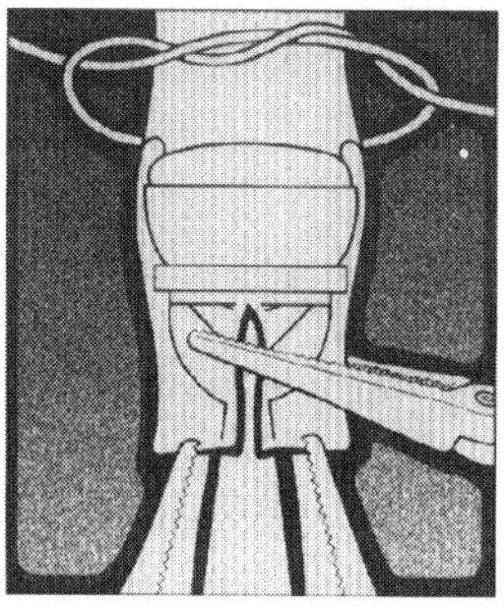

FIGURE 70.8.
To hold the bell while tying ligature, the third hemostat may be used to clamp foreskin to handle. If the slit is too long, the two hemostats should be crossed over each other to hold the bell in place. (Permission to reproduce this material has been granted by the owner, Hollister, Libertyville, IL 60048.)

ment and positioning that leave the groove in the bell well below the apex of the dorsal slit (Fig. 70.7). The bell should move freely over the glans. These relationships are maintained with hemostats and the string brought into position, resting in the groove of the bell (Fig. 70.8). The string should be pulled firmly and all aspects rechecked before the string is tightened maximally. Tension on the string is maintained for at least 30 seconds; a square knot is then placed.

Scissors are used to cut the foreskin just above the level of the string; care should be taken not to cut too close to the string or to damage the string itself (Fig. 70.9). The string is trimmed and the stem of the Plastibell broken off at its junction with the bell (Fig. 70.10). Hemostasis should be confirmed; as with the GOMCO technique, a dressing may be applied if desired. The bell may be expected to slough off in 5–8 days or it may be removed by cutting the ligature after at least 36 hours.

MOGEN CLAMP

When the Mogen clamp is used, the infant is restrained and inspected and the skin is prepared as for the other two methods. Hemostats are used to pull the foreskin upward,

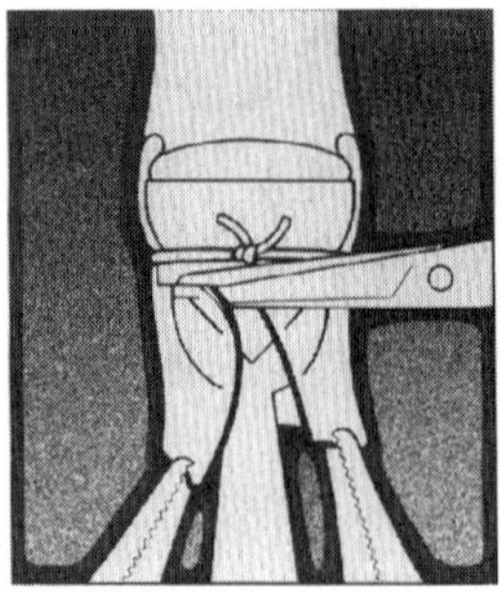

FIGURE 70.9.
After the ligature has been positioned around the bell's groove, the ligature should be drawn very tightly so it compresses foreskin into groove. A surgeon's knot is used for tying and the excess ligature is snipped off. An unobstructed urethral meatus should be visible. The foreskin is trimmed off using the outer ridge of bell as a cutting guide. Adequate traction on the foreskin should be maintained, and as much tissue as possible should be trimmed to reduce the amount of remaining necrotic tissue. If ligature is not tightly secured, oozing will occur, the bell may fall off, or the line of excision will be incomplete, thereby requiring subsequent removal of tissue tags. (Permission to reproduce this material has been granted by the owner, Hollister, Libertyville, IL 60048.)

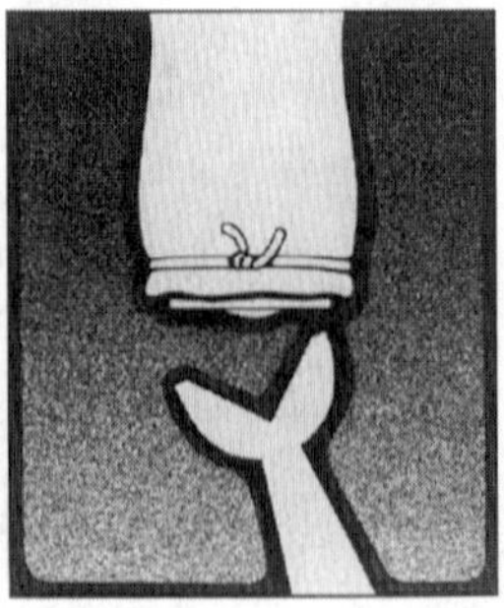

FIGURE 70.10.
The bell handle should be broken off and discarded. With the bell and ligature left in place, an unobstructed urethral meatus should be visible. No dressing is necessary. The rim of tissue under and distal to the ligature will become necrotic and separate with the bell in 5–8 days, leaving a clean, healed line of excision. If the physician desires, the bell can be removed before the infant is sent home by cutting the ligature at the knot. This may be done 36–48 hours after circumcision depending on the physician's evaluation.

and the tip of the penis is transilluminated to identify the glans. The Mogen clamp is applied with its curved side toward the glans. It is slid into place over the foreskin from dorsal to ventral in a horizontal plane, with adjustment so that the desired amount of skin is distal to the clamp. The clamp is angled so that more skin is removed from the dorsal side of the penis. The glans is again inspected and palpated to ensure it is clear of the clamp; the clamp is then tightened. A scalpel is used to cut the foreskin flush with the surface of the clamp. The clamp is left in place for roughly 1 minute before it is removed. The sides of the foreskin are separated by downward traction, inspected, and dressed. A gauze sponge may be used to help separate the sides of the foreskin if necessary, although excess bleeding may be encountered if too much force is used.

FREEHAND TECHNIQUE

The foreskin may be excised using simple surgical techniques familiar to most surgeons. The dissection of any adhesions, the exposure of the reflection for the foreskin from the glands, and the excision of the foreskin itself are well within the skills of most surgeons. Because of the small size of the tissues present, the greater risk for bleeding, and the experience needed to use the freehand method, the techniques described above are better suited in most cases.

POSTOPERATIVE CARE

After circumcision, the infant should be observed for at least 4 hours and should void before being released. The petrolatum gauze should be removed after 24 hours or if it becomes soiled. Petrolatum jelly should be applied at each diaper change until healing has occurred (about 7–10 days). At each diaper change the penile skin should be retracted to prevent adhesion formation.

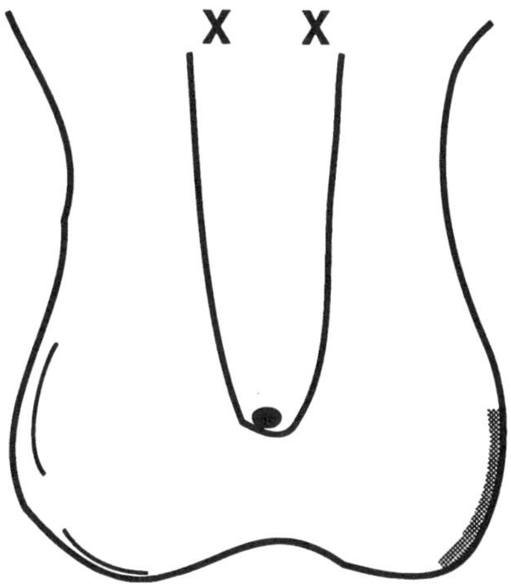

FIGURE 70.11.
Location of insertion points for dorsal penile block.

DORSAL PENILE BLOCK

Dorsal penile block is generally quick, safe, and effective. In addition to the contraindications to circumcision noted in Table 70.1, a family history of intolerance or allergy to local anesthetics should prompt reconsideration. Dorsal penile block is begun by identifying the depth of the root of the penis. This is easily accomplished by palpation using the index finger. The root is usually located 0.75–1 cm beneath the skin surface and has the size and consistency of a large blueberry.

By using aseptic technique, the penis is placed on slight downward traction and the needle inserted at the 2 o'clock position near the base (Fig. 70.11) . The needle is passed in an posteromedial direction to a depth of 3–5 mm beneath the skin, roughly 5–7 mm distal to the penile root near where the dorsal nerves branch. The tip of the needle should move freely if it is correctly located outside of the corpus cavernosum. The syringe should be aspirated to prevent intravenous injection, and 0.2–0.4 mL of anesthetic should be injected. The procedure is repeated at the 10 o'clock position. A single needle insertion point in the dorsal midline may also be used if desired. The total anesthetic dose should remain less than 0.8 mL. Full anesthesia will be achieved in 2–4 minutes.

Special Notes

When a probe or hemostat is initially inserted under the foreskin to release adhesions, care must be taken to avoid inadvertent entry into the urethra rather than the intended tissue plane. Tenting the foreskin before lateral movement of the probe or the opening of the hemostat helps ensure the correct location.

To guard against the possibility of penile rotation distorting anatomic relationships, the ventral raphe should be identified and the dorsal clamp placed directly opposite.

Persistent bleeding after circumcision suggests the presence of hemophilia. Silver nitrate should not be used for hemostasis because of the risk for permanent staining of the tissues.

If the Mogen clamp is left in place for more than a minute, the sides of the foreskin may become fused and difficult to separate. When the Mogen clamp is removed, a small ventral "dog ear" will often be present. This "dog ear" will partially necrose and heal without cosmetic defect.

Electrosurgical devices should never be used in conjunction with any of the clamp-based procedures. A bulb syringe should be kept near during circumcision as a protection against aspiration should the newborn regurgitate.

Suggested Readings

American Academy of Pediatrics. Committee statements: reports of the task force on circumcision. *Pediatrics* 1989;84:388.

Anonymous. Medical indications for childhood circumcision. *Drug Ther Bull* 1993; 31:99.

Anonymous. Neonatal circumcision revisited. Fetus and Newborn Committee, Canadian Paediatric Society. *Can Med Assoc J* 1996;154:769.

Baskin LS, Canning DA, Snyder HM, et al. Treating complications of circumcision. *Pediatr Emerg Care* 1996;12:62.

Benini F, Johnston CC, Faucher D, et al. Topical anesthesia during circumcision in newborn infants. *JAMA* 1993;270:850.

Craig JC, Grigor WG, Knight JF. Acute obstructive uropathy—a rare complication of circumcision. *Eur J Pediatr* 1994;153:369.

Flowers SW, Banks J. Anesthesia for neonatal circumcision aids hazard detection. *Am J Obstet Gynecol* 1992;167:1480.

Fontaine P, Toffler WL. Dorsal penile nerve block for newborn circumcision. *Am Fam Phys* 1991;43:1327.

Goodman JD. Plastibell circumcision. *J Roy Coll Surg Edinb* 1993;38:179.

Holman JR, Lewis EL, Ringler RL. Neonatal circumcision techniques. *Am Fam Phys* 1995;52:511.

Holton ME. Comparison of newborn circumcision pain to calcaneal heel puncture pain: is newborn circumcision pain control clinically warranted? *J Am Osteo Assoc* 1996;96:31.

Kaweblum YA, Press S, Kogan L, et al. Circumcision using the Mogen clamp. *Clin Pediatr* 1984;23:679.

Kirya C, Werthmann MW. Neonatal circumcision and penile dorsal nerve block—a painless procedure. *J Pediatr* 1978;92:998.

Kunz V. Circumcision and meatotomy. *Prim Care Clin Office Pract* 1986;13:513.

Lazim TR, Zainol J. A simple device for circumcision. *J Roy Coll Surg Edinb* 1996;41:122.

Marsh SK, Archer TJ. Bipolar diathermy haemostasis during circumcision. *Br J Surg* 1995;82:533.

McConnell RS, Boston VE, Stewart RJ. Subcuticular suture in circumcision. *Br J Urol* 1993;71:622.

Mintz MR, Ricardo G. Clinical notes: dorsal penile nerve block for circumcision. *Clin Pediatr* 1989;28:590.

Niku SD, Stock JA, Kaplan GW. Neonatal circumcision. *Urol Clin North Am* 1995;22:57.

Poland L. Sounding board: the question of routine neonatal circumcision. *N Engl J Med* 1990;322:1312.

Reynolds RD. Use of the Mogen clamp for neonatal circumcision. *Am Fam Phys* 1996;54:177.

Robson WL, Leung AK. The circumcision question. *Postgrad Med* 1992;91:237.

Ryan CA, Finer NN. Changing attitudes and practices regarding local analgesia for newborn circumcision. *Pediatrics* 1994;94:230.

Schoen J. Sounding board: the status of circumcision of newborns. *N Engl J Med* 1990;322:1308.

Smith DJ, Hamdy FC, Chapple CR. An uncommon complication of circumcision. *Br J Urol* 1994;73:459.

Snellman LW, Stang HJ. Prospective evaluation of complications of dorsal penile nerve block for neonatal circumcision. *Pediatrics* 1995;95:705.

Spach DH, Stapleton AE, Staum WE. Lack of circumcision increases the risk of urinary tract infection in young men. *JAMA* 1992;267:679.

Strimling BS. Partial amputation of glans penis during Mogen clamp circumcision. *Pediatrics* 1996;97:906.

Wisniewski PM. Mogen circumcision utilizing transillumination. *Female Patient* 1992;17:29.

Wiswell TE. Routine neonatal circumcision: a reappraisal. *Am Fam Phys* 1990;41:859.

Wiswell TE. Circumcision—an update. *Curr Prob Pediatr* 1992;22:424.

Wiswell TE, Tencer HL, Welch CA, et al. Circumcision in children beyond the neonatal period. *Pediatrics* 1993;92:791.

Wolkomir MS. Technique for freehand newborn circumcision. *J Fam Pract* 1996; 42:447.

Zafar F, Thompson JN, Pati J, et al. Sutureless circumcision. *Br J Surg* 1993;80:859.

Chapter 71

OFFICE CYSTOURETHROSCOPY

Cystourethroscopy is useful for evaluating urinary incontinence, recurrent bladder infections, or hematuria.

Equipment

- Sterile gloves, antiseptic solution and sterile cotton balls, or skin preparation swabs
- Sterile urine specimen cup (with graduations)
- 1 L of sterile saline (intravenous fluid without glucose is generally used) at room temperature
- Absorbent underpads
- 2% Xylocaine jelly in mushroom-tipped syringe (optional)
- Cystoscope (direct viewing or with a 30° or greater down angle view; the latter is better for visualizing the trigone and ureteral openings)
- Fiberoptic light source (compatible with type of cystoscope used)
- Fiberoptic light cord
- Assistant (desirable)

Training/Credentialing

Moderate experience is required; it is best to have received advanced instruction or experience before the procedure is attempted alone. No special credentialing is needed for office procedure, but many hospitals or ambulatory surgery centers have special requirements for training or proficiency.

Coding

52000 Cystoscopy

Technique

Just before testing, the patient is asked to empty her bladder (in private and in her usual manner). The patient is examined (in the lithotomy position) and the external urinary meatus is cleansed with antiseptic solution. One to three milliliters of topical anesthetic, such as 2% Xylocaine, is introduced into the urethra. With sterile technique, a straight catheter is inserted. Any residual urine is caught, measured for volume, and sent for culture to detect occult infection.

The bladder is next filled with 100–200 mL of sterile saline. Filling should be gradual to avoid inducing bladder spasm. After the light guide is attached to both the cystoscopy and light source, the tip of the cystoscope is placed at the external meatus and gently inserted. The cystoscope should initially be inserted with a slight downward angle and then gently rotated under the symphysis. The bladder wall should be inspected throughout, along with the trigone and ureteral openings. The latter is facilitated by using a cystoscope with a downward viewing angle. A direct (forward-looking) cystoscope may be used to facilitate inspection of the internal sphincter (urethral–vesical junction).

After inspection, the patient may empty her bladder or the bladder may be drained by catheter, as desired.

Normal Findings

The epithelium of the urethra and bladder should be smooth and pink, without ulceration, exudates, hemorrhages, or excrescencies. The underlying vascular pattern is usually visible.

Selected Abnormal Findings

The trigone may become irritated just inside the urethral opening because of the passage of the cystoscope; this irritation must be differentiated from the more diffuse inflammation of trigonitis. Petechial hemorrhages in the bladder wall seen after the bladder is distended, emptied, and re-distended are characteristic of interstitial cystitis.

Suggested Readings

Ostergard DR, Bent AE, eds. *Urogynecology and Urodynamics*. 4th ed. Baltimore: Williams & Wilkins, 1996.

Scotti RJ, Ostergard DR, Guillaume AA, et al. Dynamic urethroscopy: predictive value in genuine stress incontinence. *J Reprod Med* 1990;35:772.

Chapter 72

SIMPLE URODYNAMICS

Bladder function may be measured without the use of specialized equipment or techniques.

Equipment

- 12 or 14 French straight catheter
- Sterile catheter tray (may be replaced by sterile gloves, antiseptic solution and sterile cotton balls, or skin preparation swabs)
- Sterile urine specimen cup (with graduations)
- Large catheter-tip syringe (without piston) or "Asepto" surgical irrigation syringe (without bulb)
- 1 L of sterile water or saline (intravenous fluid without glucose will suffice) at room temperature
- Intravenous tubing and measuring tape or ruler, or spinal manometer
- Absorbent underpads
- Commode or toilet
- Stop watch or watch that allows counting seconds
- 2% Xylocaine jelly in mushroom-tipped syringe (optional)
- Assistant (desirable)

Training/Credentialing

Minimal experience is required; it is best to have observed or assisted on a few measurements before attempting one alone. No special credentialing is needed; office procedure only.

Coding

51725	Simple cystometrogram
51736	Simple uroflowmetry

Technique

Just before testing, the patient is asked to empty her bladder (in private and in her usual manner). The patient is examined (in the lithotomy position) and the external urinary meatus is cleansed with antiseptic solution. If anesthesia is desired, 1–3 mL of topical anesthetic, such as 2% Xylocaine, is introduced into the urethra. With sterile technique, a straight catheter is inserted. Any residual urine is caught, measured for volume, and sent for culture for determination of occult infection.

The catheter-tip or irrigation syringe is attached to the catheter to act as a funnel to fill the bladder with sterile water or saline (Fig. 72.1). With the syringe held no more than 15 cm above the level of the symphysis, fluid is placed into the syringe with the catheter pinched off. Once the measured aliquot is in the syringe, it is allowed to flow by gravity into the bladder at a rate not to exceed 1–3 mL per second. This is often best accomplished in aliquots of 50 mL at a time. The patient is asked to report her first sensation of bladder fullness; the volume infused at that point is noted. Filling continues in 25-mL aliquots until the patient cannot tolerate more; this volume is recorded as the maximal bladder capacity. Any upward movement of the fluid column, intense sensation of urgency, or leakage around the catheter is abnormal, suggests detrusor instability, and should be noted.

The catheter is then removed, and the patient is asked to cough several times. Urinary leakage at the time of cough should be noted. Leakage that occurs immediately after, is prolonged, or is of large volume suggests detrusor instability. Elevation of the urethra (Bonney test) may be attempted to evaluate the effects of urethral support when stress incontinence is demonstrated. These maneuvers may be repeated in the standing position for persons who have no urinary loss while supine.

More exact measurements of bladder function may be made by assembling intravenous tubing, a spinal manometer (or limb of extra tubing), and a three-way connector. In this configuration, filling proceeds as described above, with the exception that pressure inside the fluid column may be monitored and the presence of bladder contractions can be more easily detected and documented. When this greater degree of accuracy is required, many physicians prefer to proceed to formal urodynamics testing rather than commit to the additional tubing and time necessary to assemble this configuration.

Voiding may be assessed by filling the bladder with 200 mL of fluid and listening to the patient's voiding from outside a bathroom door or while the patient voids behind a screen. The duration of flow may be timed with a stop watch.

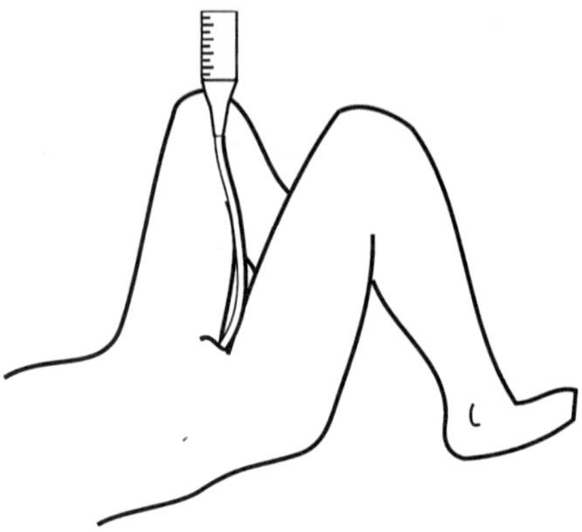

FIGURE 72.1.
Simple urodynamics testing may be done with the patient in the lithotomy position on a standard office examination table or hospital bed. A straight catheter is inserted into the bladder and attached to a catheter-tip syringe for filling.

TABLE 72.1. Anticipated Normal Values

Cystometrics	
Residual urine	< 50 mL
First sensation of fullness	150–200 mL
Maximal capacity	300–500 mL
Uroflowmetry (200 mL voided volume)	
Voiding time	< 20 sec

Normal Findings

Expected normal findings are shown in Table 72.1.

Selected Abnormal Findings

Difficulty passing the catheter or undue discomfort may indicate urethral stenosis. Very early first sensations and reduced total capacity may suggest a small-capacity, irritable bladder but may also be artificially induced by a filling rate that is too rapid or fluids that are too cold.

Bladder volumes greater than 600 mL indicate a denervated hypotonic bladder consistent with that seen in patients with diabetic neuropathy, multiple sclerosis, or neurologic injury.

Special Notes

Integral to urodynamics is an assessment of the relevant pelvic anatomy. This includes the degree of estrogen effect present in vaginal tissues, the support of the anterior and posterior vaginal walls, the presence of uterine descent or an enterocele (as applicable), and a measurement of urethral mobility, such as the Q-tip test.

Suggested Readings

Abrams P, Blaivas JG, Stanton SL, et al. The standardization of terminology of lower urinary tract function produced by the International Continence Society Committee on Standardization of Terminology. *Scand J Urol Nephrol* 1988;114:5.

American College of Obstetricians and Gynecologists. Urinary Incontinence. ACOG technical bulletin 213. Washington, DC: ACOG, 1995.

Bradley WE, Timm GW. Cystometry VI. Interpretation. *Urology* 1976;7:231.

Cardozo L, Stanton SL. Genuine stress incontinence and detrusor instability: a clinical and urodynamic review of 200 cases. *Br J Obstet Gynecol* 1980;87:184.

Consensus Conference. Urinary incontinence in adults. *JAMA* 1989;261:2685.

Fischer-Rasmussen W, Hansen RI, Stage P. Predictive values of diagnostic test in the evaluation of female urinary stress incontinence. *Acta Obstet Gynecol Scand* 1986;65:291.

Hebjorn JT, Andersen JT, Walter S, et al. Detrusor hyperreflexia. *Scand J Urol Nephrol* 1976;10:103.

Jarvis GJ, Hall S, Millar DR, et al. An assessment of urodynamic examination in incontinent women. *Br J Obstet Gynaecol* 1980;87:893.

Massey A, Abrams P. Urodynamic of the female lower urinary tract. *Urol Clin North Am* 1985;12:231.

Migliorini GD, Blenning PP. Bonney's test—fact or fiction. *Br J Obstet Gynecol* 1987;94:157.

Norton PA (ed). Urinary incontinence. *Clin Obstet Gynecol* 1990;33:293.

Ostergard DR, Bent AE, eds. *Urogynecology and Urodynamics.* 4th ed. Baltimore: Williams & Wilkins, 1996.

Ouslander J, Leach G, Staskin D. Simplified tests of lower urinary tract function in the evaluation of geriatric urinary incontinence. *J Am Geriatr Soc* 1989;37:706.

Sutherst JR, Brown MC. Comparison of single and multichannel cystometry in diagnosing bladder instability. *Br Med J* 1984;288:1720.

Urinary Incontinence Guideline Panel. Urinary incontinence in adults: clinical practice guidelines. Rockville, Maryland: Agency for Health Care Policy and Research, Public Health Service, U.S. Department of Health and Human Services, 1992; AHCPR publication no. 92–0038.

Wall LL. Diagnosis and management of urinary incontinence due to detrusor instability. *Obstet Gynecol Surv* 1990;45:1s.

Walters MD, Realini JP. The evaluation and treatment of urinary incontinence in women: a primary care approach. *J Am Board Fam Pract* 1992;5:289.

Chapter 73

COMPLEX URODYNAMICS

Bladder function can be measured with the use of specialized equipment or techniques.

Equipment

- Sterile gloves, antiseptic solution and sterile cotton balls, or skin preparation swabs
- Sterile urine specimen cup (with graduations)
- 12 or 14 French straight catheter
- 1 L of sterile saline (intravenous fluid without glucose is generally used) at room temperature
- 2% Xylocaine jelly in mushroom-tipped syringe (optional)
- Intravenous or pump tubing (based on the specifics of the equipment used)
- Absorbent underpads
- Urodynamics testing unit (includes recording device, fluid pump, catheter puller, and uroflowmetry commode)
- Printer for urodynamics reports
- Assistant (desirable)

Training/Credentialing

Moderate experience is required; it is best to have received advanced instruction or experience before measurement is attempted alone. Special credentialing may be needed depending on the local custom and location of testing.

Coding

51726	Complex urodynamics
51772	Urethral profilometry
51741	Complex uroflowmetry

Technique

Just before testing, the patient is asked to empty her bladder (in private and in her usual manner). The patient is examined (in the lithotomy position), and the external urinary meatus is cleansed with antiseptic solution. If anesthesia is desired, 1–3 mL of topical anesthetic, such as 2% Xylocaine, is introduced into the urethra. With sterile technique, a straight catheter is inserted. Any residual urine is caught, measured for volume, and sent for culture for determination of occult infection. The catheter is then removed.

Catheter-tip microtransducer catheters are introduced into the bladder to record bladder and urethral pressure (Fig. 73.1). A reference catheter is placed in either the vaginal or rectal canal (Fig. 73.2). This pressure is used to infer intra-abdominal pressure. These catheters are secured and attached to the urodynamics unit; bladder filling proceeds in a controlled manner using the pumping system supplied with the urodynamics equipment (Fig. 73.3). The usual filling rate is approximately 50 mL per minute. The first sensation of bladder fullness, the occurrence of a sense of urgency, and maximal bladder capacity are noted using the method appropriate for the specific equipment being used. The patient is asked to cough several times and this is entered into the record maintained by the urodynamics machine. Urinary leakage at the time of cough should be noted. Leakage that occurs immediately after, is prolonged, is associated with an increase in true bladder pressure, or is of large volume suggests detrusor instability. These maneuvers may be repeated in the standing position for persons who have no urinary loss while supine.

If leak point pressures are to be measured, the volume of the bladder must be adjusted to 200 mL and the pressure catheter must be no greater than 10 French. Pressures are recorded from both the urethra and bladder; the true detrusor pressure is calculated by subtraction of the reference pressure obtained from the vagina or rectum. The patient is asked to strain and the pressure at which leakage occurs (if any) is noted.

The reference pressure catheter is removed and urethral profilometry is performed using the machine's catheter puller to removed the bladder catheter at a known rate. Pressure profiles are thus compiled by the urodynamics equipment and may be repeated while the patient coughs to obtain a dynamic profile.

Cystoscopy is commonly performed as a part of complex urodynamics testing (see Chapter 71, Office Cystourethroscopy).

Uroflowmetry is done using the urodynamic equipment's commode, which is equipped to measure flow rate, volume, and time. These variables are automatically recorded and displayed in formats that are determined by the specific equipment used.

Electromyography of the pelvic floor and urinary system have fallen out of favor. These studies should only be performed by specialized consultants, and even then only infrequently.

Normal Findings

Complex urodynamics testing can generate a long list of objective or semi-objective values that describe urinary tract structure and function. In the primary care context of the tests described in this book, one need only be concerned with the most common values measured. Normal values for these are shown in Table 73.1. When more complex values are required, consultation or referral should be considered.

Selected Abnormal Findings

High resting tone or poor compliance of the bladder represents a significant risk to renal function. These conditions require aggressive evaluation and treatment. A

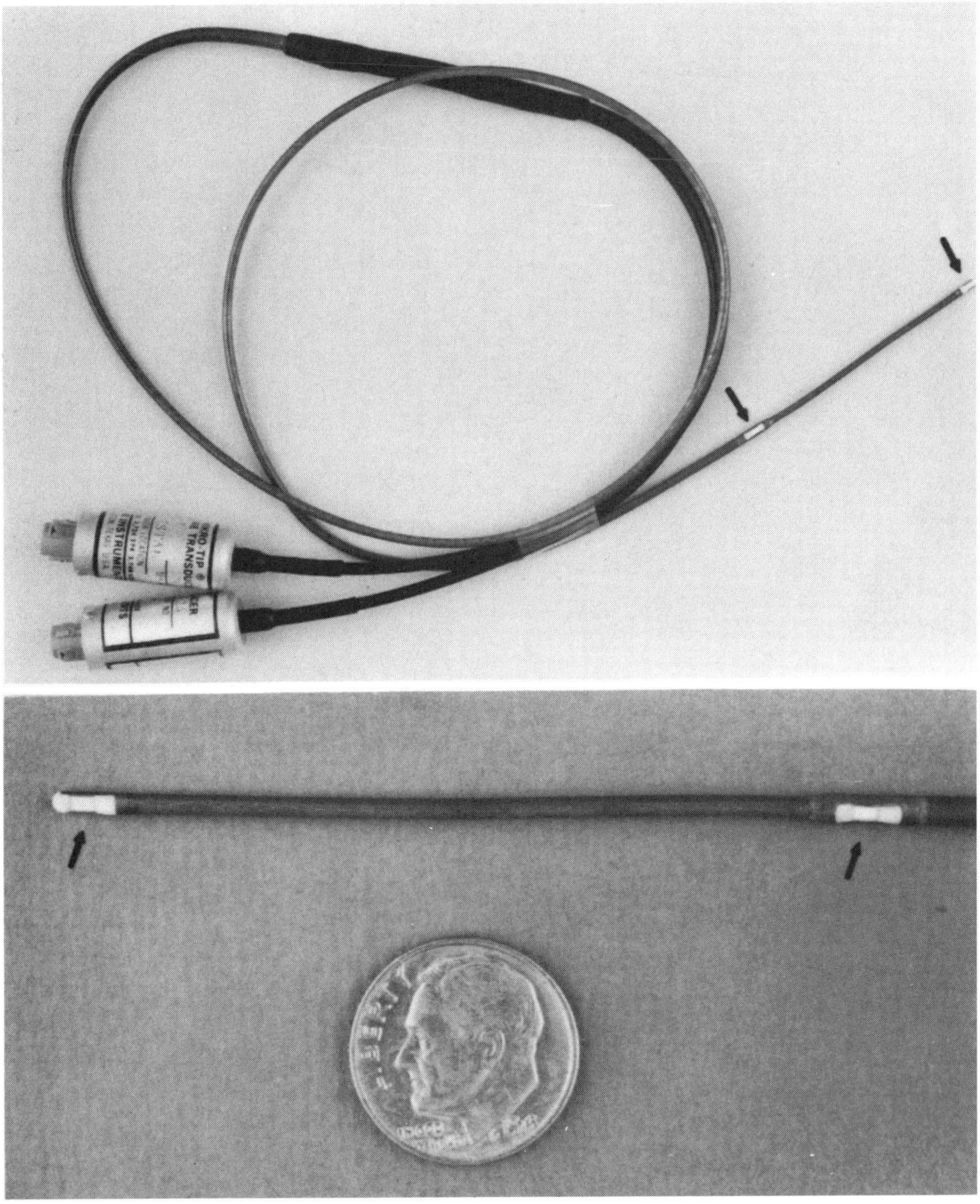

FIGURE 73.1.
The microtransducer catheter. The two microtransducers (arrows) measure intravesical and intraurethral pressures. (Reproduced with permission from Ostergard DR, Bent AE. Urogynecology and Urodynamics. *3rd ed. Baltimore: Williams & Wilkins, 1991:130.)*

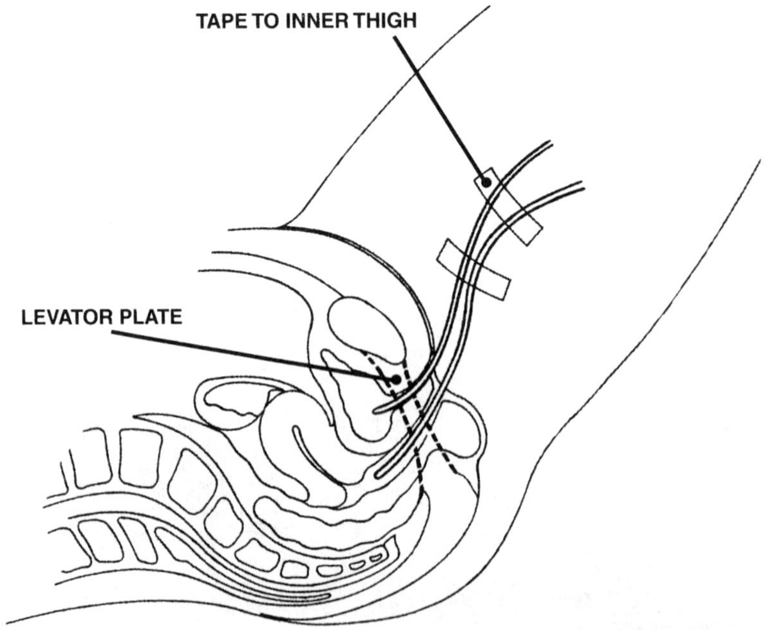

FIGURE 73.2.
The pressure transducers used for complex urodynamics must be positioned as shown to ensure accurate readings. (Courtesy of MedAmicus, Minneapolis, MN 55447.)

TABLE 73.1. Anticipated Normal Values

Cystometrics	
Residual urine	< 50 mL
Resting pressure	20–30 cm H_2O
Maximal capacity	300–500 mL
Compliance (increase in pressure)	< 10 cm H_2O
First urge (sensation of fullness)	150–200 mL
Profilometry	
Maximum urethral pressure	50–100 cm H_2O
Maximum closure pressure	50–80 cm H_2O
Functional urethral length	> 3 cm
Uroflowmetry (200 mL voided volume)	
Voiding time	< 20 sec
Peak flow rate	> 15 mL/sec
Average flow rate	> 10 mL/sec
Flow pressure (range)	20–60 cm H_2O
Mean maximal flow pressure	58 cm H_2O

Reproduced with permission from Smith RP. *Gynecology in Primary Care.* Baltimore: Williams & Wilkins, 1996:590.

denervated bladder generally demonstrates high resting tone and high urethral pressures.

Special Notes

Cystometrics are associated with a false-negative rate of approximately 50% and a false-positive rate of 15% in cases of urge incontinence.

Urethral pressure profiles are poorly correlated with the presence or absence of incontinence.

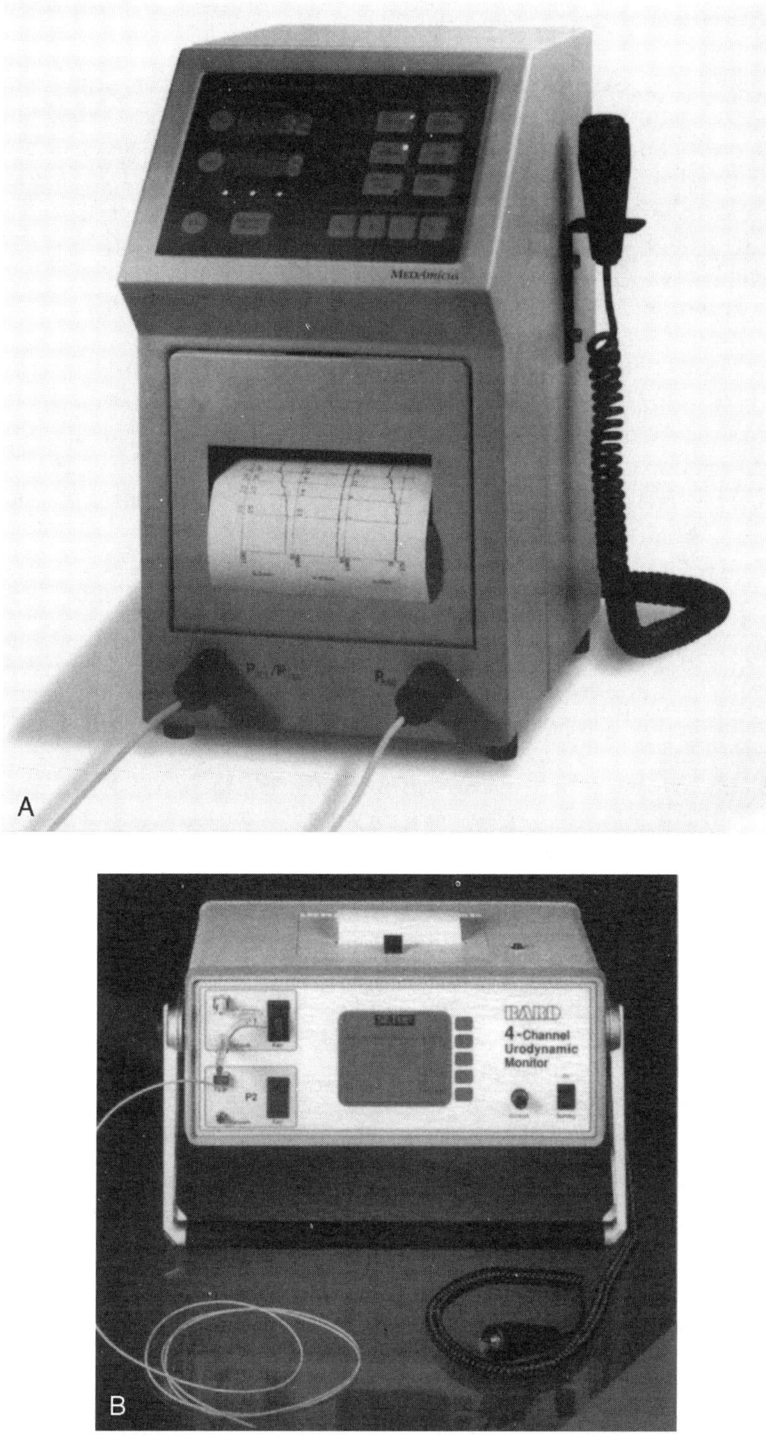

FIGURE 73.3.
*Several types of urodynamics equipment are available for office use. (**A,** Courtesy of MedAmicus, Minneapolis, MN 55447. **B,** Courtesy of C.R. Bard, Bard Urological Division, Covington, GA 30209.)*

Suggested Readings

Abrams P, Blaivas JG, Stanton SL, et al. The standardization of terminology of lower urinary tract function produced by the International Continence Society Committee on Standardization of Terminology. *Scand J Urol Nephrol* 1988;114:5.

American College of Obstetricians and Gynecologists. *Urinary Incontinence.* ACOG technical bulletin 213. Washington, DC: ACOG, 1995.

Bergman A, Bhatia NN. Urodynamics: the effect of urinary tract infection on urethral and bladder function. *Obstet Gynecol* 1985;66:366.

Bhatia NN, Bergman A. Urodynamic appraisal of the Bonney test in women with stress urinary incontinence. *Obstet Gynecol* 1983;62:696.

Bradley WE, Timm GW. Cystometry VI. Interpretation. *Urology* 1976;7:231.

Cardozo L, Stanton SL. Genuine stress incontinence and detrusor instability: a clinical and urodynamic review of 200 cases. *Br J Obstet Gynecol* 1980;87:184.

Consensus Conference. Urinary incontinence in adults. *JAMA* 1989;261:2685.

Decter RM, Harpster L. Pitfalls in determination of leak point pressure. *J Urol* 1992;148:588.

Fischer-Rasmussen W, Hansen RI, Stage P. Predictive values of diagnostic test in the evaluation of female urinary stress incontinence. *Acta Obstet Gynecol Scand* 1986;65:291.

Gilmour RF, Churchill BM, Steckler RE, et al. A new technique for dynamic analysis of bladder compliance. *J Urol* 1993;150:1200.

Massey A, Abrams P. Urodynamic of the female lower urinary tract. *Urol Clin North Am* 1985;12:231.

Norton PA (ed). Urinary incontinence. *Clin Obstet Gynecol* 1990;33:293.

Ostergard DR, Bent AE, eds. *Urogynecology and Urodynamics.* 4th ed. Baltimore: Williams & Wilkins, 1996.

Song JT, Rozanski TA, Belville WD. Stress leak point pressure: a simple and reproducible method utilizing a fiberoptic microtransducer. *Urology* 1995;46:81.

Sutherst JR, Brown MC. Comparison of single and multichannel cystometry in diagnosing bladder instability. *Br Med J* 1984;288:1720.

Urinary Incontinence Guideline Panel. Urinary incontinence in adults: clinical practice guidelines. Rockville, Maryland: Agency for Health Care Policy and Research, Public Health Service, U.S. Department of Health and Human Services, 1992; AHCPR publication no. 92–0038.

Wall LL, Hewitt JK, Helms MJ. Are vaginal and rectal pressures equivalent approximations of one another for the purpose of performing subtracted cystometry? *Obstet Gynecol* 1995;85:488.

Wall LL. Diagnosis and management of urinary incontinence due to detrusor instability. *Obstet Gynecol Surv* 1990;45:1s.

Walters MD, Realini JP. The evaluation and treatment of urinary incontinence in women: a primary care approach. *J Am Board Fam Pract* 1992;5:289.

INDEX

Page numbers preceded by a *t* or *f* indicate tables or figures, respectively.

A

D

E

F